High-Yield

Gross Anatomy

3RD EDITION

High-Yield

Gross Anatomy

3RD EDITION

Ronald W. Dudek, PhD
Professor
Brody School of Medicine
East Carolina University
Department of Anatomy and Cell Biology
Greenville, North Carolina

Thomas M. Louis, PhD
Professor
Brody School of Medicine
East Carolina University
Department of Anatomy and Cell Biology
Greenville, North Carolina

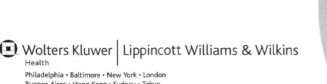

Wolters Kluwer | Lippincott Williams & Wilkins
Health
Philadelphia • Baltimore • New York • London
Buenos Aires • Hong Kong • Sydney • Tokyo

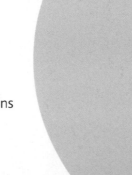

Acquisitions Editor: Crystal Taylor
Managing Editor: Grace R. Caputo
Development Editor: Kathleen H. Scogna
Marketing Manager: Emilie Linkins
Production Editor: Eve Malakoff-Klein
Designer: Terry Mallon
Compositor: Maryland Composition, Inc.
Printer: Data Reproductions Corporation

351 West Camden Street
Baltimore, MD 21201

530 Walnut Street
Philadelphia, PA 19106

Printed in the United States of America

First Edition, 1997
Second Edition, 2002

Library of Congress Cataloging-in-Publication Data
Dudek, Ronald W., 1950-
   High-yield gross anatomy / Ronald W. Dudek, Thomas Louis. — 3rd ed.
      p. ; cm. — (High-yield series)
   Includes index.
   ISBN-13: 978-0-7817-7015-6
   ISBN-10: 0-7817-7015-7
   1. Human anatomy—Outlines, syllabi, etc. 2. Anatomy, Surgical and topographical—
Outlines, syllabi, etc. I. Louis, Thomas. II. Title. III. Series.
   [DNLM: 1. Anatomy—Outlines. QS 18.2 D845h 2007]
   QM31.D83 2007
   611—dc22

                                                                                    2006017306

The publishers have made every effort to trace the copyright holders for borrowed material. If they have inadvertently overlooked any, they will be pleased to make the necessary arrangements at the first opportunity.

To purchase additional copies of this book, call our customer service department at **(800) 638-3030** or fax orders to **(301) 223-2320**. International customers should call **(301) 223-2300**.

Visit Lippincott Williams & Wilkins on the Internet: http://www.LWW.com. Lippincott Williams & Wilkins customer service representatives are available from 8:30 am to 6:00 pm, EST.

                                                                06 07 08 09 10
                                                          1 2 3 4 5 6 7 8 9 10

Preface

High Yield Gross Anatomy addresses many of the recurring clinical themes of the USMLE Step 1. The information presented in *High Yield Gross Anatomy* prepares you to handle not only the clinical vignettes found on the USMLE Step 1 but also questions concerning basic gross anatomy concepts.

Like the USMLE Step 1, the discussions are comprehensively illustrated with a combination of drawings, MRIs, CT scans, radiographs, and cross-sectional anatomy. In addition, *High Yield Gross Anatomy* directly addresses clinical issues that require a knowledge of basic gross anatomy to deduce the correct answer. Also included are a number of common clinical techniques (e.g. liver biopsy, tracheostomy, and lumbar puncture) that require a knowledge of the accompanying gross anatomy relationships.

For *High Yield Gross Anatomy*, 3rd edition, I have invited Dr. Thomas Louis to serve as a coauthor. Dr. Louis has taught gross anatomy for about 30 years in both cadaver-dissection and computer-assisted distance-learning gross anatomy courses. Dr. Louis has been a leader in developing computer-assisted distance learning at the Brody School of Medicine and has received national recognition for his efforts. Dr. Louis has used *High Yield Gross Anatomy* in his physician assistant gross anatomy course for about 3 years with excellent success. Dr. Louis supplemented the clinical anatomy presented in *High Yield Gross Anatomy* with critical basic anatomy figures and diagrams to assist his students in learning the gross anatomy relationships of these clinically relevant areas. In this new edition, Dr. Louis and I have added some of his suggested basic anatomy figures and diagrams that he has found crucial for student understanding of these clinically relevant areas. Unfortunately, we were not able to include all the basic anatomy figures due to page limitations. In addition, Dr. Louis has compiled a plethora of clinical vignettes that he uses in his physician assistant gross anatomy course. We have added a number of clinical vignettes in this new edition. Finally, we have added new chapters on the Autonomic Nervous System, Lymphatic System, Eye, and Ear.

I would like to thank Dr. Edward A. Monaco III for his suggestions and contributions to many of the chapters (especially the chapters on the Lymphatic System and Eye). Dr. Monaco has a PhD in Neuroscience from SUNY Upstate Medical University and is currently completing his medical studies at Columbia University College of Physicians and Surgeons in New York City.

I would appreciate your comments or suggestions about this book, especially after you have taken the USMLE Step 1, so that future editions can be improved and made more relevant to the USMLE Step 1. You may contact me at dudekr@ecu.edu.

Contents

Chapter 1

Vertebral Column

I **The Vertebral Column (Figure 1-1)** consists of 33 vertebrae (cervical C1–C7, thoracic T1–T12, lumbar L1–L5, sacral S1–S5 [sacrum], and coccygeal Co1–Co4 [coccyx]). The **vertebral canal** contains the spinal cord, dorsal rootlets, ventral rootlets, dorsal nerve root, ventral nerve root, and meninges. The spinal nerve is located outside the vertebral canal by exiting through the **intervertebral foramen.**

II **Curves (Figure 1-1)**

A. **Primary curves** are the thoracic and sacral curvatures that form during the fetal period.

B. **Secondary curves** are the cervical and lumbar curvatures that form after birth as a result of lifting the head and walking, respectively.

C. **Kyphosis** is an exaggeration of the thoracic curvature that may occur in the aged as a result of osteoporosis or disk degeneration.

D. **Lordosis** is an exaggeration of the lumbar curvature that may occur as a result of pregnancy, spondylolisthesis, or "pot-belly."

E. **Scoliosis** is a complex lateral deviation or torsion that may occur as a result of poliomyelitis, a short leg, or hip disease.

III **Joints**

A. **Atlanto-occipital joints** are the articulations between the superior articular surfaces of atlas (C1) and the occipital condyles. The actions of **nodding the head (as in indicating "yes")** and **sideways tilting of the head** occur at these joints. These are synovial joints and have **no** intervertebral disk. The **anterior and posterior atlanto-occipital membranes** limit excessive movement at this joint.

B. **Atlanto-axial joints** are the articulations between atlas (C1) and axis (C2), which include two **lateral atlanto-axial joints** between the inferior facets of C1 and superior facets of C2 and one **median atlanto-axial joint** between the anterior arch of C1 and dens of C2. The action of **turning the head side-to-side (as in indicating "no")** occurs at these joints. These are synovial joints and have **no** intervertebral disk. The **alar ligaments** that extend from the sides of the dens to the lateral margins of the foramen magnum limit excessive movement at this joint.

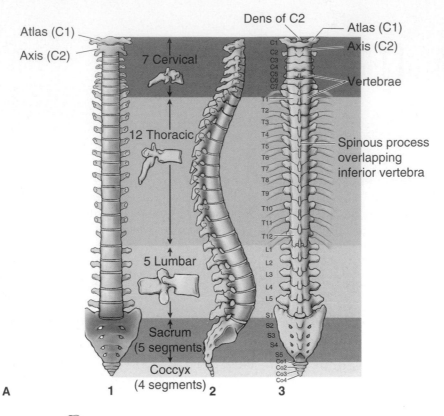

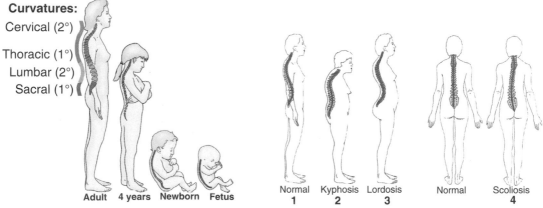

● **Figure 1-1 (A) Vertebral Column. (1)** Anterior view. **(2)** Right lateral view. **(3)** Posterior view with vertebral ends of the ribs. **(B) Curvatures of the Vertebral Column from Fetus to Adult. (C) Curvatures of the Vertebral Column. (1)** Normal. **(2)** Kyphosis. **(3)** Lordosis. **(4)** Scoliosis. **(D) Vertebral Levels.** Vertebral levels are used to reference the location of important anatomic structures.

VERTEBRAL LEVELS FOR REFERENCE

Knowledge of these vertebral levels will assist in deciphering clinical vignette questions. For example, a clinical vignette question may describe a pulsatile swelling located at vertebral level T2. Knowledge that the arch of the aorta is found at T2 will allow you to deduce an aortic arch aneurysm.

Anatomic Structure	Vertebral Level
Hyoid bone, bifurcation of common carotid artery	C4
Thyroid cartilage, carotid pulse palpated	C5
Cricoid cartilage, start of trachea, start of esophagus	C6
Sternal notch, arch of aorta	T2
Sternal angle, junction of superior and inferior mediastinum, bifurcation of trachea	T4
Pulmonary hilum	T5–T7
Inferior vena cava hiatus	T8
Xiphisternal joint	T9
Esophageal hiatus	T10
Aortic hiatus	T12
Duodenum	T12–L1
Celiac artery, upper pole of left kidney	T12
Superior mesenteric artery, upper pole of right kidney, end of spinal cord in adult (conus medullaris) and pia mater	L1
Renal artery	L2
End of spinal cord in newborn, inferior mesenteric artery, umbilicus	L3
Iliac crest, bifurcation of aorta	L4
Sacral promontory, start of sigmoid colon	S1
End of dural sac, dura, arachnoid, subarachnoid space, and cerebrospinal fluid	S2
End of sigmoid colon	S3

D

● **Figure 1-1 (Continued).**

   C. Clinical Consideration (Figure 1-2). Atlanto-axial dislocation (subluxation) is caused by the **rupture of the transverse ligament of atlas** as a result of trauma (e.g. Jefferson fracture) or rheumatoid arthritis. This allows mobility of the **dens** (part of C2) within the vertebral canal, which places at risk the cervical spinal cord (leading to quadriplegia) or the medulla (respiratory paralysis leading to sudden death). The **dens** is secured in its position by the **transverse ligament of atlas**, which together with the **superior longitudinal band** and **inferior longitudinal band** form the **cruciate ligament**; **alar ligaments**; and **tectorial membrane**, which is a continuation of the posterior longitudinal ligament. A widening of the atlantodental interval (distance from the anterior arch of C1 to the dens) suggests tearing of the transverse ligament.

Ⅳ Vasculature of the Vertebral Column

   A. Arterial Supply. The vertebrae are supplied by **periosteal branches, equatorial branches**, and **spinal branches** from larger parent arteries that include the vertebral arteries, ascending cervical arteries, segmental arteries of the trunk, posterior intercostal arteries, subcostal and lumbar arteries in the abdomen, iliolumbar arteries, and lateral and medial sacral arteries in the pelvis. The periosteal and equatorial branches arise from these parent arteries as they travel along the anterolateral surface of the vertebrae. The spinal branches enter the intervertebral foramina and divide into the **anterior vertebral canal branch**, which sends **nutrient arteries** into the vertebral bodies, and the **posterior vertebral canal branch**. The spinal branches terminate as the **segmental medullary arteries** or **radicular arteries**, which supply the spinal cord.

Posterior view

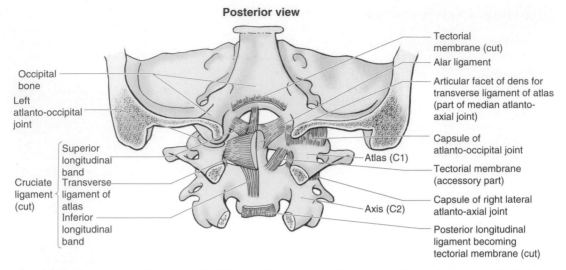

● **Figure 1-2 Ligaments of the Atlanto-Occipital and Atlanto-Axial Joints (posterior view).** The tectorial membrane and the right side of the cruciate ligament have been removed to show the attachment of the right alar ligament to the dens of C2.

B. **Venous Drainage.** Spinal veins draining the vertebrae form the **internal vertebral venous plexus** and the **external vertebral venous plexus**. The **basivertebral veins** form within the vertebral bodies, exit via foramina on the vertebral surface, and drain into the internal vertebral venous plexus (anterior portion). The **intervertebral veins** receive veins from the spinal cord and the vertebral venous plexuses as they accompany spinal nerves through the intervertebral foramina.

Ⓥ Clinical Considerations

A. **Denervation of Zygapophyseal (facet) Joints.** The zygapophyseal (facet) joints are synovial joints between **inferior and superior articular processes**. These joints are located near the intervertebral foramen. If these joints are traumatized or diseased (e.g. rheumatoid arthritis), a spinal nerve may be impinged and cause severe pain. To relieve the pain, medial branches of the dorsal primary ramus are severed (i.e. dorsal rhizotomy).

B. **Dislocations without fracture** occur only in the cervical region because the articular surfaces are inclined horizontally. Cervical dislocations will stretch the posterior longitudinal ligament.

C. **Dislocations with fracture** occur in the thoracic and lumbar region because the articular surfaces are inclined vertically.

D. **Stability of the vertebral column** is mainly determined by four ligaments: anterior longitudinal ligament, posterior longitudinal ligament, ligamentum flavum, and interspinous ligament.

E. **A route of metastasis** for breast, lung, and prostate cancer to the brain exists because the **internal vertebral venous plexus, basivertebral veins**, and **external vertebral venous plexus** surrounding the vertebral column communicate with the cranial dural sinuses and veins of the thorax, abdomen, and pelvis.

F. **Spina bifida occulta** is a common congenital malformation in which the **vertebral arch** is absent. The defect is covered by skin and is usually marked by a tuft of hair. This condition is not associated with any neurologic deficit.

G. **Hemivertebrae** occurs when a portion of the **vertebral body** fails to develop and can lead to scoliosis.

H. **Sickle cell anemia** is associated with "**fish mouth vertebra**" (as observed radiographically) in which central depressions occur in the **vertebral body.**

I. **Osteomyelitis** is a bacterial infection that may occur within vertebral bodies. *Staphylococcus aureus* and *Pseudomonas aeruginosa* (in immunosuppressed patients and intravenous drug users) are causative agents. Osteomyelitis in sickle cell anemia patients is often associated with *Salmonella.*

J. **Protrusion of the nucleus pulposus (Figure 1-3).** An intervertebral disk consists of the **annulus fibrosus** (fibrocartilage) and **nucleus pulposus** (remnant of the embryonic notochord). The nucleus pulposus generally herniates in a **posterolateral direction** and compresses a nerve root.

K. **Spondylolysis (Figure 1-4A, B)** is a stress fracture of the **pars interarticularis** (an area between the pedicle and lamina of a vertebra). It is often seen in adolescent athletes, most commonly at the L4 or L5 vertebra. On an oblique radiograph of the lumbar vertebrae, the fracture appears as a **radiolucent "collar" around the neck of the Scottie dog.**

L. **Spondylolisthesis (Figure 1-4 C)** (Greek: spondylo = vertebra; listhesis = to slide on an incline) is the anterior subluxation of the vertebral body so that the body of the vertebra moves anterior with respect to the vertebrae below it, causing lordosis. This occurs when the **pedicles** of a lumbar vertebra degenerate or fail to develop properly, or as a sequela of spondylolysis. Consequently, this may result in a **degenerative spondylolisthesis,** which usually occurs at L4 to L5 vertebral level, or a **congenital spondylolisthesis,** which usually occurs at L5 to S1 vertebral level. A **traumatic spondylolisthesis of C2** (also called a **hangman fracture**) occurs when a force is applied with the neck <u>hyperextended</u> (e.g. extension component of whiplash, car accident when chin or forehead strikes dashboard, head-on collision in football, or hanging) and places the spinal cord at risk. A traumatic spondylolisthesis of C2 includes the following pathology: fracture of the pars interarticularis bilateral to C2 vertebra, anterior subluxation of C2 vertebra, tear of anterior longitudinal ligament, and posterior fractured portion of C2 remains attached to C3 (in a legal drop hanging).

M. **Spondylosis** is a very common degenerative process of the vertebral column that occurs in the cervical region of elderly patients. The extent of degeneration may range from mild disk space narrowing and bone spur formation to severe **spondylosis deformans** (which include disk space narrowing, facet joint narrowing, and bone spur formation [**Figure 1-4D**]).

N. **Ankylosing spondylosis** (**rheumatoid spondylitis** or **Marie-Strümpell disease**) is an inflammatory osteoarthritis generally affecting the lumbar vertebrae and sacroiliac joint. The **annulus fibrosus** of the intervertebral disks may become ossified, producing severe spinal immobility. The ossification bridges the disks at various levels, forming a "**bamboo spine.**" A majority of these patients are positive for histocompatibility antigen HLA-B27.

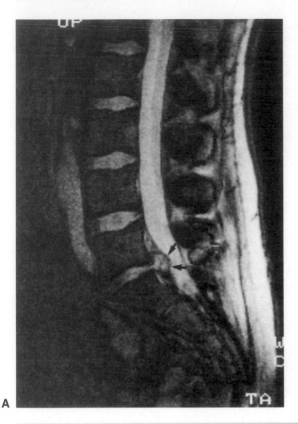

A

● **Figure 1-3 Herniated Disk. (A)** MRI (sagittal view) shows a herniated disk (arrows) between L5 and S1. **(B)** Important features of a herniated disk at various vertebral levels. From various clinical signs, you should be able to deduce which nerve root is compressed and then identify the appropriate intervertebral disk on a radiograph or MRI.

Herniated Disk Between	Compressed Nerve Root	Dermatome Affected	Muscles Affected	Movement Weakness	Nerve and Reflex Involved
C4 and C5	*C5*	C5 Shoulder Lateral surface of upper limb	Deltoid	Abduction of arm	Axillary nerve ↓ Biceps jerk
C5 and C6	*C6*	C6 Thumb	Biceps Brachialis Brachioradialis	Flexion of forearm Supination/pronation	Musculocutaneous nerve ↓ Biceps jerk ↓ Brachioradialis jerk
C6 and C7	*C7*	C7 Posterior surface of upper limb Middle and index fingers	Triceps Wrist extensors	Extension of forearm Extension of wrist	Radial nerve ↓ Triceps jerk
L3 and L4	*L4*	L4 Medial surface of leg Big toe	Quadriceps	Extension of knee	Femoral nerve ↓ Knee jerk
L4 and L5	*L5*	L5 Lateral surface of leg Dorsum of foot	Tibialis anterior Extensor hallucis longus Extensor digitorum longus	Dorsiflexion of ankle (patient cannot stand on heels) Extension of toes	Common fibular nerve No reflex loss
L5 and S1 (most common)	*S1*	S1 Posterior surface of lower limb Little toe	Gastrocnemius Soleus	Plantar flexion of ankle (patient cannot stand on toes) Flexion of toes	Tibial nerve ↓ Ankle jerk

Note the correspondence between the dermatome affected and the compressed nerve root (bold italic).

B

O. Teardrop fracture (see Figure 1-7A) is caused by **hyperflexion of the cervical region** (e.g. diving into shallow water, rebound flexion component of whiplash from a rear-end car accident, head-on collision in football) and places the spinal cord at risk. A triangular fragment ("teardrop body") is sheared off of the anterior-inferior corner of the dislocating vertebral body. The result is a complete disruption of the cervical spine, with the upper portion of the vertebra displaced posteriorly and angulated anteriorly. A teardrop fracture includes the following pathology: avulsion fracture of the vertebral body ("teardrop body"), fracture of spinous process, posterior subluxation of vertebrae, compression of spinal cord, tear of anterior longitudinal ligament, and tear or disruption of the posterior longitudinal ligament, ligamentum flavum, interspinous ligament, or supraspinous ligament.

P. Jefferson fracture (see Figure 1-7B) is caused by **compression of the cervical region** (e.g. force applied to top of head) and places the spinal cord at risk. A Jefferson fracture includes the following pathology: fracture of C1 vertebra at multiple sites, lateral displacement or C1 vertebra beyond margins of C2 vertebra, and tear of the transverse ligament.

Q. Hyperextension (whiplash) injury (see Figure 1-7C) is caused by **hyperextension of the cervical region** (e.g. extension component of whiplash from a rear-end car accident, car accident when chin or forehead strikes dashboard, head-on collision in football). The usual whiplash injury is a strain of the paravertebral and neck muscles. In more severe injuries, tear of the anterior longitudinal ligament, tear of the anterior attachment of the intervertebral disk, and widening of the intervertebral space may occur (bony fractures and dislocations are uncommon). However, in more violent hyperextension injuries (e.g. head-on collision in football), fracture of the posterior portion of the cervical vertebrae may occur.

R. Chance fracture (see Figure 1-7D) is caused by **hyperflexion of the thoracic or lumbar region** (e.g. "seat belt injury" most commonly at vertebral level L2 or L3 when a car occupant is thrown forward against a restraining seat belt during sudden deceleration and associated with intraabdominal injuries) and generally does not place the spinal cord at risk. A Chance fracture includes the following pathology: transverse fracture of vertebral body and arch, rupture of intervertebral disk, and tear of posterior longitudinal ligament, ligamentum flavum, interspinous ligament, and supraspinous ligament.

Ⓥ Radiology

A. Radiographs and Diagrams of Spondylolysis with Spondylolisthesis, Traumatic Spondylolisthesis (Hangman Fracture), Legal Drop Hanging, and a Severe Cervical Spondylosis (Figure 1-4)

B. Median Sagittal MRI of the Cervical Region and Anteroposterior Radiograph of the Thoracic Region (Figure 1-5, A and B)

C. Lateral Radiograph of the Lumbosacral Region and Oblique Radiograph of the Lumbosacral Region ("Scottie dog" projection) (Figure 1-6, A and B)

D. Radiographs and Diagrams of Teardrop Hyperflexion Injury, Jefferson Fracture, Hyperextension (whiplash) Injury, and Chance Fracture (Figure 1-7)

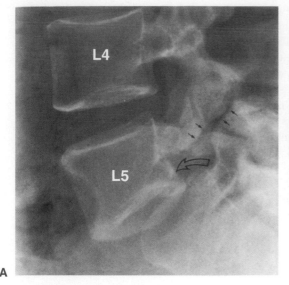

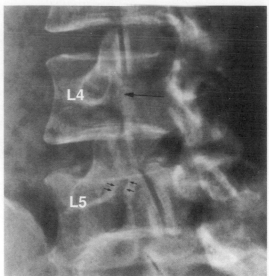

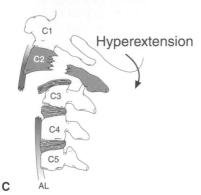

Hyperextension

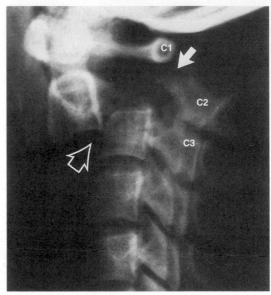

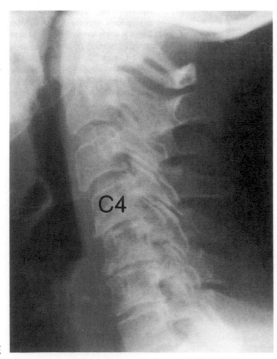

● **Figure 1-4 (A, B) Spondylolysis with Spondyolisthesis.**
(A) Lateral radiograph shows spondylolysis at L5 (small arrows) with a spondylolisthesis where L5 vertebra is subluxed anteriorly with respect to S1. **(B)** Oblique radiograph shows the bony defect at the pars interarticularis with sclerotic margins (small arrows). Note that the pars interarticularis at L4 vertebra is normal (large arrow). **(C, D)** Traumatic spondylolisthesis (Hangman fracture): **(C)** Diagram shows the classical components of a traumatic spondylolisthesis: fracture of the pars interarticularis bilaterally of C2 vertebra, anterior subluxation of C2 vertebra with respect to C3 vertebra, tear of anterior longitudinal ligament (AL). **(D)** Lateral radiograph of a traumatic spondylolisthesis. Note the fracture of the pars interarticularis of C2 vertebra (solid arrow) and the anterior subluxation of C2 vertebra with respect to C3 vertebra (open arrow). **(E) Severe Cervical Spondylosis.** Lateral radiograph shows narrowing of all the disk spaces below C4. Bone spurs encroach the vertebral canal. The disk level and sclerosis of the facet joints are apparent.

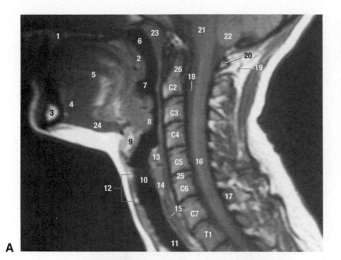

1 Hard palate	14 Cricoid cartilage
2 Soft palate	15 Esophagus
3 Mandible	16 Spinal cord
4 Genioglossus	17 Spinous process
5 Tongue	18 Cerebrospinal fluid in
6 Nasopharynx	subarachnoid space
7 Oropharynx	19 Nuchal ligament
8 Epiglottis	20 Posterior arch of atlas
9 Hyoid bone	21 Medulla oblongata
10 Vestibule	22 Tonsil of cerebellum
11 Trachea	23 Pharyngeal tonsil (adenoid)
12 Thyroid cartilage	24 Geniohyoid
13 Arytenoid cartilage	25 Intervertebral disk
	26 Dens of axis

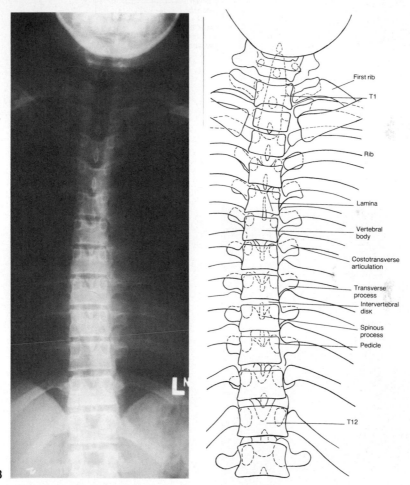

● **Figure 1-5 Cervical and Thoracic Regions. (A)** Median sagittal MRI of the cervical region. Note the superior projection of the dens axis (26) and its relationship to atlas, spinal cord (16), and medulla (21). The dens axis is secured in its position predominately by the transverse ligament, the rupture of which will place the spinal cord and possibly the medulla in jeopardy. **(B) AP Radiograph of the Thoracic Region.**

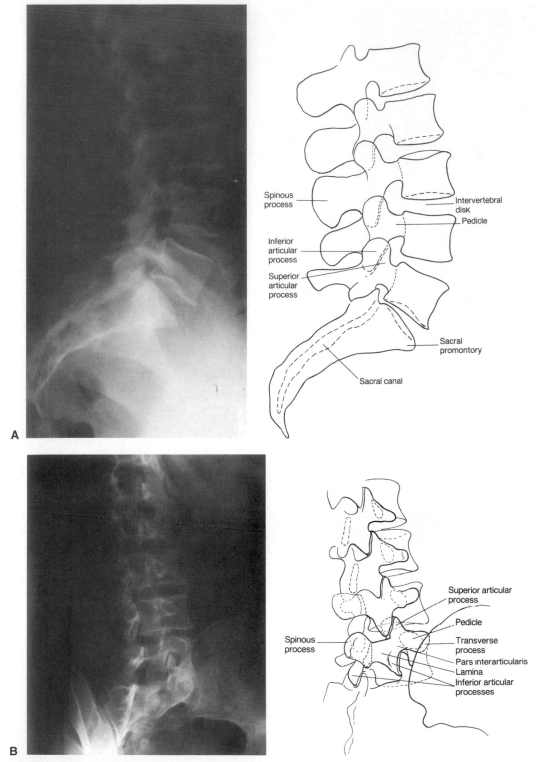

● **Figure 1-6 Lumbosacral Region. (A) Lateral radiograph of the lumbosacral region. (B) Oblique radiograph of the lumbosacral region ("Scottie dog" projection).** The anatomic structures of lumbar vertebrae portray a "Scottie dog" appearance in an oblique view. The ears of the Scottie dog are the superior articular process. The legs of the Scottie dog are the inferior articular process The nose of the Scottie dog is the transverse process. The neck of the Scottie dog is the pars interarticularis. The eye of the Scottie dog is the pedicle.

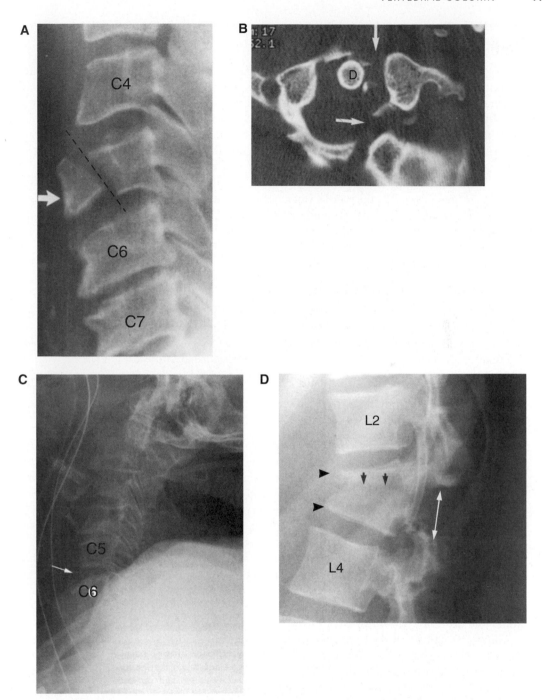

● **Figure 1-7 (A) Lateral Radiograph of a Teardrop Hyperflexion Injury.** Note the avulsion fracture of the C5 vertebral body ("teardrop body": arrow and dotted line) and the posterior subluxation of the C5 vertebra. **(B) CT of a Jefferson Fracture.** D = dens. **(C) Lateral Radiograph of a Hyperextension (Whiplash) Injury.** Note the anterior widening of the intervertebral space at C5–C6 (arrow). **(D) Lateral Radiograph of a Chance Fracture.** Note the compressed L3 vertebral body (arrowheads) as a result of the transverse fracture (arrows). Note the increased distance between the spinous processes as a result of the tear of LF, IS, and SS ligaments (long double-headed arrow). LF = ligamentum flavum; LS = interspinous ligament; SS = supraspinous ligament.

Case Study

A 35-year-old construction worker who frames homes experienced a pain in his lower back on trying to move a beam from one side of the construction site to another site 100 feet away. The man explains the pain as being "sudden" and "sharp" and states that during the last several days the pain has begun to move from his lower back into his right leg. The patient also states that he has been experiencing some numbness and tingling over the posterior surface of his right leg, foot, and little toe. The patient states that he had experienced intermittent back pain for the last couple of years but has never experienced the leg pain.

On examination the patient presents with antalgic gait and appears uncomfortable as he sits. The patient states that the pain is worsened by straining and coughing. Raising his right extended leg is painful, and there is tenderness along his posterior thigh on palpation. The patient is experiencing some weakness in plantar flexion of his right foot ("cannot stand on his toes"), has loss of sensation over the dorsal side of the right fourth and fifth toes, and a reduced ankle jerk reflex.

Musculoskeletal Examination

- The SLR (straight leg raise) test exacerbates right lower limb pain at 45 degrees elevation and the crossed SLR test exacerbates the pain at 40 degrees elevation.
- Pain restricts active flexion of the lumbosacral spine to 20 degrees.
- Palpation of the lower back shows a flattening of the normal lordosis.

The patient has been taking an over-the-counter pain medicine but finds that the only thing that helps is lying in bed.

Explanation

Pain is associated with improper body mechanics because of the weakening of the muscles and ligaments that help support the spine. This man has probably not used proper body mechanics for a while, and picking up the heavy beam as mentioned above has worsened his condition.

The patient has weakness on plantar flexion and he is experiencing loss of sensation on his foot because there is compression of the tibial nerve (L4 through S3). This nerve is motor to the posterior compartment muscles of the thigh (except for the short head of the biceps femoris), leg, and the sole of the foot. The muscles that produce plantar flexion of the foot are posterior compartment muscles of the leg (i.e. gastrocnemius, soleus, and plantaris). When the tibial nerve is compressed, weakness of plantar flexion occurs. A branch of the tibial nerve, the **medial sural cutaneous nerve**, is usually joined by the **sural communicating branch of the common fibular nerve** to form the **sural nerve**. The sural nerve supplies the skin of the lateral and posterior part of the inferior one third of the leg and the lateral side of the foot.

About 95% of lumbar disk protrusions occur at the L4–L5 or L5–S1 levels. Protrusions of the nucleus pulposus usually occur posterolaterally. This is because the nucleus pulposus is pushed further posteriorly during flexion. The anulus fibrosus is weaker posteriorly and laterally, and the posterior longitudinal ligament does not completely support the disks. The diagnosis of this man's injury is a herniated disk at L5–S1. The nucleus pulposus is protruding through the anulus fibrosus at this level on the right side. It is compressing the right spinal nerve root at S1, causing acute low back pain and sciatica.

Chapter 2

Spinal Cord and Spinal Nerves

I   Components of the Spinal Cord (Figure 2-1)

A. **Gray matter** of the spinal cord consists of neuronal cell bodies and is divided into the dorsal horn, ventral horn, and **lateral horn**.

B. **White matter** of the spinal cord consists of neuronal fibers and is divided into the dorsal funiculus, ventral funiculus, and **lateral funiculus**.

C. **Ventral median fissure** is a distinct surface indentation present at all spinal cord levels and is related to the anterior spinal artery.

D. **Dorsal median fissure** is a less distinct surface indentation present at all spinal cord levels.

E. **Dorsal intermediate septum** is a surface indentation present only **at and above T6** that distinguishes ascending fibers within the **gracile fasciculus** (from the lower extremity) from ascending fibers within the **cuneate fasciculus** (from the upper extremity).

F. **Conus medullaris** is the end of the spinal cord that occurs at vertebral level **L1 in the adult** and vertebral level **L3 in the newborn**.

G. **Cauda equina** consists of the dorsal and ventral nerve roots of L2 through coccygeal 1 spinal nerves traveling in the subarachnoid space below the conus medullaris.

H. **Filum terminale** is a prolongation of the **pia mater** from the conus medullaris to the end of the dural sac at vertebral level S2 where it blends with the dura. The dura continues caudally as the **filum of the dura mater** (or coccygeal ligament), which attaches to the dorsum of the coccyx bone.

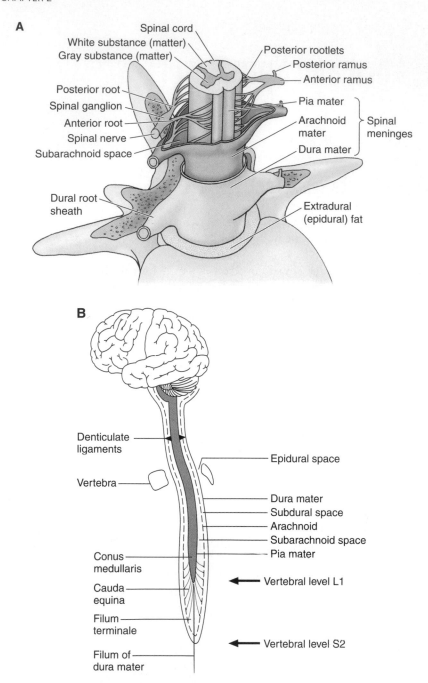

● **Figure 2-1 Spinal Cord Anatomy. (A)** A diagram of the spinal cord, spinal nerves, and meninges. **(B)** A diagram indicating craniocaudal extent of the spinal cord and meninges.

II Meninges and Spaces (Figure 2-1)

A. **Epidural space** is located between the vertebra and dura mater. This space contains fat and the **internal vertebral venous plexus.**

B. **Dura mater** is the tough, outermost layer of the meninges.

C. **Subdural space** is located between the dura mater and arachnoid.

D. **Arachnoid** is a filmlike, transparent layer connected to the pia mater by **trabeculations.**

E. **Subarachnoid space** is located between the arachnoid and pia mater and is filled with **cerebrospinal fluid.**

F. **Pia mater** is a thin layer that is closely applied to the spinal cord and has lateral extensions called **denticulate ligaments**, which attach to the dura mater and thereby suspend the spinal cord within the dural sac.

III Arterial Supply of the Spinal Cord

A. **Anterior Spinal Artery and Posterior Spinal Arteries.** There is only one anterior spinal artery, which arises from the vertebral arteries and runs in the anterior median fissure. The anterior spinal artery gives rise to **sulcal arteries**, which supply the **ventral two-thirds** of the spinal cord. There are two posterior spinal arteries, which arise from either the vertebral arteries or the posterior inferior cerebellar arteries. The posterior spinal arteries supply the **dorsal one-third** of the spinal cord. The anterior and posterior spinal arteries supply only the short superior part of the spinal cord. The circulation to much of the spinal cord depends on the segmental medullary arteries and radicular arteries.

B. **Anterior and Posterior Medullary Segmental Arteries.** These arteries arise from the spinal branches of the ascending cervical, deep cervical, vertebral, posterior intercostal, and lumber arteries. The anterior and posterior medullary segmental arteries occur irregularly in place of radicular arteries and are located mainly in the cervical and lumbosacral spinal enlargements. They enter the vertebral canal through the intervertebral foramina. The medullary segmental arteries are actually "large radicular arteries" that connect with the anterior and posterior spinal arteries, whereas the radicular arteries do not.

C. **Great Anterior Segmental Medullary (of Adamkiewicz).** This artery generally arises on the left side from a posterior intercostal artery or a lumbar artery and enters the vertebral canal through the intervertebral foramen at the lower thoracic or upper lumbar level. This artery is clinically important as it makes a major contribution to the anterior spinal artery and the lower part of the spinal cord. If this artery is ligated during resection of an **abdominal aortic aneurysm**, **anterior spinal artery syndrome** may result. Clinical symptoms include paraplegia, impotence, loss of voluntary control of the bladder and bowel (incontinence), and loss of pain and temperature sensation but preservation of vibration and proprioception sensation.

D. Anterior and Posterior Radicular Arteries. These arteries are small and supply only the dorsal and ventral roots of spinal nerves and superficial parts of the gray matter. They enter the vertebral canal through the intervertebral foramina.

Ⅳ Components of a Spinal Nerve (Figure 2-2). There are 31 pairs of spinal nerves: 8 cervical, 12 thoracic, 5 lumbar, 5 sacral, and 1 coccygeal. Small bundles of nerve fibers called the **dorsal (posterior) rootlets** and **ventral (anterior) rootlets** arise from the dorsal and ventral surfaces of the spinal cord, respectively. The dorsal rootlets converge to form the **dorsal (posterior) root** (containing afferent or sensory fibers), and the ventral rootlets converge to form the **ventral (anterior) root** (containing efferent or motor fibers). The dorsal root and ventral root join to form the **mixed spinal nerve** near the intervertebral foramen. Each spinal nerve divides into a **dorsal (posterior) primary ramus** (which innervates the skin and deep muscles of the back) and **ventral (anterior) primary ramus** (which innervates the remainder of the body). Spinal nerves are connected to the paravertebral ganglia (sympathetic chain ganglia) and prevertebral ganglia by the **white communicating rami** (containing myelinated preganglionic sympathetic nerve fibers present in spinal nerves T1 to L3) and **gray communicating rami** (containing unmyelinated postganglionic sympathetic nerve fibers present in all spinal nerves).

● **Figure 2-2 (A) Basic Organization of the Nervous System.** Note that each spinal nerve bears the same letter and numerical designation as the vertebra forming the superior boundary of its exit from the vertebral column, except in the cervical region. In the cervical region, each spinal nerve bears the same letter and numerical designation as the vertebra forming the inferior boundary of its exit from the vertebral column. Note that spinal nerve C8 exits between vertebrae C7 and T1. **(B) Components of a Typical Thoracic Spinal Nerve.** The four functional components are indicated: general somatic afferent (GSA), general somatic efferent (GSE), general visceral afferent (GVA), and general visceral efferent (GVE). The muscle stretch (myotactic) reflex includes the neuromuscular spindle, GSA dorsal root ganglion cell, GSE ventral horn motor neuron, and the neuromuscular junction. DRG = dorsal root ganglion, DPR = dorsal primary ramus, VPR = ventral primary ramus, WR = white communicating ramus, GR = gray communicating ramus, PARA = paravertebral (sympathetic chain) ganglion, PRE = prevertebral ganglion, SpN = splanchnic nerve.

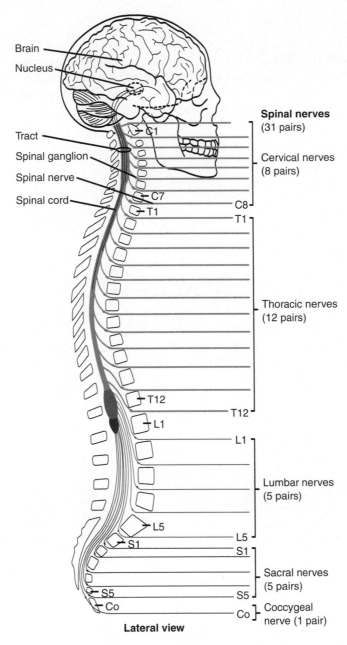

A

Brain

Nucleus

Tract

Spinal ganglion

Spinal nerve

Spinal cord

Spinal nerves
(31 pairs)

Cervical nerves
(8 pairs)

C1

C7

C8

T1

T1

T12

T12

L1

L1

Thoracic nerves
(12 pairs)

Lumbar nerves
(5 pairs)

L5

L5

S1

S1

S5

S5

Co

Co

Sacral nerves
(5 pairs)

Coccygeal
nerve (1 pair)

Lateral view

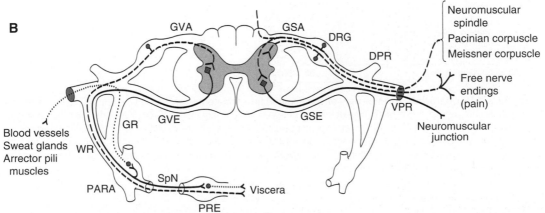

B

GVA

GSA

DRG

DPR

Neuromuscular
spindle
Pacinian corpuscle
Meissner corpuscle

GVE

GSE

VPR

Free nerve
endings
(pain)

Blood vessels
Sweat glands
Arrector pili
muscles

GR

WR

PARA

SpN

PRE

Neuromuscular
junction

Viscera

V **Dermatomes (Figure 2-3)** are strips of skin extending from the posterior midline to the anterior midline that are supplied by sensory branches of dorsal and ventral rami of a single spinal nerve. A clinical finding of sensory deficit in a dermatome is important to assess what spinal nerve, nerve root, or spinal cord segment may be damaged.

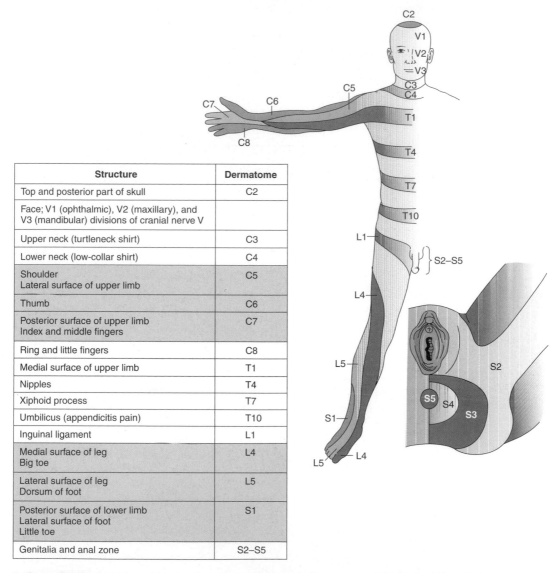

Structure	Dermatome
Top and posterior part of skull	C2
Face; V1 (ophthalmic), V2 (maxillary), and V3 (mandibular) divisions of cranial nerve V	
Upper neck (turtleneck shirt)	C3
Lower neck (low-collar shirt)	C4
Shoulder Lateral surface of upper limb	C5
Thumb	C6
Posterior surface of upper limb Index and middle fingers	C7
Ring and little fingers	C8
Medial surface of upper limb	T1
Nipples	T4
Xiphoid process	T7
Umbilicus (appendicitis pain)	T10
Inguinal ligament	L1
Medial surface of leg Big toe	L4
Lateral surface of leg Dorsum of foot	L5
Posterior surface of lower limb Lateral surface of foot Little toe	S1
Genitalia and anal zone	S2–S5

● **Figure 2-3 Dermatomes.** Anterior view of some important dermatomes of the body. Although dermatomes are shown as distinct segments, in reality, there is overlap between any two adjacent dermatomes. Note that the sensory innervation of the face does not involve dermatomes but is carried by cranial nerves (CN) V, V1 (ophthalmic division), V2 (maxillary division), and V3 (mandibular division). Shaded areas in the table indicate dermatomes affected by a herniated disk (see Chapter 1, Section V. J. and Figure 1-3). Knowledge of dermatomes is important because clinical vignette questions will include a description of sensory loss at a specific dermatome level.

Clinical Procedures (Figure 2-4)

A. **Lumbar puncture** can be done to either withdraw cerebrospinal fluid (CSF) or inject an anesthetic (e.g. spinal anesthesia). A needle is inserted above or below the spinous process of the **L4 vertebra.** The needle will pass through the following structures: skin → superficial fascia → supraspinous ligament → interspinous ligament → ligamentum flavum → epidural space containing the internal vertebral venous plexus → dura mater → arachnoid → subarachnoid space containing CSF. The pia mater is not pierced.

B. **Spinal anesthesia (spinal block or saddle block)** is produced by injecting anesthetic into the subarachnoid space and may be used during childbirth. Sensory nerve fibers for pain from the uterus travel with the (1) pelvic splanchnic nerves (parasympathetic) to S2 through S4 spinal levels from the cervix (may be responsible for referred pain to the gluteal region and legs) and (2) hypogastric plexus and lumbar splanchnic nerves (sympathetic) to L1 through L3 spinal levels from the fundus and body of the uterus and oviducts (may be responsible for referred pain to the back). Spinal anesthesia up to **spinal nerve T10** is necessary to block pain from vaginal childbirth and up to **spinal nerve T4** for Caesarean. Pregnant women require a smaller dose of anesthetic (than nonpregnant patients) because the subarachnoid space is compressed because the **internal vertebral venous plexus** is engorged with blood as a result of the pregnant uterus compressing the inferior vena cava. Complications may include **hypotension** as a result of sympathetic blockade and vasodilation, **respiratory paralysis** involving the phrenic nerve as a result of high spinal blockade, and **spinal headache** as a result of CSF leakage.

C. **Lumbar epidural anesthesia** is produced by injecting anesthetic into the **epidural space** and may be used during childbirth. Complications may include **respiratory paralysis** as a result of high spinal blockage if the dura and arachnoid are punctured and the usual amount of anesthetic is injected in the subarachnoid space by mistake, and **central nervous system (CNS) toxicity** (slurred speech, tinnitus, convulsions, cardiac arrest) as a result of injection of the anesthetic into the **internal vertebral venous plexus** (intravenous injection versus epidural application).

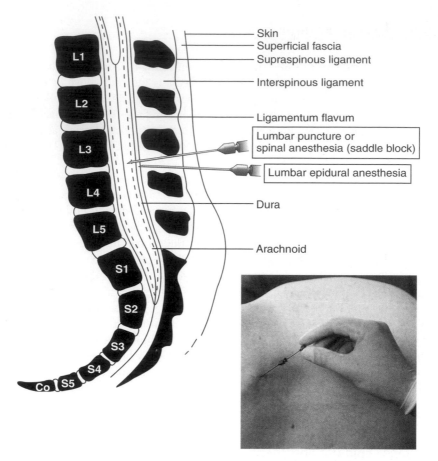

● **Figure 2-4 Lumbar Vertebral Column and Spinal Cord.** A needle is shown inserted into the subarachnoid space above the spinous process of L4 (L3–L4 interspace) to withdraw cerebrospinal fluid (CSF) as in a lumbar puncture or to administer spinal anesthesia (saddle block). A second needle is shown inserted into the epidural space to administer lumbar epidural anesthesia. Note the sequence of layers (superficial to deep) that the needle must penetrate. Co = coccyx.

VII Major Tracts of the Spinal Cord

A. Dorsal column–medial lemniscus pathway mediates tactile discrimination, vibration sensation, and form recognition, along with joint and muscle sensation (proprioception).

B. Lateral spinothalamic pathway mediates pain and temperature sensation.

C. Lateral corticospinal tract mediates voluntary skilled motor activity.

D. Dorsal and ventral spinocerebellar tracts transmit proprioceptive and muscle reflex activity information from the spinal cord to the cerebellum.

E. Hypothalamospinal tract influences preganglionic sympathetic neurons of the intermediolateral cell column and preganglionic parasympathetic neurons of the sacral parasympathetic nucleus. Interruption of this tract above T1 results in **Horner syndrome**.

Clinical Considerations

A. **Lesions of the Spinal Cord**

1. **Poliomyelitis and Werdnig-Hoffmann disease** are caused by damage to alpha motor neurons within the ventral gray horn. These lesions are classified as lower motor neuron (LMN) lesions. Clinical findings include those characteristic of an LMN lesion: flaccid paralysis, areflexia, atrophy, fasciculations and fibrillations, and no Babinski sign.

2. **Amyotrophic lateral sclerosis (ALS; Lou Gehrig disease)** is caused by damage to alpha motor neurons within the ventral gray horn and the lateral corticospinal tract. This lesion is classified as a lower motor neuron (LMN) and upper motor neuron (UMN) lesion. Clinical findings include those characteristic of an LMN lesion (see above) and UMN lesion: spastic paralysis or paresis, no atrophy, hyperreflexia, no fasciculations or fibrillations, and positive Babinski sign.

3. **Tabes dorsalis (dorsal column disease)** is caused by damage to dorsal column sensory pathways. Clinical findings include loss of tactile discrimination, vibration sensation, and proprioception; it is associated with tertiary syphilis.

4. **Brown-Sequard syndrome (incomplete spinal cord injury; hemisection)** is caused by damage attributable to a penetrating blow to the dorsal columns, lateral corticospinal tract, lateral spinothalamic tract, hypothalamospinal tract, and ventral gray horn. Clinical findings include ipsilateral loss of tactile discrimination, vibration sensation, and proprioception; ipsilateral spastic paresis with pyramidal signs below the lesion; contralateral loss of pain and temperature sensation one segment below the lesion; ipsilateral Horner syndrome; and ipsilateral flaccid paralysis.

5. **Anterior spinal artery occlusion** results in damage to the lateral corticospinal tracts, lateral spinothalamic tracts, hypothalamospinal tracts, ventral gray horns, and corticospinal tracts to sacral parasympathetic centers at S2 through S4. Clinical findings include bilateral spastic paresis with pyramidal signs below the lesion, bilateral loss of pain and temperature sensation below the lesion, bilateral Horner syndrome, bilateral flaccid paralysis, and loss of voluntary bladder and bowel control.

6. **Vitamin B$_{12}$ neuropathy** is caused by pernicious anemia (megaloblastic anemia) and results in damage to the dorsal columns, lateral corticospinal tracts, and spinocerebellar tracts. Clinical findings include bilateral loss of tactile discrimination, vibration sensation, and proprioception; bilateral spastic paresis with pyramidal signs; and bilateral arm and leg dystaxia.

7. **Syringomyelia** is a central cavitation of the cervical spinal cord of unknown origin and results in damage to ventral white commissure, involving the decussating lateral spinothalamic axons, and ventral gray horns. Clinical findings include bilateral loss of pain and temperature sensation and flaccid paralysis of the intrinsic muscles of the hand.

B. **Spinal Cord Injury (SCI)**

1. **Complete SCI (transection of spinal cord)** results in loss of sensation and motor function below the lesion. There are two types of complete SCI:

   a. **Paraplegia** (i.e. paralysis of lower limbs) occurs if the transection occurs anywhere between the cervical and lumbar enlargements of the spinal cord.

   b. **Quadriplegia** (i.e. paralysis of all four limbs) occurs if the transection occurs above C3. These individuals may die quickly as a result of respiratory failure if the phrenic nerve is compromised.

2. **Incomplete SCI** can be ameliorated somewhat by rapid surgical intervention. There are three situations that may lead to an incomplete SCI: a concussive blow, anterior spinal artery occlusion, or a penetrating blow (e.g. Brown-Sequard syndrome).

3. **Complications of any SCI** include hypotension in the acute setting, ileus (bowel obstruction as a result of lack of motility), renal stones, pyelonephritis, renal failure, and deep venous thrombosis. **Methylprednisolone** may be of benefit if administered within 8 hours of injury.

C. **Tumors of the spinal cord** are classified as follows:
   1. **Intramedullary Tumors (within the spinal cord)**
      a. **Ependymomas** typically arise within or adjacent to the ependymal lining of the ventricular system. In children, most ependymomas are found in the posterior fossa of the cranial vault; the fourth ventricle is the most common infratentorial site. In adults, most ependymomas are found in the spinal cord and may occur in the cervical region near the obliterated central canal where tumor cells align themselves around pathologic tubular cavities (**syrinx**) or in the lumbosacral region associated with the conus medullaris. Ependymomas are usually well demarcated with frequent areas of calcification, hemorrhage, and cysts; ependymal rosettes are diagnostic. Clinical presentation is dependent on tumor location. Patients with posterior fossa tumors present with increased intracranial pressure, headache, nausea, vomiting, ataxia, vertigo, papilledema, cranial nerve (CN) VI to CN X cranial nerve palsies. Patients with spinal cord tumors present with deficits related to involvement of ascending and descending tracts and deficits related to exiting peripheral nerves.
      b. **Astrocytomas** (account for 70% of all neuroglial tumors) typically arise from astrocytes and are composed of cells with elongated or irregular, hyperchromatic nuclei and an eosinophilic glial fibrillary acidic protein (GFAP)-positive cytoplasm. Astrocytomas are divided into grade I (benign), grade II (benign), grade III (anaplastic astrocytomas; malignant), and grade IV (glioblastoma multiforme; malignant). Grade II astrocytomas are associated with missense mutations in the *p53* tumor suppressor gene and loss of chromosome 22q. The transition from a low-grade to a high-grade astrocytoma is associated with the inactivation of tumor suppressor genes on chromosomes 9p, 13q, and 19q (appears to be unique to glial tumors and not other human cancers). The transition to a malignant glioblastoma is associated with the inactivation of *PTEN/MMAC1* tumor suppressor gene on chromosome 10 and amplification of the epidermal growth factor receptor (*EGFR*) gene.
         i. **Fibrillary (pilocytic) astrocytomas.** In children, most astrocytomas are low-grade (benign) and involve the cerebellum and brainstem. Fibrillary astrocytomas of the cerebellum are the most common primary brain tumor in children and have an excellent prognosis. These tumors produce a cystic cavity and have characteristic Rosenthal fibers. Other sites of benign astrocytomas include the optic nerve, spinal cord (cervical and thoracic regions), and the brainstem (which has a very poor prognosis because of its location).
         ii. **Glioblastoma multiforme (GBM).** GBMs are the most common primary brain tumor in adults (men 40 to 70 years of age), are highly malignant, and pursue a rapidly fatal course. GBMs have histologic features that include hemorrhagic necrosis with proliferation of blood vessels in areas of necrosis; pseudopalisading of neoplastic cells around foci of necrosis and blood vessels; and highly pleomorphic neoplastic cells (bizarre tumor giant cells) with frequent atypical mitotic figures. A common site of GBMs is the frontal lobe, where the tumor commonly crosses the corpus callosum and produces a butterfly appearance on MRI.

2. **Intradural Tumors (within the meninges)**

   a. **Meningiomas** (90% are benign) arise from arachnoid cap cells of the arachnoid villi of the meninges and are found at the skull vault, sites of dural reflection (e.g. falx cerebri, tentorium cerebelli), optic nerve sheath, and choroid plexus. The most common presentation of a symptomatic meningioma is a focal or generalized seizure or gradually worsening neurologic defect. Meningiomas occur more commonly in women, may increase in size during pregnancy, have an increased incidence in women taking postmenopausal hormones, and are associated with breast cancer; all of which suggest a potential involvement of steroid hormones. In 50% of meningiomas, mutations in the *NF2* gene (neurofibromatosis type II) and *DAL-1* gene have been documented as an early event in tumorigenesis.

   b. **Schwannomas** are benign, well-circumscribed, encapsulated tumors that arise from Schwann cells located on cranial nerves, spinal nerve roots (presents as a dumbbell-shaped tumor protruding through the intervertebral foramen), or spinal nerves. The most common intracranial site is the cerebellopontine angle with involvement of CN VIII (acoustic neuroma), in which expansion of the tumor results in tinnitus and sensorineural deafness. Multiple Schwannomas may occur associated with neurofibromatosis type II. Schwannomas have histologic features that include a very compact, wavy, palisading pattern of interlacing bundles (Antoni type A areas) interspersed with loosely structured myxomatous-appearing areas of stellate-shaped cells with long processes (Antoni type B areas) that resemble a zebra's stripes.

   c. **Neurofibromas** have a clinical presentation that is nearly identical to that of a Schwannoma, as indicated above. Neurofibromas may occur within any nerve in the body. Involvement of a peripheral spinal nerve is manifest as a firm, rubbery, subcutaneous lesion.

3. **Extradural Tumors (outside the meninges)**

   a. **Metastatic Tumors.** Primary cancers of the lung, breast, and prostate generally metastasize to the **vertebral bodies** of vertebrae and are the most common extradural tumor.

   b. **Chordomas** are malignant, midline, lobulated, mucoid tumors that arise from remnants of the embryonic notochord and usually occur in the sacral (most common site) or clival region. Chordomas have histologic features that include physaliphorous (bubble-bearing) cells with mucoid droplets in the cytoplasm.

ⓧ Radiology

A. **MRIs of an Astrocytoma, Meningioma, and Schwannoma (Figure 2-5)**

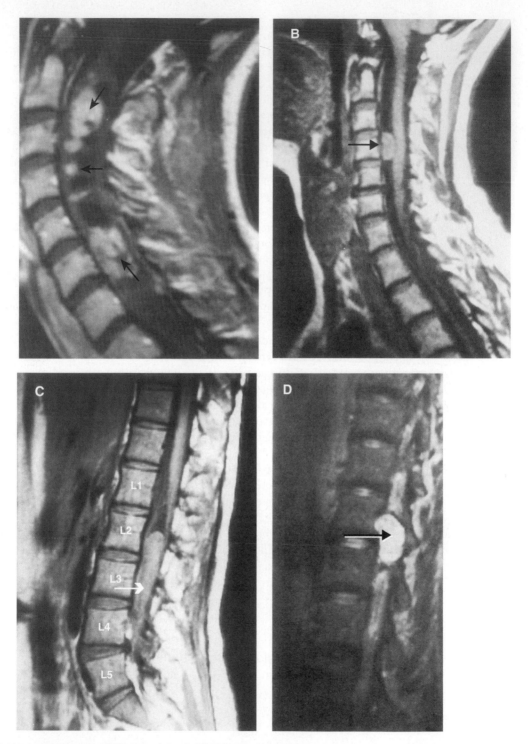

● **Figure 2-5 Tumors of the Spinal Cord. (A) MRI of an Astrocytoma.** An astrocytoma is an excellent example of an intramedullary (within the spinal cord) tumor. Note the astrocytoma (arrows) within the substance of the spinal cord that has a cystic appearance. **(B) MRI of a Meningioma.** A meningioma is an example of an intradural (within the meninges) tumor. Note the meningioma (arrow) outside of the spinal cord causing some compression of the spinal cord. **(C, D) MRIs of a Schwannoma. (C)** A Schwannoma is another example of an intradural (within the meninges) tumor. Note the Schwannoma (arrow) within the dural sac at about vertebral level L3 involving the cauda equina. The key to interpreting this MRI is to remember that the spinal cord in the adult ends at vertebral level L1. So, at L3 the spinal cord is not present so this tumor CANNOT be intramedullary. **(D)** An MRI of the intervertebral foramen shows the Schwannoma protruding through the intervertebral foramen (arrow), which is a clear characteristic of a Schwannoma (or neurofibroma).

Chapter 3

Autonomic Nervous System

(I) **General Features of the Nervous System.** The nervous system can be anatomically divided into the **central nervous system (CNS)**, which consists of the brain and spinal cord, and the **peripheral nervous system (PNS)**, which consists of 12 pairs of cranial nerves and 31 pairs of spinal nerves along with their associated ganglia. In addition, the nervous system can be functionally divided into the **somatic nervous system**, which controls voluntary activities by innervating skeletal muscle, and the **visceral (or autonomic) nervous system**, which controls involuntary activities by innervating smooth muscle, cardiac muscle, and glands. The autonomic nervous system (ANS) is divided into the **sympathetic (thoracolumbar) division** and the **parasympathetic (craniosacral) division**. The **hypothalamus** has central control of the ANS, whereby the hypothalamus coordinates all ANS actions. The ANS has a **visceromotor component** and a **viscerosensory component** (although traditionally only the visceromotor component has been emphasized).

(II) **Sympathetic Division of the ANS (Thoracolumbar)**

A. **Motor (Efferent) Component (Figures 3-1 and 3-2).** The motor component of the sympathetic nervous system has a "fight or flight" or catabolic function that is necessary in emergency situations in which the body needs a sudden burst of energy. In a controlled environment, the sympathetic nervous system is not necessary for life but is essential for any stressful situation. The whole motor component of the sympathetic nervous system tends to "go off" together in an emergency situation. The motor component of the sympathetic nervous system is a two-neuron chain that consists of a **preganglionic sympathetic neuron** and a **postganglionic sympathetic neuron** that follows this general pattern: CNS → short preganglionic neuron → ganglion → long postganglionic neuron → smooth muscle, cardiac muscle, and glands.

1. **Preganglionic Sympathetic Neuron.** The preganglionic neuronal cell bodies are located in the gray matter of the T1 through L2 or L3 spinal cord (i.e. intermediolateral cell column). Preganglionic sympathetic neurons use acetylcholine as a neurotransmitter. Preganglionic axons have a number of fates:

   a. Preganglionic axons enter the paravertebral chain ganglia through white communicating rami where they synapse with postganglionic neurons at that level.

   b. Preganglionic axons travel up or down the paravertebral chain ganglia where they synapse with postganglionic neurons at upper or lower levels, respectively.

   c. Preganglionic axons pass through the paravertebral chain ganglia (i.e. no synapse) as thoracic splanchnic nerves (greater, lesser, and least), lumbar splanchnic nerves (L1 through L4), and sacral splanchnic nerves (L5 and S1 through S3), which synapse with postganglionic neurons in prevertebral ganglia (i.e. celiac ganglion, aorticorenal ganglion, superior mesenteric ganglion, inferior mesenteric ganglion) as well as in the superior hypogastric plexus and inferior hypogastric plexus.

d. Preganglionic axons pass through the paravertebral chain ganglia (i.e. no synapse) as thoracic splanchnic nerves, which synapse with modified postganglionic sympathetic neurons in the adrenal medulla called **chromaffin cells**.

2. **Postganglionic Sympathetic Neuron.** The postganglionic neuronal cell bodies are located in the paravertebral chain ganglia and the prevertebral ganglia. Postganglionic sympathetic neurons use **norepinephrine** as a neurotransmitter (except for those innervating eccrine sweat glands, which use acetylcholine), which binds to α_1, α_2, β_1, β_2, **and** β_3 **adrenergic receptors** located on the cell membrane of smooth muscle, cardiac muscle, and glands. Postganglionic axons have a number of fates:

a. Postganglionic axons leave the paravertebral chain ganglia through gray communicating rami and join all 31 pairs of spinal nerves to innervate smooth muscle of blood vessels, arrector pili smooth muscle of the hair follicle, and sweat glands of the skin.

b. Postganglionic axons leave the superior cervical ganglion of the prevertebral chain ganglia and follow the carotid arterial system into the head and neck to innervate smooth muscle of blood vessels, dilator pupillae muscle, superior tarsal muscle, lacrimal gland, submandibular gland, sublingual gland, and parotid gland.

c. Postganglionic axons leave the paravertebral chain ganglia (from the superior cervical ganglion through T4 levels) to enter complex cardiac and pulmonary nerve plexuses to innervate the heart and lung, respectively.

d. Postganglionic axons leave prevertebral ganglia and the superior and inferior hypogastric plexus to innervate smooth muscle of various visceral organs.

e. Modified postganglionic sympathetic neurons called chromaffin cells within the adrenal medulla release epinephrine (the majority product; 90%) and norepinephrine (the minority product; 10%) into the bloodstream, both of which are potent sympathetic neurotransmitters.

B. **Sensory (Afferent) Component (Figure 3-3).** The sensory component of the sympathetic nervous system carries **visceral pain sensation** from **nociceptors** located in viscera to the CNS. Nociceptors are free nerve endings that respond to pathologic stimuli such as myocardial infarction, appendicitis, and gastrointestinal cramping or bloating. Visceral pain sensation is carried almost exclusively by the sensory (afferent) component of the sympathetic nervous system. Visceral pain sensation is **poorly localized** because nociceptor density is low, nociceptor fields are large, and its projection to higher CNS levels is widespread. The sensory component of the sympathetic nervous system is a three- or four-neuron chain.

1. The first neuron in the chain has its neuronal cell body located in the dorsal root ganglia at T1 through L2 or L3 spinal cord levels. This neuron sends a peripheral process to the viscera that ends as a free nerve ending (or nociceptor) and sends a central process into the spinal cord that synapses with the second neuron in **laminae I and V** or **laminae VII and VIII**.

2. The second neuron in the chain (in laminae I and V) projects axons to the **anterolateral system (ALS)** both contralaterally and ipsilaterally, where they synapse with the third neuron in the **ventral posterolateral (VPL) nucleus** of the thalamus. The second neuron in the chain (in laminae VII and VIII) projects axons to the **spinoreticular tract** both contralaterally and ipsilaterally, where they synapse in the **reticular formation**.

3. The third neuron in the chain (in the VPL nucleus) projects axons to the **postcentral gyrus** and the **insula** of the cerebral cortex. The third neuron in the chain (from the reticular system) projects axons to the **hypothalamus** and the **intralaminar nuclei** of the thalamus.

4. The fourth neuron in the chain (in the intralaminar nuclei) projects axons to **diverse areas of the cerebral cortex.**

Ⅲ Parasympathetic Division of the ANS (Craniosacral)

A. Motor (Efferent) Component (Figures 3-4 and 3-5). The motor component of the parasympathetic nervous system has a "rest and digest" or anabolic function that is necessary to conserve energy, restore body resources, and get rid of wastes. The whole motor component of the parasympathetic nervous system does not "go off" together but instead specific activities are initiated when appropriate. The motor component of the parasympathetic nervous system is a two-neuron chain that consists of a **preganglionic parasympathetic neuron** and a **postganglionic parasympathetic neuron** that follows this general pattern: CNS → long preganglionic neuron → ganglion → short postganglionic neuron → smooth muscle, cardiac muscle, and glands.

1. **Preganglionic Parasympathetic Neuron.** The preganglionic neuronal cell bodies are located in the Edinger-Westphal nucleus, lacrimal nucleus, superior salivatory nucleus, inferior salivatory nucleus, the dorsal motor nucleus of the vagus nerve, and gray mater of the S2 through S4 spinal cord. Preganglionic parasympathetic neurons use acetylcholine as a neurotransmitter. Preganglionic axons have a number of fates:

    a. Preganglionic axons from the Edinger-Westphal nucleus run with cranial nerve (CN) III and enter the ciliary ganglia where they synapse with postganglionic neurons.

    b. Preganglionic axons from the lacrimal nucleus run with CN VII and enter the pterygopalatine ganglion where they synapse with postganglionic neurons.

    c. Preganglionic axons from the superior salivatory nucleus run with CN VII and enter the submandibular ganglion where they synapse with postganglionic neurons.

    d. Preganglionic axons from the inferior salivatory nucleus run with CN IX and enter the otic ganglion where they synapse with postganglionic neurons.

    e. Preganglionic axons from the dorsal motor nucleus of the vagus nerve run with CN X and travel to various visceral organs (up to the splenic flexure of the transverse colon) where they synapse with postganglionic neurons.

    f. Preganglionic axons from the gray matter of the S2 through S4 spinal cord run as **pelvic splanchnic nerves**, which interact with the inferior hypogastric plexus and travel to various visceral organs (distal to the splenic flexure of the transverse colon) where they synapse with postganglionic neurons.

2. **Postganglionic Parasympathetic Neuron.** The postganglionic neuronal cells bodies are located in the ciliary ganglion, pterygopalatine ganglion, submandibular ganglion, and otic ganglion, and within various visceral organs. Postganglionic parasympathetic neurons use **acetylcholine** as a neurotransmitter, which binds to M_1, M_2, **and** M_3 **muscarinic acetylcholine receptors** located on the cell membrane of smooth muscle, cardiac muscle, and glands. Postganglionic axons have a number of fates:

    a. Postganglionic axons leave the ciliary ganglion to innervate the sphincter pupillae muscle and ciliary muscle.

   b. Postganglionic axons leave the pterygopalatine ganglion to innervate the lacrimal glands and nasal glands.
   c. Postganglionic axons leave the submandibular ganglion to innervate the submandibular glands and sublingual glands.
   d. Postganglionic axons leave the otic ganglion to innervate the parotid gland.
   e. Postganglionic axons associated with CN X innervate smooth muscle of various visceral organs and cardiac muscle.
   f. Postganglionic axons associated with the pelvic splanchnic nerves innervate various visceral organs.

B. Sensory (Afferent) Component (Figure 3-6). The sensory component of the parasympathetic nervous system carries **visceral pressure and movement sensation** from **rapidly adapting mechanoreceptors, visceral stretch sensation** from **slowly adapting mechanoreceptors, arterial oxygen tension (PaO_2)** and **arterial pH** information from **chemoreceptors** (i.e. carotid bodies located at the bifurcation of the common carotid artery and aortic bodies located in the aortic arch), **blood pressure** information from **baroreceptors** (i.e. carotid sinus located in the walls of the common carotid artery and baroreceptors located in the great veins, atria, and aortic arch), **osmolarity** information from **osmoreceptors**, and **temperature** from **internal thermal receptors**. The sensory component of the parasympathetic nervous system is a three-neuron chain.

   1. The first neuron in the chain has its neuronal cell body located in the geniculate ganglion of CN VII, inferior (petrosal) ganglion of CN IX, inferior (nodose) ganglion of CN X, and the dorsal root ganglia of the S2 through S4 spinal cord. These neurons send a peripheral process to the viscera that ends at the rapidly adapting mechanoreceptors, slowly adapting mechanoreceptors, chemoreceptors, baroreceptors, osmoreceptors, and internal thermal receptors. These neurons also send a central process into the brainstem or spinal cord, which synapses with a second neuron in the **solitary nucleus,** in the **dorsal horn of the spinal cord,** or in the **gray matter of the S2 through S4 spinal cord.**
   2. The second neuron in the chain (in the solitary nucleus) projects axons to the **dorsal motor nucleus of the vagus nerve** and the **rostral ventrolateral medulla,** where they synapse with a third neuron. The second neuron in the chain (in the dorsal horn of the spinal cord) projects axons to the **anterolateral system** and the **spinoreticular tract.** The second neuron in the chain (in the gray matter of the S2 through S4 spinal cord) is actually a preganglionic parasympathetic motor neuron of a pelvic splanchnic nerve (forming a sensorimotor reflex arc).
   3. The third neuron in the chain (in the dorsal motor nucleus of the vagus nerve) is actually a preganglionic parasympathetic motor neuron of CN X (forming a sensorimotor reflex arc). The third neuron in the chain (in the rostral ventrolateral medulla) projects axons to the intermediolateral cell column of the spinal cord and thereby controls the activity of preganglionic sympathetic motor neurons (forming a sensorimotor reflex arc).

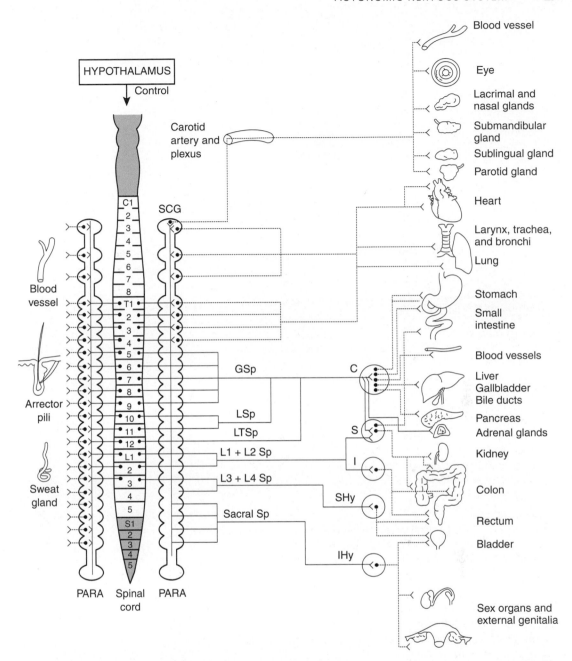

● **Figure 3-1 Diagram of the Motor Component of the Sympathetic Nervous System.** Solid lines = preganglionic sympathetic neurons, dashed lines = postganglionic sympathetic neurons, PARA = paravertebral chain ganglia, C = celiac ganglion, S = superior mesenteric ganglion, I = inferior mesenteric ganglion, SHy = superior hypogastric plexus, IHy = inferior hypogastric plexus, GSp = greater thoracic splanchnic nerve, LSp = lesser thoracic splanchnic nerve, LTSp = least thoracic splanchnic nerve, Sp = splanchnic nerve, SCG = superior cervical ganglion.

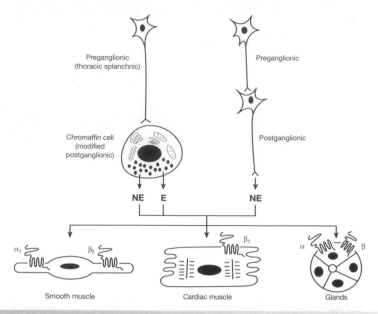

SPECIFIC SYMPATHETIC MOTOR ACTIONS

Smooth Muscle
Contracts dilator pupillae muscle causing dilation of pupil (mydriasis)
Contracts arrector pili muscle in skin
Contracts smooth muscle in skin, skeletal muscle, and visceral blood vessels
Relaxes smooth muscle in skeletal muscle blood vessels
Relaxes bronchial smooth muscle in lung (bronchodilation)
Relaxes smooth muscle in gastrointestinal tract wall
Contracts smooth muscle in gastrointestinal tract sphincters
Relaxes smooth muscle in urinary bladder
Contracts smooth muscle in urinary tract sphincter
Contracts smooth muscle of ductus deferens causing ejaculation (emission); "shoot"
Female reproductive tract?*

Cardiac Muscle
Accelerates sinoatrial node (increases heart rate); positive chronotropism
Increases conduction velocity in atrioventricular node; positive dromotropism
Increases contractility of cardiac muscle; positive inotropism

Glands
Increases secretion from salivary glands
Increases eccrine sweat gland secretion (thermoregulation)
Increases apocrine sweat gland secretion (stress)
Stimulates seminal vesicle and prostate secretion during ejaculation (emission)

Other
Stimulates gluconeogenesis and glycogenolysis in hepatocytes (hyperglycemia)
Stimulates lipolysis in adipocytes
Stimulates renin secretion from juxtaglomerular cells in kidney (increases blood pressure)
Inhibits insulin secretion from pancreatic beta cells (hyperglycemia)

*Despite numerous studies, specific sympathetic actions on the female reproductive tract remain inconclusive.

● **Figure 3-2 Specific Motor Actions of the Sympathetic Nervous System.** The postganglionic sympathetic axons release norepinephrine, which binds to α_1, α_2, β_1, β_2, and β_3 adrenergic receptors located on the cell membrane of smooth muscle, cardiac muscle, and glands. This elicits specific sympathetic actions that are indicated in the table. In addition, note that the chromaffin cells (modified postganglionic sympathetic neurons) of the adrenal medulla (which is technically an endocrine gland) are functionally a part of the sympathetic nervous system. The chromaffin cells release epinephrine (the majority product; 90%) and norepinephrine (the minority product; 10%) into the bloodstream. NE = norepinephrine, E = epinephrine.

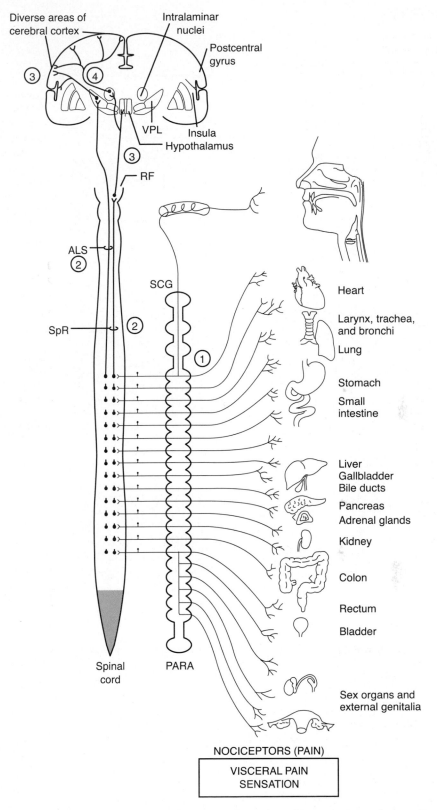

● **Figure 3-3 Diagram of the Sensory Component of the Sympathetic Nervous System (Visceral Pain Sensation).** The circled numbers indicate the three- or four-neuron chain involved in visceral pain sensation. ALS = anterolateral system, SpR = spinoreticular tract, VPL = ventral posterolateral nucleus of the thalamus, PARA = paravertebral chain ganglia, RF = reticular formation.

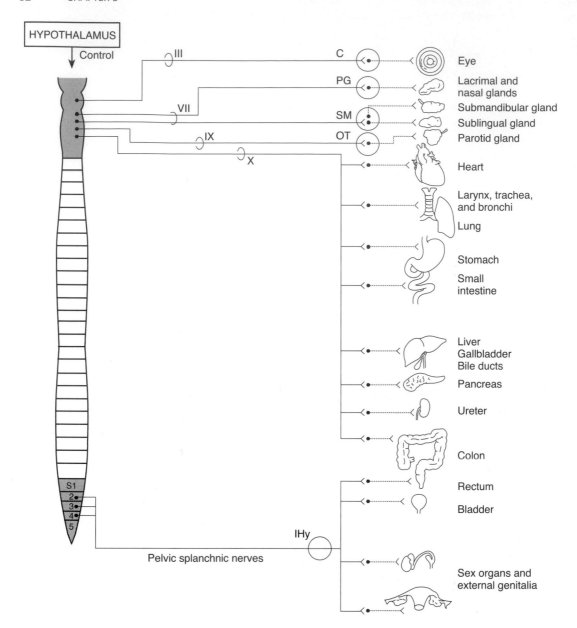

● **Figure 3-4 Diagram of the Motor Component of the Parasympathetic Nervous System.** Solid lines = preganglionic parasympathetic neurons, dashed lines = postganglionic parasympathetic neurons, C = ciliary ganglion, PG = pterygopalatine ganglion, SM = submandibular ganglion, OT = otic ganglion, IHy = inferior hypogastric plexus.

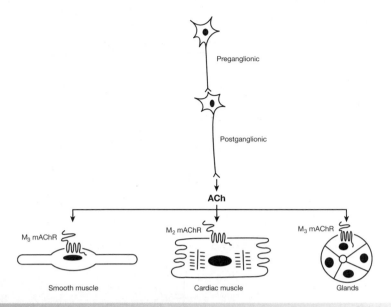

SPECIFIC PARASYMPATHETIC MOTOR ACTIONS

Smooth Muscle
Contracts sphincter pupillae muscle causing constriction of pupil (miosis)
Contracts ciliary muscle causing accommodation for near vision
Contracts bronchial smooth muscle in lung (bronchoconstriction)
Contracts smooth muscle in gastrointestinal tract wall
Relaxes smooth muscle in gastrointestinal tract sphincters
Contracts smooth muscle in urinary bladder
Relaxes smooth muscle in urinary tract sphincter
Relaxes smooth muscle in penile blood vessels causing dilation (erection of penis); "point"
Female reproductive tract?? *

Cardiac Muscle
Decelerates sinoatrial node (decrease heart rate; vagal arrest); negative chronotropism
Decreases conduction velocity in atrioventricular node; negative dromotropism
Decreases contractility of cardiac muscle (atrial); negative inotropism

Glands
Increases watery secretion from salivary glands
Increases secretion from lacrimal gland
Increases secretion from mucosal and submucosal glands of gastrointestinal tract

*Despite numerous studies, specific parasympathetic actions on the female reproductive tract remain inconclusive.

● **Figure 3-5 Specific Motor Actions of the Parasympathetic Nervous System.** The postganglionic parasympathetic axons release acetylcholine, which binds to M_1, M_2, and M_3 muscarinic acetylcholine receptors located on the cell membrane of smooth muscle, cardiac muscle, and glands. This elicits specific parasympathetic actions that are indicated in the table. ACh = acetylcholine, mAChR = muscarinic acetylcholine receptor.

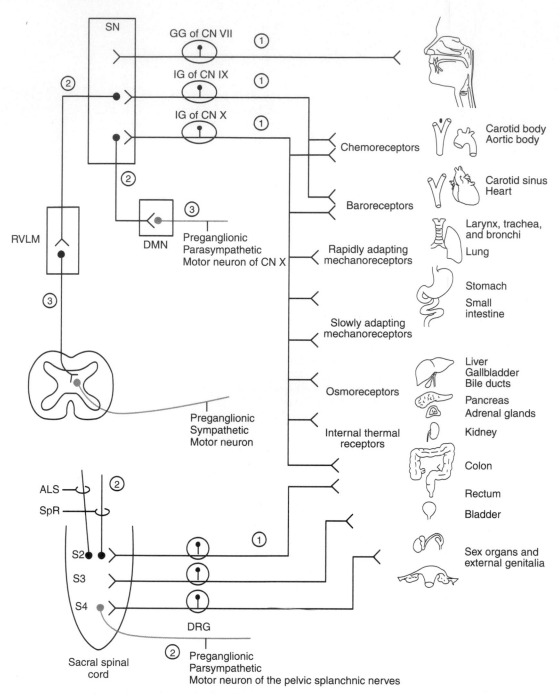

● **Figure 3-6 Diagram of the Sensory Component of the Parasympathetic Nervous System (Visceral Pressure and Movement Sensation, Visceral Stretch Sensation, Arterial Oxygen Tension and Arterial pH, Blood Pressure, Osmolarity, and Temperature).** The circled numbers indicate the three-neuron chain involved in visceral sensation. DRG = dorsal root ganglion, ALS = anterolateral system, SpR = spinoreticular tract, RVLM = rostral ventrolateral medulla, DMN = dorsal motor nucleus of the vagus nerve, SN = solitary nucleus, GG = geniculate ganglion of CN VII, IG of CN IX = inferior (petrosal) ganglion of the glossopharyngeal nerve, IG of CN X = inferior (nodose) ganglion of the vagus nerve.

Chapter 4

Lymphatic System

❶ Central Lymphatic Drainage (Figure 4-1)

A. General Features. The lymphatic system is a collection of vessels that function to drain extracellular fluid from tissues of the body and return it to the venous system. All regions of the body possess lymphatic drainage except for the brain and spinal cord. A knowledge of the lymphatic system plays a key role in determining the prognosis of cancer and in cancer staging.

B. Thoracic Duct. The thoracic duct begins in a majority of individuals as the **abdominal confluence of lymph trunks** at the L1 to L2 vertebral level, which receives lymph from four main lymphatic trunks: the **right and left lumbar lymph trunks** and the **right and left intestinal lymph trunks**. In a small percentage of individuals, the abdominal confluence of lymph trunks is represented as a dilated sac (called the **cisterna chyli**). The thoracic duct ascends to the right of the midline between the azygos vein and the thoracic aorta. The thoracic duct traverses the aortic aperture of the diaphragm. The thoracic duct inclines to the left side at the T5 vertebral level and ascends along the left border of the esophagus. The thoracic duct terminates at the junction of the left internal jugular vein and left subclavian vein (i.e. **left brachiocephalic vein**) at the base of the neck. As a general rule, the thoracic duct drains lymph from the **left side of the head and neck, left breast, left upper limb and superficial thoracoabdominal wall, and all the body below the diaphragm**. Along its course, the thoracic duct receives lymph from the following tributaries:
1. **Right and left descending thoracic lymph trunks** convey lymph from the lower intercostal spaces 6 through 11.
2. **Upper intercostal lymph trunks** convey lymph from the upper intercostal spaces 1 through 5.
3. **Mediastinal lymph trunks.**
4. **Left subclavian lymph trunk.**
5. **Left jugular lymph trunk.**
6. **Left bronchomediastinal lymph trunk.**

C. Right Lymphatic Duct. The right lymphatic duct (a short vessel) begins with a high degree of variability as a convergence of the **right subclavian lymph trunk, right jugular lymph trunk**, and **right bronchomediastinal lymph trunk**. The right lymphatic duct terminates at the junction of the right internal jugular vein and right subclavian vein (i.e. **right brachiocephalic vein**) at the base of the neck. As a general rule, the right lymphatic duct drains lymph from the **right side of the head and neck, right breast, and right upper limb and superficial thoracoabdominal wall**.
1. **Right subclavian lymph trunk** conveys lymph from the right upper extremity and the right superficial thoracoabdominal wall up to the umbilicus.

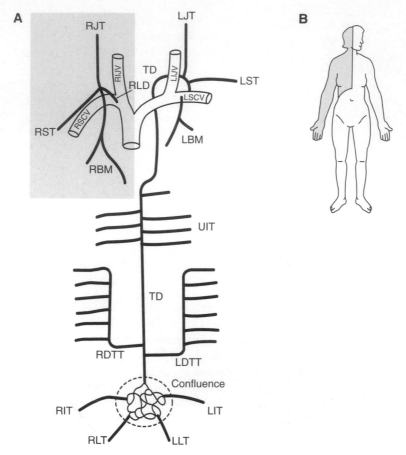

● Figure 4-1 (A) Diagram of the Lymphatic System. (B) General Body Pattern of Lymph Drainage. Shaded area = lymph drainage into the right lymphatic duct, unshaded area = lymph drainage into the thoracic duct. LJT = left jugular lymph trunk, LST = left subclavian lymph trunk, LBM = left bronchomediastinal lymph trunk, LIJV = left internal jugular vein, UIT = upper intercostal lymph trunks, LDTT = left descending thoracic lymph trunk, LIT = left intestinal lymph trunk, LLT = left lumbar lymph trunk, LSCV = left subclavian vein, RJT = right jugular lymph trunk, RST = right subclavian lymph trunk, RBM = right bronchomediastinal lymph trunk, RDTT = right descending thoracic lymph trunk, RIT = right intestinal lymph trunk, RLT = right lumbar lymph trunk, RSCV = right subclavian vein, RIJV = right internal jugular vein, RLD = right lymphatic duct, TD = thoracic duct.

2.   **Right jugular lymph trunk** conveys lymph from the right side of the head and neck.
3.   **Right bronchomediastinal lymph trunk** conveys lymph from the right side of the diaphragm and liver; right lung, bronchi, and trachea; and right breast.

Ⅱ **Head and Neck.** Lymph from the right side of the head and neck ultimately drains into the right lymphatic duct. Lymph from the left side of the head and neck ultimately drains into the thoracic duct. The head and neck has a **paracervical collar of superficial lymph nodes** and **deep cervical lymph nodes**.

A.   The paracervical collar of superficial lymph nodes includes **submental nodes, submandibular nodes, parotid nodes, buccal nodes, mastoid nodes, occipital nodes, superficial cervical nodes**, and **anterior cervical nodes**. The lymph from these superficial nodes drains into the deep cervical lymph nodes: **perivascular collar of superficial lymph nodes → deep cervical lymph nodes**.

B.   The deep cervical lymph nodes are found alongside the carotid sheath associated with the internal jugular vein and deep to the sternocleidomastoid muscle. The deep cervical nodes receive lymph not only from the paracervical collar of superficial lymph nodes but also from the **retropharyngeal nodes, paratracheal nodes, infrahyoid nodes, prelaryngeal nodes, pretracheal nodes**, and **lingual nodes.** Lymph from the head and neck drains directly or indirectly into the deep cervical nodes. Efferent lymphatic vessels from the deep cervical lymph nodes join to form the right jugular lymph trunk and left jugular lymph trunk. Lymph from the head and neck drains as follows: **perivascular collar of superficial lymph nodes** → **retropharyngeal nodes, paratracheal nodes, infrahyoid nodes, prelaryngeal nodes, pretracheal nodes, and lingual nodes** → **deep cervical lymph nodes** → **right jugular lymph trunk (for the right side of the head and neck)** or **left jugular lymph trunk (for the left side of the head and neck).** On the right side, the right jugular lymph trunk joins with the right subclavian lymph trunk and the right bronchomediastinal lymph trunk to form the right lymphatic duct. On the left side, the left jugular lymph trunk joins the thoracic duct.

III Thorax

A. Breast. Lymph from the right breast ultimately drains into the right lymphatic duct. Lymph from the left breast ultimately drains into the thoracic duct. The breast has lymphatic plexuses that communicate freely called the **circumareolar plexus, perilobular plexus**, and **interlobular plexus.** All drain into the deep **subareolar plexus.** From the subareolar plexus, lymph flows as indicated below:

1. A majority of the lymph (>75%) from the lateral quadrant of the right and left breast drains as follows: **axillary nodes (humeral, subscapular pectoral, central, and apical)** → **infraclavicular and supraclavicular nodes** → **right subclavian lymph trunk (for the right breast)** or **left subclavian lymph trunk (for the left breast).** On the right side, the right subclavian lymph trunk joins with the right jugular lymph trunk and the right bronchomediastinal lymph trunk to form the right lymphatic duct. On the left side, the left subclavian lymph trunk joins the thoracic duct. The remaining lateral drainage (approximately 25%) occurs via the interpectoral, deltopectoral, supraclavicular, and inferior deep cervical nodes.

2. The lymph from the medial quadrant of the right and left breast drains as follows: **parasternal nodes** → **right bronchomediastinal lymph trunk (for the right breast)** or **left bronchomediastinal lymph trunk (for the left breast).** On the right side, the right bronchomediastinal lymph trunk joins with the right subclavian lymph trunk and the right jugular lymph trunk to form the right lymphatic duct. On the left side, the left bronchomediastinal lymph trunk joins the thoracic duct. The lymph from the medial quadrant may also **drain into the opposite breast.**

3. The lymph from the inferior quadrant of the right and left breast drains into the nodes of the upper abdomen (e.g. **inferior phrenic lymph nodes**).

4. **Clinical Considerations**
   a. Clinically, three levels of axillary lymph nodes are described: **level 1**, lateral to pectoral minor; **level 2**, deep to pectoral minor; and **level 3**, medial to pectoral minor. A higher level of involvement is correlated with a worse prognosis. More important to prognosis is the number of lymph nodes involved, which in part determines staging.
   b. Surgical treatment of breast cancer commonly involves a **modified radical mastectomy.** This surgical procedure involves, in part, removal of the level 1 and 2 axillary lymph nodes. One of the possible complications of this surgical procedure is disruption of lymphatic drainage from the arm and resultant **lymphedema.**

c. Skin dimpling, edema, and erythema can sometimes be seen on physical examination of the breast. This orange peel appearance of the skin, known as **peau d'orange,** can be indicative of infection or inflammatory breast cancer. When caused by cancer, it is caused by the invasion of dermal lymphatics by malignant cells.

B. Lung. Lymph from the right lung ultimately drains into the right bronchomediastinal trunk. Lymph from the left lung ultimately drains into the left bronchomediastinal trunk (except for the left lower lobe, which drains to the right side). The lung has two lymphatic plexuses that communicate freely called the **superficial plexus** and **deep plexus.**

   1. The **superficial plexus** of lymphatic vessels lies just deep to the visceral pleura and drains lymph to the **bronchopulmonary lymph nodes** → **inferior and superior tracheobronchial lymph nodes** → **paratracheal lymph nodes** → **right bronchomediastinal lymph trunk (for the right lung) or left bronchomediastinal lymph trunk (for the left lung, except the left lower lobe, which drains to the right side).** On the right side, the right bronchomediastinal lymph trunk joins with the right subclavian lymph trunk and the right jugular lymph trunk to form the right lymphatic duct. On the left side, the left bronchomediastinal lymph trunk joins the thoracic duct.

   2. The **deep plexus** of lymphatic vessels lies in the submucosa and connective tissue of the bronchi and drains lymph into the **pulmonary lymph nodes** → **bronchopulmonary lymph nodes** → **inferior and superior tracheobronchial lymph nodes** → **paratracheal lymph nodes** → **right bronchomediastinal lymph trunk (for the right lung) or left bronchomediastinal lymph trunk (for the left lung, except the left lower lobe, which drains to the right side).** On the right side, the right bronchomediastinal lymph trunk joins with the right subclavian lymph trunk and the right jugular lymph trunk to form the right lymphatic duct. On the left side, the left bronchomediastinal lymph trunk joins the thoracic duct.

C. Heart. The heart has lymphatic plexuses that communicate freely called the **subendocardial plexus, myocardial plexus,** and **subepicardial plexus.** The subendocardial and myocardial plexuses drain into the subepicardial plexus, which coalesces into the **right cardiac collecting trunk** and **left cardiac collecting trunk.** The right and left cardiac collecting trunks predominately drain into the **left bronchomediastinal trunk,** which empties into the junction of the left internal jugular vein and left subclavian vein.

   1. Right cardiac collecting trunk drains the right atrium and part of the right ventricle (right border and inferior surface), travels in the coronary sulcus near the right coronary artery, and ascends anterior to the ascending aorta to empty into the **anterior mediastinal nodes** → **left brachiocephalic nodes (most commonly)** → **left bronchomediastinal trunk.**

   2. Left cardiac collecting trunk drains the left atrium, part of the right ventricle, and left ventricle. One branch of the left cardiac collecting trunk travels in the anterior interventricular sulcus. Another branch of the left cardiac collecting trunk travels in the posterior interventricular sulcus. The two branches join in the coronary sulcus to form a large unnamed lymphatic vessel. The unnamed lymphatic vessel ascends between the pulmonary trunk and left atrium to empty into the **inferior tracheobronchial nodes** → **superior tracheobronchial nodes** → **paratracheal nodes** → **left bronchomediastinal trunk.**

D. Posterior Mediastinum. Posterior mediastinal lymph nodes sit behind the pericardium and are related to the esophagus and thoracic aorta. These nodes drain the esophagus, posterior pericardium, diaphragm, and middle posterior intercostals spaces.

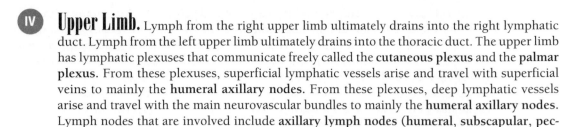

IV **Upper Limb.** Lymph from the right upper limb ultimately drains into the right lymphatic duct. Lymph from the left upper limb ultimately drains into the thoracic duct. The upper limb has lymphatic plexuses that communicate freely called the **cutaneous plexus** and the **palmar plexus.** From these plexuses, superficial lymphatic vessels arise and travel with superficial veins to mainly the **humeral axillary nodes.** From these plexuses, deep lymphatic vessels arise and travel with the main neurovascular bundles to mainly the **humeral axillary nodes.** Lymph nodes that are involved include **axillary lymph nodes (humeral, subscapular, pectoral, central, and apical), supratrochlear nodes,** and **infraclavicular nodes.**

A. **Lymph Drainage of the Superficial Upper Limb.** Lymph from this region drains as follows: **humeral axillary nodes → apical axillary nodes → right subclavian lymph trunk (for the right upper limb) or left subclavian lymph trunk (for the left upper limb).** On the right side, the right subclavian lymph trunk joins with the right jugular lymph trunk and the right bronchomediastinal lymph trunk to form the right lymphatic duct. On the left side, the left subclavian lymph trunk joins the thoracic duct.

B. **Lymph Drainage of the Deep Upper Limb.** Lymph from this region drains as follows: **humeral axillary nodes → apical axillary nodes → right subclavian lymph trunk (for the right upper limb) or left subclavian lymph trunk (for the left upper limb).** On the right side, the right subclavian lymph trunk joins with the right jugular lymph trunk and the right bronchomediastinal lymph trunk to form the right lymphatic duct. On the left side, the left subclavian lymph trunk joins the thoracic duct.

V **Abdominal Viscera.** Lymph from the abdominal viscera drains into the **celiac nodes, superior mesenteric nodes,** and **inferior mesenteric nodes.**

A. The celiac nodes receive lymph from the **superior mesenteric nodes, inferior mesenteric nodes, gastric nodes (i.e. left gastric nodes, right gastroepiploic nodes, and pyloric nodes), hepatic nodes (i.e. cystic node, node of the epiploic foramen), pancreaticoduodenal nodes,** and **pancreaticosplenic nodes.** Efferent lymphatic vessels from the celiac nodes join to the form the **right intestinal lymph trunk** and **left intestinal lymph trunk,** both of which empty into the abdominal confluence of lymph trunks and finally into the thoracic duct.

1. **Lymph Drainage of the Stomach and Duodenum.** Lymph from these regions drains as follows: left gastric nodes, right gastroepiploic nodes, pancreaticosplenic nodes, pyloric nodes, hepatic nodes → celiac nodes → right intestinal lymph trunk and left intestinal lymph trunk → abdominal confluence of lymph trunks → thoracic duct.

2. **Lymph Drainage of the Liver.** The hepatocytes of the liver produce 50% of the lymph found in the thoracic duct. Lymph in the perisinusoidal space of Disse drains into **deep lymphatic vessels** found in the parenchymal connective tissue (i.e. associated with the portal triads). The liver also has **superficial lymphatic vessels** found in the fibrous liver capsule. Lymph from the liver drains as follows: (1) deep lymphatic vessels and superficial lymphatic vessels from the anterior surface of the liver converge at the porta hepatis → hepatic nodes → celiac nodes → right intestinal lymph trunk → abdominal confluence of lymph trunks → thoracic duct; and (2) superficial lymphatic vessels from the posterior surface of the liver → phrenic nodes → posterior mediastinal nodes → thoracic duct.

3. **Lymph Drainage of the Gallbladder and Bile Ducts.** The gallbladder and bile ducts have lymphatic plexuses that communicate freely called the **submucosal lymph plexus** and **subserosal lymph plexus.** These plexuses drain lymph into the

hepatic nodes, especially the cystic node and node of the epiploic foramen. Lymph from the gallbladder and bile ducts drains as follows: hepatic nodes, cystic node, node of the epiploic foramen → celiac nodes → right and intestinal lymph trunks → abdominal confluence of lymph trunks → thoracic duct.

4. **Lymph Drainage of the Pancreas.** Lymph from the pancreas drains as follows: pancreaticoduodenal nodes, pancreaticosplenic nodes, pyloric nodes → celiac nodes → right and left intestinal lymph trunks → abdominal confluence of lymph trunks → thoracic duct.

5. **Lymph Drainage of the Spleen.** Lymph from the spleen drains as follows: pancreaticosplenic nodes → celiac nodes → right and left intestinal lymph trunks → abdominal confluence of lymph trunks → thoracic duct.

B. The superior mesenteric nodes and inferior mesenteric nodes receive lymph from the **mesenteric nodes, ileocolic nodes (i.e. ileal nodes, anterior ileocolic nodes, posterior ileocolic nodes, appendicular nodes), colic nodes (i.e. epicolic nodes, paracolic nodes, intermediate colic nodes, preterminal colic nodes), and pararectal nodes.** Efferent lymphatic vessels from the superior and inferior mesenteric nodes empty into the celiac nodes.

1. **Lymph Drainage of the Jejunum and Ileum.** The jejunum and ileum have lymphatic plexuses that communicate freely called the **periglandular plexus** and **submucosal lymph plexus.** In addition, specialized lymphatic vessels called **lacteals** lie within the intestinal villi and drain their lipid-rich fluid into the lymph plexuses. Lymph from the jejunum and ileum drains as follows: mesenteric nodes → superior mesenteric nodes → celiac nodes → right and left intestinal lymph trunks → abdominal confluence of lymph trunks → thoracic duct.

2. **Lymph Drainage of the Appendix and Cecum.** Lymph from the appendix and cecum drains as follows: ileocolic nodes → superior and inferior mesenteric nodes → celiac nodes → right and left intestinal lymph trunks → abdominal confluence of lymph trunks → thoracic duct.

3. **Lymph Drainage of the Colon.** Lymph from the colon drains as follows: colic nodes → superior and inferior mesenteric nodes → celiac nodes → right and left intestinal lymph trunks → abdominal confluence of lymph trunks → thoracic duct.

4. **Lymph Drainage of the Upper Part of the Rectum.** Lymph from the **upper part of the rectum** drains as follows: pararectal nodes → superior and inferior mesenteric nodes → celiac nodes → right and left intestinal lymph trunks → abdominal confluence of lymph trunks → thoracic duct.

VI   **Pelvic Viscera.** Lymph from the pelvic viscera ultimately drains into **lateral aortic nodes** (also called **lumbar nodes**), which are located along the lateral border of the abdominal aorta. The lateral aortic nodes receive lymph from the **common iliac nodes, external iliac nodes, internal iliac nodes, inferior epigastric and circumflex iliac nodes, and sacral nodes.** Efferent lymphatic vessels from the lateral aortic nodes join to form the **right lumbar lymph trunk** and **left lumbar lymph trunk**, both of which empty into the abdominal confluence of lymph trunks and finally into the thoracic duct.

A. **Lymph Drainage of the Lower Part of the Rectum and Anal Canal above the Pectinate Line.** Lymph from these regions drains as follows: internal iliac nodes → common iliac nodes → lateral aortic nodes → right and left lumbar lymph trunks → abdominal confluence of lymph trunks → thoracic duct.

B. **Lymph Drainage of the Anal Canal below the Pectinate Line.** Lymph from this region drains as follows: superficial inguinal nodes → deep inguinal nodes → external iliac nodes → common iliac nodes → lateral aortic nodes → right and left lumbar lymph trunks → abdominal confluence of lymph trunks → thoracic duct.

C. **Lymph Drainage of the Kidney.** The kidney has three lymphatic plexuses called the **intrarenal plexus, subcapsular plexus**, and **perirenal plexus**. The subcapsular plexus and the perirenal plexus communicate freely with each other. The intrarenal plexus forms **4 to 5 collecting trunks** that follow the course of the renal veins. As the 4 to 5 collecting trunks leave the renal hilum, they are joined by **lymphatics from the subcapsular plexus**. The 4 to 5 collecting trunks drain into the **lateral aortic nodes**. The perirenal plexus also drains directly into the **lateral aortic nodes**. Lymph from the kidney drains as follows: 4 to 5 collecting trunks → lymphatics from the subcapsular plexus → lymphatics from the perirenal plexus → lateral aortic nodes → right and left lumbar lymph trunks → abdominal confluence of lymphatic trunks → thoracic duct.

D. **Lymph Drainage of the Ureter.** The ureter has three lymphatic plexuses called the **submucosal plexus, muscular plexus**, and **adventitial plexus**, all of which communicate freely with each other.
   1. **Lymph Drainage of the Upper Part of the Ureter.** Lymph from this region drains as follows: upper ureter lymphatic vessels → lateral aortic nodes → right and left lumbar lymph trunks → abdominal confluence of lymphatic trunks → thoracic duct.
   2. **Lymph Drainage of the Middle Part of the Ureter.** Lymph from this region drains as follows: middle ureter lymphatic vessels → common iliac nodes → lateral aortic nodes → right and left lumbar lymph trunks → abdominal confluence of lymphatic trunks → thoracic duct.
   3. **Lymph Drainage of the Lower Part of the Ureter.** Lymph from this region drains as follows: lower ureter lymphatic vessels → external and internal iliac nodes → common iliac nodes → lateral aortic nodes → right and left lumbar lymph trunks → abdominal confluence of lymphatic trunks → thoracic duct.

E. **Lymph Drainage of the Urinary Bladder.** The bladder has three lymphatic plexuses called the **submucosal plexus, muscular plexus**, and **adventitial plexus**, all of which communicate freely with each other. Lymph from the urinary bladder drains as follows: bladder lymphatic vessels → external and internal iliac nodes → common iliac nodes → lateral aortic nodes → right and left lumbar lymph trunks → abdominal confluence of lymphatic trunks → thoracic duct.

F. **Male Reproductive Organs**
   1. **Lymph Drainage of the Testes.** The testes have two lymphatic plexuses that communicate freely called the **superficial plexus** and **deep plexus**. These plexuses form **4 to 8 collecting trunks** that ascend in the spermatic cord. Lymph from the testes drains as follows: lymphatics from the superficial and deep plexus → 4 to 8 collecting trunks → lateral aortic nodes → right and left lumbar lymph trunks → abdominal confluence of lymphatic trunks → thoracic duct.
   2. **Lymph Drainage of the Ductus Deferens, Seminal Vesicle, and Ejaculatory Duct.** Lymph from these regions drains as follows: external and internal iliac nodes → common iliac nodes → lateral aortic nodes → right and left lumbar lymph trunks → abdominal confluence of lymphatic trunks → thoracic duct.
   3. **Lymph Drainage of the Prostate Gland.** Lymph from the prostrate gland drains as follows: internal iliac nodes and sacral nodes → common iliac nodes → lateral aortic nodes → right and left lumbar lymph trunks → abdominal confluence of lymphatic trunks → thoracic duct.

4. **Lymph Drainage of the Penile Erectile Tissue and Penile Urethra.** Lymph from these regions drains as follows: internal iliac nodes → common iliac nodes → lateral aortic nodes → right and left lumbar lymph trunks → abdominal confluence of lymphatic trunks → thoracic duct.

5. **Lymph Drainage of the Scrotum and Skin of the Penis.** Lymph from these regions drains as follows: superficial inguinal nodes → deep inguinal nodes → external iliac nodes → common iliac nodes → lateral aortic nodes → right and left lumbar lymph trunks → abdominal confluence of lymphatic trunks → thoracic duct.

G. **Female Reproductive Organs**
1. **Lymph Drainage of the Ovary.** The ovary has lymphatic plexuses that communicate freely. These plexuses form lymphatics vessels that ascend along the ovarian artery. Lymph from the ovary drains as follows: lymphatics vessels along the ovarian artery → lateral aortic nodes → right and left lumbar lymph trunks → abdominal confluence of lymphatic trunks → thoracic duct.

2. **Lymph Drainage of the Upper Part of the Uterus and Uterine Tube.** Lymph from these regions drains as follows: lateral aortic nodes → right and left lumbar lymph trunks → abdominal confluence of lymphatic trunks → thoracic duct.

3. **Lymph Drainage of the Lower Part of the Uterus and Cervix.** Lymph from these regions drains as follows: external iliac nodes, internal iliac nodes, and sacral nodes → common iliac nodes → lateral aortic nodes → right and left lumbar lymph trunks → abdominal confluence of lymphatic trunks → thoracic duct.

4. **Lymph Drainage of the Upper Part of the Vagina.** Lymph from this region drains as follows: external iliac nodes and internal iliac nodes → common iliac nodes → lateral aortic nodes → right and left lumbar lymph trunks → abdominal confluence of lymphatic trunks → thoracic duct.

5. **Lymph Drainage of the Middle Part of the Vagina.** Lymph from this region drains as follows: internal iliac nodes → common iliac nodes → lateral aortic nodes → right and left lumbar lymph trunks → abdominal confluence of lymphatic trunks → thoracic duct.

6. **Lymph Drainage of the Lower Part of the Vagina (below the hymen).** Lymph from this region drains as follows: superficial inguinal nodes → deep inguinal nodes → external iliac nodes → common iliac nodes → lateral aortic nodes → right and left lumbar lymph trunks → abdominal confluence of lymphatic trunks → thoracic duct.

7. **Lymph Drainage of the Clitoris and Labia Minora.** Lymph from this region drains as follows: deep inguinal nodes → external iliac nodes → common iliac nodes → lateral aortic nodes → right and left lumbar lymph trunks → abdominal confluence of lymphatic trunks → thoracic duct.

8. **Lymph Drainage of the Vulva and Perineal Skin.** Lymph from this region drains as follows: superficial inguinal nodes → deep inguinal nodes → external iliac nodes → common iliac nodes → lateral aortic nodes → right and left lumbar lymph trunks → abdominal confluence of lymphatic trunks → thoracic duct.

H. **Lower Limb.** Lymph from the right and left lower limb ultimately drains into the thoracic duct. The lower limb has lymphatic plexuses that communicate freely called the **cutaneous plexus** and the **plantar plexus**. From these plexuses, **medial superficial lymphatic vessels** (travel with the great saphenous vein) and **lateral superficial lymphatic vessels** (travel with the small saphenous vein) arise and travel with superficial veins to mainly the **superficial inguinal nodes**. The deep lymphatic vessels arise and travel with the main neurovascular bundles to mainly the **deep inguinal nodes**. Lymph nodes that are involved include **superficial inguinal nodes, deep inguinal nodes,** and **popliteal nodes.**

1. **Lymph Drainage of the Superficial Lower Limb.** Lymph from this region drains as follows: superficial inguinal nodes → external iliac nodes → common iliac nodes → lateral aortic nodes → right and left lumbar lymph trunks → abdominal confluence of lymphatic trunks → thoracic duct.

2. **Lymph Drainage of the Deep Lower Limb.** Lymph from this region drains as follows: deep inguinal nodes → external iliac nodes → common iliac nodes → lateral aortic nodes → right and left lumbar lymph trunks → abdominal confluence of lymphatic trunks → thoracic duct.

I. **Gluteal Region.** Lymph from the gluteal region drains into the **superficial inguinal nodes, superior gluteal nodes,** and **inferior gluteal nodes.**

1. **Lymph Drainage of the Superficial Gluteal Region.** Lymph from this region drains as follows: superficial inguinal nodes → external iliac nodes → common iliac nodes → lateral aortic nodes → right and left lumbar lymph trunks → abdominal confluence of lymphatic trunks → thoracic duct.

2. **Lymph Drainage of the Deep Gluteal Region.** Lymph from this region drains as follows: superior gluteal nodes and inferior gluteal nodes → internal iliac nodes → common iliac nodes → lateral aortic nodes → right and left lumbar lymph trunks → abdominal confluence of lymphatic trunks → thoracic duct.

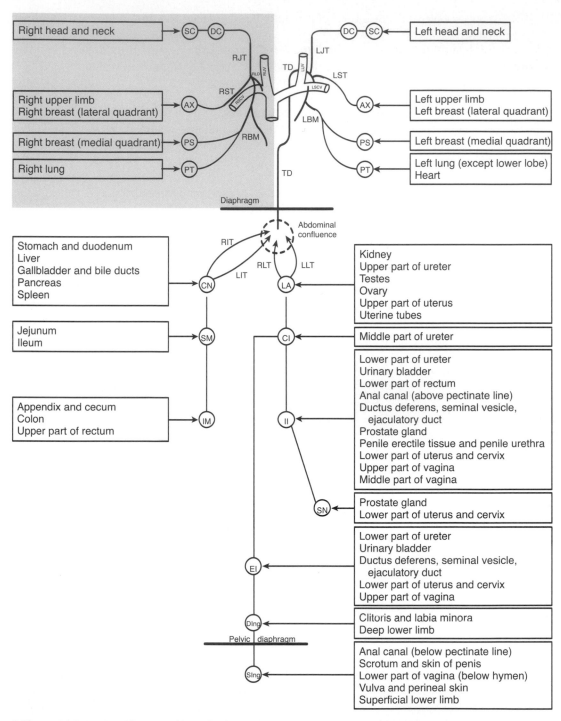

● **Figure 4-2 Summary Diagram of Lymphatic Drainage.** CI = common iliac nodes, DIng = deep inguinal nodes, EI = external iliac nodes, II = internal iliac nodes, LA = lateral aortic nodes, LLT = left lumbar lymph trunk, RLT = right lumbar lymph trunk, SIng = superficial inguinal nodes, TD = thoracic duct, RIT = right intestinal lymph trunk, LIT = left intestinal lymph trunk, SN = sacral nodes, CN = celiac nodes, SM = superior mesenteric nodes, IM = inferior mesenteric nodes, PT = paratracheal nodes, PS = parasternal nodes, AX = axillary nodes, SC = superficial cervical nodes, DC = deep cervical nodes, RBM = right bronchomediastinal lymph trunk, LBM = left bronchomediastinal lymph trunk, RST = right subclavian lymph trunk, LST = left subclavian lymph trunk, RJT = right jugular lymph trunk, LJT = left jugular lymph trunk, RSCV = right subclavian vein, RIJV = right internal jugular vein, LSCV = left subclavian vein, LIJV = left internal jugular vein, RLD = right lymphatic duct.

Chapter 5

Chest Wall

I **General Features of the Thorax.** The thorax extends from the top of the sternum to the diaphragm and is encased in an expandable cage of ribs and other bones. It is bounded by the sternum, ribs, and thoracic vertebrae. The thorax resembles a beehive or inverted cone. The entrance to the thorax (called the **thoracic inlet**) is small and kidney-shaped. The boundaries of the thoracic inlet are the manubrium anteriorly, rib 1 laterally, and the thoracic vertebrae posteriorly. The outlet from the thorax (called the **thoracic outlet**) is large and is separated from the abdomen by the diaphragm. The boundaries of the thoracic outlet are the xiphoid process anteriorly, costal cartilages 7 through 10 and rib 12 laterally, and T12 vertebra posteriorly.

II **Bones of the Thorax (Figure 5-1)**

A. Thoracic Vertebrae. There are 12 thoracic vertebrae that have facets on their bodies (**costal facets**) for articulation with the heads of ribs, facets on their transverse processes for articulation with the tubercles of rib 9 (except for ribs 11 and 12), and long spinous processes.

B. Ribs. There are 12 pairs of ribs that articulate with the thoracic vertebrae. A rib consists of a **head, neck, tubercle,** and **body**. The head articulates with the body of adjacent thoracic vertebrae and the intervertebral disk at the **costovertebral joint.** The tubercle articulates with the transverse process of a thoracic vertebra at the **costotransverse joint.**
  1. **True (vertebrosternal) ribs** are **ribs 1 through 7** that articulate individually with the sternum by their costal cartilages.
  2. **False (vertebrochondral) ribs** are **ribs 8 through 12**. Ribs 8 through 10 articulate with more superior costal cartilage and form the **anterior costal margin.** Ribs 11 and 12 (often called **floating ribs**) articulate with vertebral bodies but do not articulate with the sternum.

C. Sternum consists of the following:
  1. The **manubrium** forms the **jugular notch** at its superior margin, has a **clavicular notch** that articulates with the clavicle at the **sternoclavicular joint,** and articulates with the costal cartilages of ribs 1 and 2.
  2. The **body** articulates with the manubrium at the **sternal angle of Louis,** articulates with the costal cartilages of ribs 2 through 7, and articulates with the **xiphoid process** at the **xiphosternal joint.**
  3. The **xiphoid process** articulates with the body of the sternum and attaches to the diaphragm and abdominal musculature via the **linea alba.**
  4. The **sternal angle of Louis** marks the junction between the manubrium and body of the sternum at vertebral level T4. This is the site where rib 2 articulates with the

45

sternum, the aortic arch begins and ends, the trachea bifurcates, and the superior mediastinum ends.

III   Muscles of the Thorax

A. Diaphragm (most important muscle of inspiration) elevates the ribs and increases the vertical, transverse ("bucket handle" movement), and anteroposterior ("pump handle" movement) diameters of the thorax. The diaphragm is innervated by the **phrenic nerves** (ventral primary rami of C3 through C5), which provide motor and sensory innervation. Sensory innervation to the periphery of the diaphragm is provided by the **intercostal nerves**. A lesion of the phrenic nerve may result in **paralysis** and **paradoxical movement** of the diaphragm. The paralyzed dome of the diaphragm does not descend during inspiration and is consequently forced upward because of increased abdominal pressure.

B. The **intercostal muscles** are thin multiple layers of muscle that occupy the **intercostal spaces (1 through 11)** and keep the intercostal space rigid during inspiration or expiration. The **external intercostal muscles** elevate the ribs and play a role in inspiration during exercise or lung disease. The **internal intercostal muscles** play a role in expiration during exercise or lung disease. The **innermost intercostal muscles** are presumed to act with the internal intercostal muscles. The intercostal vein, artery, and nerve run between the internal intercostal muscles and innermost intercostal muscles.

C. The **serratus posterior superior muscle** attaches from the nuchal ligament to the upper borders of ribs 2 through 4 and elevates the ribs. The **serratus posterior inferior muscle** attaches from the T1 through L2 vertebrae to the lower borders of ribs 8 through 12 and lowers the ribs. The **levator costarum muscle** attaches from the T7 through T11 vertebrae to the subjacent ribs and elevates the ribs. The **transverse thoracic muscle** attaches from the posterior surface of the lower sternum to the internal surface of costal cartilages 2 through 6 and weakly lowers the ribs.

D. The **sternocleidomastoid, pectoralis major** and **minor**, and **scalene muscles** attach to the ribs and play a role in inspiration during exercise or lung disease.

E. The **external oblique, internal oblique, transverse abdominal**, and **rectus abdominis muscles** (i.e. abdominal muscles) play a role in expiration during exercise, lung disease, or the Valsalva maneuver.

IV   Nerves of the Thorax.

The **intercostal nerves** are the ventral primary rami of T1 through T11 and run in the **costal groove** between the internal intercostal muscles and innermost intercostal muscles. The **subcostal nerve** is the ventral primary ramus of T12. Intercostal nerve injury is evidenced by a sucking in (on inspiration) and bulging out (on expiration) of the affected intercostal space.

V   Arteries of the Thorax

A. Internal thoracic artery is a branch of the **subclavian artery** that descends just lateral to the sternum and terminates at intercostal space 6 by dividing into the **superior epigastric artery** and **musculophrenic artery**.

B. **Anterior Intercostal Arteries.** The anterior intercostal arteries that supply intercostal spaces 1 through 6 are branches of the **internal thoracic artery**. The anterior intercostal arteries that supply intercostal spaces 7 through 9 are branches of the **musculophrenic artery**. There are two anterior intercostal arteries within each intercostal space that anastomose with the posterior intercostal arteries.

C. **Posterior Intercostal Arteries.** The posterior intercostal arteries that supply intercostal spaces 1 and 2 are branches of the **superior intercostal artery** that arises from the **costocervical trunk** of the subclavian artery. The posterior intercostal arteries that supply intercostal spaces 3 through 11 are branches of the **thoracic aorta**. The **subcostal artery** is also a branch of the thoracic aorta. All posterior intercostal arteries give off a posterior branch that travels with the dorsal primary ramus of a spinal nerve to supply the spinal cord, vertebral column, back muscles, and skin. The posterior intercostal arteries anastomose anteriorly with the anterior intercostal arteries.

VI Veins of the Thorax

A. **Anterior Intercostal Veins.** The anterior intercostal veins drain the anterior thorax and empty into the **internal thoracic veins**, which then empty into the **brachiocephalic veins**.

B. **Posterior Intercostal Veins.** The posterior intercostal veins drain the lateral and posterior thorax and empty into the **hemiazygos veins** on the left side and the **azygos vein** on the right side. The hemiazygos veins empty into the azygos vein, which empties into the superior vena cava.

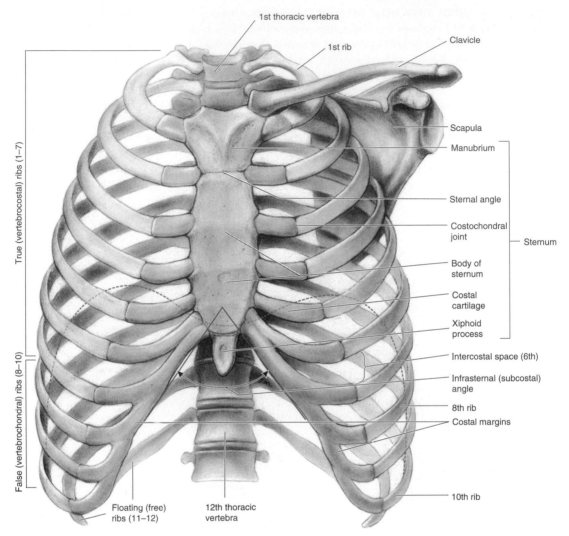

● **Figure 5-1 The Thoracic Skeleton (anterior view).** The osteocartilaginous thoracic cage includes the sternum, 12 pairs of ribs and costal cartilages, and 12 thoracic vertebrae with their intervertebral disks. The clavicles and scapulae form the pectoral (shoulder) girdle. The dotted line indicates the position of the diaphragm separating the thoracic cavity from the abdominal cavity.

Breast (Figure 5-2). The breast lies in the superficial fascia of the anterior chest wall overlying the **pectoralis major** and **serratus anterior muscles** and extends into the **superior lateral quadrant** of the axilla as the **axillary tail** where a high percentage of tumors occur. In a well-developed woman, the breast extends vertically from **rib 2 to rib 6** and laterally from the **sternum to the midaxillary line.** At the greatest prominence of the breast is the **nipple,** which is surrounded by a circular pigmented area of skin called the **areola.** The **retromammary space** lies between the breast and the **pectoral (deep) fascia** and allows free movement of the breast. If breast carcinoma invades the retromammary space and pectoral fascia, contraction of the pectoralis major may cause the **whole breast to move superiorly.** **Suspensory ligaments (Cooper's)** extend from the dermis of the skin to the pectoral fascia and provide support for the breast. If breast carcinoma invades the suspensory ligaments, the ligaments may shorten and cause **dimpling of the skin** or **inversion of the nipple.** **Adipose tissue** within the breast contributes largely to the contour and size of the breast.

A. Nipple and Areola

1. The nipple is a round, raised area of modified skin in the center of the **areola.** The skin has a lightly **keratinized stratified squamous epithelium** and a dermis of **connective tissue with elastic fibers and smooth muscle fibers** arranged circularly around the base of the nipple and longitudinally parallel to the lactiferous ducts. Contraction of the smooth muscles as a result of cold, tactile, or emotional stimulation results in **erection of the nipple.** The base of the epithelium is invaded by deep dermal papillae containing numerous capillaries that bring blood close to the surface and impart a **pinkish color** to the nipple in children and blonde individuals. At puberty, the epithelium becomes pigmented (melanin) and changes the color to **light to dark brown.**

2. The skin around nipple is called the **areola,** which is modified skin that contains large sebaceous glands that form small nodular elevations in the areola called **Montgomery tubercles.** The color of the areola is initially pinkish (like the nipple) but during pregnancy the color changes to light to dark brown as a result of increased pigmentation (melanin). After delivery, the areola may lighten in color but rarely returns to its original shade. The **sensory innervation** of the nipple and areola is important because stimulation of the nipple and areola by the suckling infant triggers a sequence of neurohormonal events that result in **ejection of milk (oxytocin)** and **production of milk (prolactin).**

3. **Clinical Considerations.** Nipple secretion typically contains exfoliated duct cells, α-lactalbumin, immunoglobulins, lactose, cholesterol, steroids, and fatty acids, along with ethanol, caffeine, nicotine, barbiturates, pesticides, and technetium. A nipple discharge that is green, milky, yellow, or brown, not spontaneous, and bilateral and affects multiple ducts is usually a **benign situation.** A milky discharge (galactorrhea) along with a headache and peripheral vision loss may indicate a **pituitary adenoma (prolactinoma,** an adenoma in the sella turcica that may cause a disruption of the inhibitory hypothalamic dopaminergic control of mammotrophs in the adenohypophysis causing unimpeded secretion of prolactin, i.e. the **"stalk effect").** A nipple discharge that is bloody or clear (serous), spontaneous, and unilateral and affects a single duct usually indicates a **malignant situation.**

B. Mammary Gland. In general, the mammary gland is a compound, tubuloalveolar gland that develops as downgrowths of the epidermis along the **milk line,** which runs from the axilla to the groin on each side. The mammary gland consists of epithelial cells arranged as **alveoli,** which are ultimately drained by **15 to 20 lactiferous ducts** that open onto the tip of the **nipple arranged in a ring**. Just deep to the surface of the nipple, each lactiferous duct expands into a **lactiferous sinus**, which serves as a reservoir for milk during lactation. In the nonpregnant or nonlactating woman, these structures are rudimentary. The histology of the mammary gland changes as the woman progresses through prepuberty, puberty, pregnancy, and lactation.

1. **Prepuberty.** At birth and prepuberty, the nipple and a simple system of ducts (or epithelial downgrowths) embedded in connective tissue are present. The full development of epithelial downgrowths begins at puberty.

2. **At Puberty.** The development of breasts at puberty is one of the secondary sex characteristics of women. Under the influence of **estrogen** from the ovary, the breast accumulates **adipose tissue**, which is largely responsible for variations in breast size. In addition, epithelial downgrowths begin in earnest and branch into the connective tissue to form a system of ducts. There are no alveoli present, only **solid masses of epithelial cells**.

3. **During Pregnancy.** Under the influence of estrogen and progesterone, the duct system grows prolifically in length and branching. Eventually, the characteristic structure of the mammary gland takes shape: **15 to 20 lobules** drained by **intralobular ducts** that empty into **interlobular ducts** and eventually into the **lactiferous ducts**. In addition, the solid masses of epithelial cells grow and form **alveoli**, which are surrounded by **myoepithelial cells**. This proliferation of glandular tissue takes place at the expense of the adipose tissue, which concurrently decreases as glandular tissue increases. Ducts and alveoli distend as alveoli secrete **colostrum**. Colostrum is a creamy white to yellowish premilk fluid that is secreted from the breast during the first 72 hours after the birth of an infant. This "first food of life" actually precedes the production of breast milk. Colostrum contains substances such as immunoglobulins and lactoferrin that play key roles in fighting viruses, bacteria, fungi, allergens, and toxins. Colostrum also stimulates maturation of B lymphocytes and increases the activity of macrophages, thereby enhancing the immune system.

4. **During Lactation.** The epithelial cells of the alveoli become active in **milk production**. Numerous fat droplets and secretory vacuoles containing dense aggregates of milk proteins can be observed ultrastructurally at the apical end of the alveolar epithelial cells. Human breast milk is produced 1 to 3 days after childbirth. Breast milk contains a substantial amount of lipid, protein, lactose, vitamins, and secretory IgA (which affords temporary enteric passive immunity). Although milk is produced continuously by the alveoli (milk production), it is delivered only in response to suckling (**milk letdown**). Suckling stimulates afferent neurons, which relay the information to the hypothalamus such that the following actions occur: (1) **oxytocin** is released from the posterior hypophysis, which causes the contraction of myoepithelial cells and milk letdown, (2) **prolactin-inhibiting hormone (PIH; dopamine)** is inhibited, which causes the release of **prolactin** from the adenohypophysis and further milk production.

C. **Arterial Supply.** The arterial supply of the breast is from the medial mammary branches from the **internal thoracic artery**, lateral mammary branches from the **lateral thoracic artery**, pectoral branches from the **thoracoacromial artery**, perforating branches from the **anterior intercostal arteries**, and **posterior intercostal arteries**.

D. **Venous Drainage.** The venous drainage from the breast is mainly to the **axillary vein** via lateral mammary veins and the lateral thoracic vein, with additional drainage to the **internal thoracic vein** via medial mammary veins, **anterior intercostal veins**, and **posterior intercostal veins** (drain into the azygos system). Metastasis of breast carcinoma to the brain may occur by the following route: cancer cells enter an intercostal vein → external vertebral venous plexuses → internal vertebral venous plexus → cranial dural sinuses.

E. Innervation. The nerves of the breast are derived from anterior and lateral cutaneous branches of **intercostal nerves 4 through 6** (i.e. **T4, T5, and T6 dermatomes**). These nerves convey sensory nerve fibers to the skin of the breast and sympathetic nerve fibers to blood vessels and smooth muscle of the nipple.

F. Clinical Considerations

1. **Fibroadenoma** is a benign proliferation of connective tissue such that the mammary glands are compressed into cords of epithelium. A fibroadenoma presents clinically as a sharply circumscribed, spherical nodule that is freely movable. It is the most common benign neoplasm of the breast.

2. **Infiltrating duct carcinoma** is a malignant proliferation of duct epithelium in which the tumor cells are arranged in cell nests, cords, anastomosing masses, or a mixture of all these. It is the most common type of breast cancer, accounting for 65 to 80% of all breast cancers. An infiltrating duct carcinoma presents clinically as a jagged density, fixed in position, with dimpling of skin, inversion of the nipple, and thick, leathery skin.

   The presence of **estrogen receptors** or **progesterone receptors** within the carcinoma cells indicates a good prognosis for treatment. **Tamoxifen** is an estrogen receptor blocker and is a drug of choice for treatment. The presence of the **c-erb B2 oncoprotein** (a protein similar to the epidermal growth factor [EGF] receptor) on the surface of the carcinoma cells indicates a poor prognosis for treatment. *BRCA1* (breast cancer susceptibility gene) is an anti-oncogene (tumor suppressor gene) located on chromosome 17 (17q21) that encodes for BRCA protein (a zinc-finger gene-regulatory protein) containing phosphotyrosine that will suppress the cell cycle. A mutation of the *BRCA1* gene is present in 5 to 10% of women with breast cancer and confers a very high lifetime risk of breast and ovarian cancer.

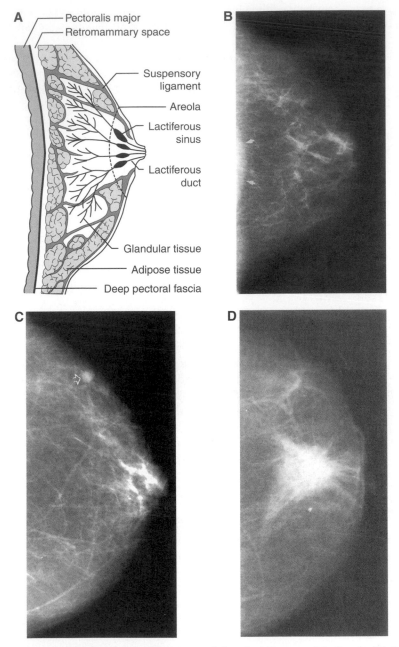

● **Figure 5-2 Diagram and Mammograms of the Breast. (A)** Sagittal diagram of the breast**. (B)** Craniocaudal (CC) mammogram of a normal left breast. The pectoralis major muscle (arrows) is seen. **(C)** CC mammogram of a benign mass (arrow). A benign mass has the following characteristics: **shape** is round or oval, **margins** are well-circumscribed, **density** is low-medium contrast, it becomes smaller over time, and **calcifications** are large, smooth, and uniform. **(D)** CC mammogram of a malignant mass. A malignant mass has the following characteristics: **shape** is irregular with many lobulations, **margins** are irregular or spiculated, **density** is medium-high, breast architecture may be distorted, it becomes larger over time, and **calcifications** (not shown) are small, irregular, variable, and found within ducts (ductal casts).

VIII   Anterior Chest Wall

A. **Insertion of a Central Venous Catheter (Figure 5-3A).** In clinical practice, access to the superior vena cava (SVC) and right side of the heart is required to monitor blood pressure or for long-term feeding or administration of drugs. The internal jugular vein and subclavian vein are generally used.

   1. **Internal Jugular Vein (central or anterior approach).** The needle is inserted at the apex of a triangle formed by the two heads of the sternocleidomastoid muscle and the clavicle of the right side.

   2. **Subclavian Vein (infraclavicular approach).** Place index finger at sternal notch and thumb at the intersection of the clavicle and first rib as anatomic landmarks. The needle is inserted below the clavicle and lateral to your thumb on the right side.

   3. **Complications of a central venous catheter** may include the following: puncture of subclavian artery or subclavian vein, pneumothorax, hemothorax, trauma to trunks of brachial plexus, arrhythmias, venous thrombosis, erosion of catheter through the SVC, damage to tricuspid valve, and infections.

B. **Postductal coarctation of the aorta (Figure 5-3B)** is a congenital malformation associated with increased blood pressure to the upper extremities, diminished and delayed femoral artery pulse, and high risk of cerebral hemorrhage and bacterial endocarditis. A postductal coarctation of the aorta is generally located distal to the left subclavian artery and the ligamentum arteriosum. The **internal thoracic artery** → **intercostal arteries** → **superior epigastric artery** → **inferior epigastric artery** → **external iliac arteries** are involved in the collateral circulation to bypass the constriction and become dilated. Dilation of the intercostal arteries causes erosion of the lower border of the ribs, termed "**rib notching.**" A **preductal coarctation** is less common and occurs proximal to the ductus arteriosus; blood reaches the lower part of the body via a patent ductus arteriosus.

C. **Aneurysm of the aorta (Figure 5-3C)** may compress the trachea or tug on the trachea with each cardiac systole such that it can be felt by palpating the trachea at the sternal notch (T2).

D. **Aortic dissection (Figure 5-3D)** is a result of a deceleration injury in which the aorta tears just distal to the left subclavian artery. The tear is through the tunica intima and tunica media.

E. **Thoracic outlet syndrome (Figure 5-3E)** may be the result of an anomalous cervical rib that compresses the lower trunk of the brachial plexus, subclavian artery, or both. Clinical findings include atrophy of thenar and hypothenar eminences, atrophy of interosseous muscles, sensory deficits on medial side of forearm and hand, diminished radial artery pulse on moving head to the opposite side, and a bruit over the subclavian artery.

F. **Knife wound to chest wall above the clavicle** may damage structures at the root of the neck. The **subclavian artery** may be cut. The **lower trunk of the brachial plexus** may be cut, causing loss of hand movements (ulnar nerve involvement) and loss of sensation over the medial aspect of the arm, forearm, and last two digits (C8 and T1 dermatomes). The **cervical pleura** and **apex of the lung** may be cut, causing an open pneumothorax and collapse of the lung. These structures project superiorly into the neck through the thoracic inlet and posterior to the sternocleidomastoid muscle.

G. Projections of the Diaphragm on the Chest Wall. The central tendon of the diaphragm lies directly posterior to the xiphosternal joint. The **right dome** of the diaphragm arches superiorly to the <u>upper</u> border of rib 5 in the midclavicular line. The **left dome** of the diaphragm arches superiorly to the <u>lower</u> border of rib 5 in the midclavicular line.

H. Scalene Lymph Node Biopsy. Scalene lymph nodes are located behind the clavicle surrounded by pleura, lymph ducts, and the phrenic nerve. Inadvertent damage to these structures will cause the following clinical findings: pneumothorax (pleura), lymph leakage (lymph ducts), and diaphragm paralysis (phrenic nerve).

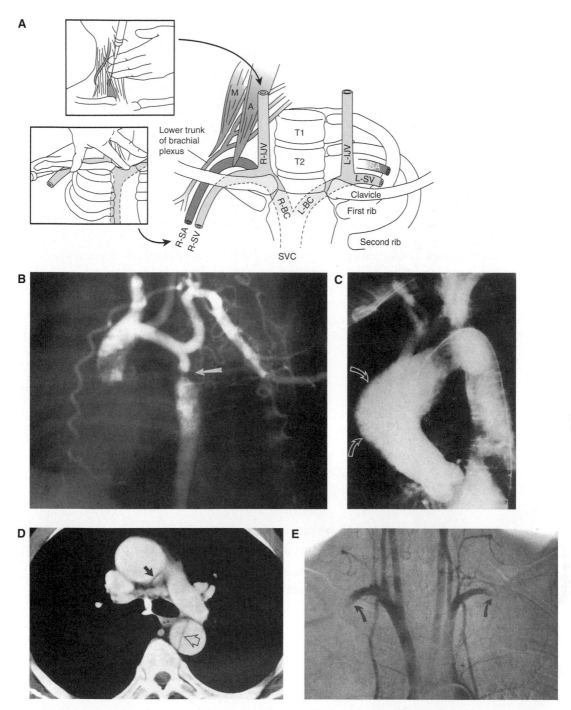

● **Figure 5-3 (A) Anterior Chest Wall.** The first pair of ribs is shown with their articulation with the T1 vertebra and manubrium of the sternum. On the right, structures crossing rib 1 are shown (subclavian vein, subclavian artery, and brachial plexus). Note the relationship of these structures to the clavicle. Note also the arrangement of the large veins in this area and their use in a placing a central venous catheter (internal jugular vein approach or subclavian approach). L-IJV = left internal jugular vein, L-SV = left subclavian vein, L-BC = left brachiocephalic vein, R-BC = right brachiocephalic vein, SVC = superior vena cava, R-IJV = right internal jugular vein, R-SV = right subclavian vein, L-SA = left subclavian artery, R-SA = right subclavian artery, M = middle scalene muscle, A = anterior scalene muscle. **(B) Postductal Coarctation of the Aorta.** Angiogram demonstrates a narrowing (arrow) just distal to the prominent left subclavian artery. The aortic arch is hypoplastic. Note the tortuous internal thoracic artery. **(C) Aortic Aneurysm.** Angiogram shows an atherosclerotic aneurysm (curved arrows) protruding from the ascending aorta. **(D) Aortic Dissection.** CT scan shows a tunica intima flap within the ascending (closed arrow) and descending (open arrow) aorta. The larger false lumen compresses the true lumen. **(E) Thoracic Outlet Syndrome.** Angiogram taken with abduction of both arms shows blood flow is partially occluded in the subclavian arteries (arrows).

IX   Lateral Chest Wall (Figure 5-4)

A. **Tube thoracostomy** is performed to evacuate ongoing production of air or fluid into the pleural cavity. A tube is inserted through intercostal space 5 in the anterior axillary line (i.e. posterior approach) close to the <u>upper</u> border of the rib to avoid the **intercostal vein, artery, and nerve**, which run in the costal groove between the internal intercostal muscle and innermost intercostal muscle. An incision is made at intercostal space 6 lateral to the nipple but medial to the latissimus dorsi muscle. The tube will penetrate **skin → superficial fascia → serratus anterior muscle → external intercostal muscle → internal intercostal muscle → innermost intercostal muscle → parietal pleura.**

B. **Intercostal nerve block** may be necessary to relieve pain associated with a rib fracture or herpes zoster (shingles). A needle is inserted at the posterior angle of the rib along the <u>lower</u> border of the rib to bathe the nerve in anesthetic. The needle penetrates the following structures: **skin → superficial fascia → serratus anterior muscle → external intercostal muscle → internal intercostal muscle.** Several intercostal nerves must be blocked to achieve pain relief because of the presence of nerve collaterals (i.e. overlapping of contiguous dermatomes).

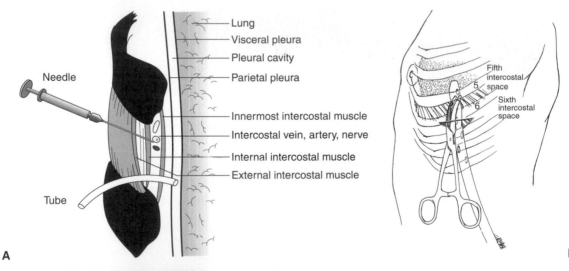

A

B

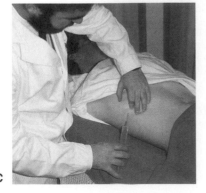

C

● **Figure 5-4 Lateral Chest Wall. (A)** A schematic diagram of an intercostal space and layers. Note their relationship to pleura and lung. The needle indicates the positioning for an intercostal nerve block. The tube indicates the positioning for thoracocentesis. **(B)** Diagram shows surgical approach for a tube thoracostomy. **(C)** Photograph shows approach for an intercostal nerve block.

X Posterior Chest Wall (Figure 5-5A)

A. Fractures of the Lower Ribs. A rib fracture on the right side may damage the **right kidney** and **liver**. A rib fracture on the left side may damage the **left kidney** and **spleen**. A rib fracture on either side may damage the **pleura** as it crosses rib 12.

XI Mediastinum (Figure 5-5B, C) is defined as the space between the pleural cavities in

the thorax. It is bounded laterally by the pleural cavities, anteriorly by the sternum, and posteriorly by the vertebral column. The mediastinum is artificially divided into a **superior division** and **inferior division** by a line from the sternal angle of Louis to the T4–T5 intervertebral disk. The inferior division is then further divided into the **anterior**, **middle**, and **posterior** divisions.

A. Superior Mediastinum. The contents of the superior mediastinum include the trachea, esophagus, thymus, phrenic nerves, azygos vein, SVC, brachiocephalic artery and veins, aortic arch, left common carotid artery, left subclavian artery, and thoracic duct. Common pathologies found in this area include **aortic arch aneurysm, esophageal perforation from either endoscopy or invading malignancy,** or **traumatic rupture of the trachea.**

B. Anterior Mediastinum. The anterior mediastinum lies in front of the pericardium and middle mediastinum. The contents of the anterior mediastinum include the thymus, fat, lymph nodes, and connective tissue. Common pathologies found in this area include **thymoma associated with myasthenia gravis and red blood cell (RBC) aplasia, thyroid mass, germinal cell neoplasm,** or **lymphomas (Hodgkin or non-Hodgkin).**

C. Middle Mediastinum. The middle mediastinum lies in the midline. The contents of the middle mediastinum include the heart, pericardium, phrenic nerves, ascending aorta, SVC, and coronary arteries and veins. Common pathologies found in this area include **pericardial cysts, bronchiogenic cysts,** or **sarcoidosis.** The surface anatomy of the middle mediastinum is important because one can draw an imaginary outline of the heart on the surface of the thorax of the patient as follows:
   1. The superior line runs from the inferior border of left costal cartilage 2 to the superior border of right costal cartilage 3.
   2. The right line runs from costal cartilage 3 to costal cartilage 6 and is slightly convex.
   3. The inferior line runs from the inferior end of the right border to a point in the middle of intercostal space 5 at the midclavicular line.
   4. The left line runs from the ends of the superior and inferior borders on the left.

D. Posterior Mediastinum. The posterior mediastinum is located anterior to the T5 through T12 vertebrae, posterior to the pericardium, and between the parietal pleura of the two lungs. The contents of the posterior mediastinum include the descending aorta, esophagus, thoracic duct, azygos vein, splanchnic nerves, and vagus nerves (cranial nerve [CN] X). Common pathologies found in this area include **ganglioneuromas, neuroblastomas,** or **esophageal diverticula or neoplasms.**

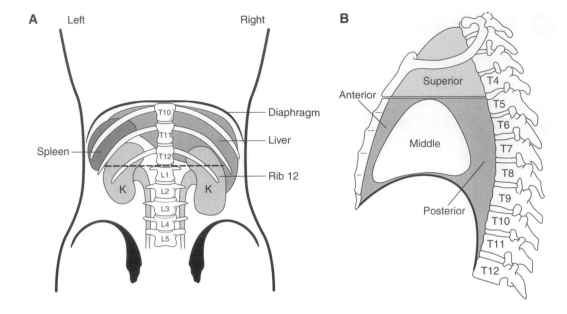

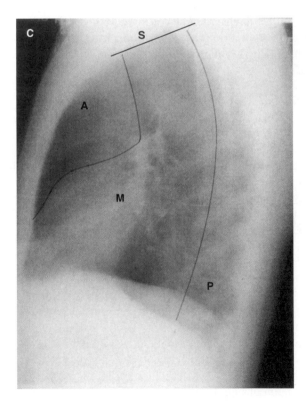

● **Figure 5-5 Posterior Chest Wall and Mediastinum. (A) Posterior Chest Wall.** Note that the kidneys are located from T12 to L3 vertebrae and that the right kidney is lower than the left. The pleura extend across rib 12 (dotted line). Note the structures that may be injured by fractures to the lower ribs. During a splenectomy, the left kidney may be damaged because of its close anatomic relationship and connection via the splenorenal ligament. K = kidney. **(B, C) Mediastinum. (B)** Diagram indicating the superior, anterior, middle, and posterior divisions of the mediastinum. **(C)** A lateral radiograph demarcating the superior (S), anterior (A), middle (M), and posterior (P) divisions of the mediastinum.

XII Radiology

A. **Posteroanterior (PA) Chest Radiograph (Figure 5-6)**

B. **Lateral Chest Radiograph (Figure 5-7)**

C. **Aortic Angiogram (Figure 5-8)**

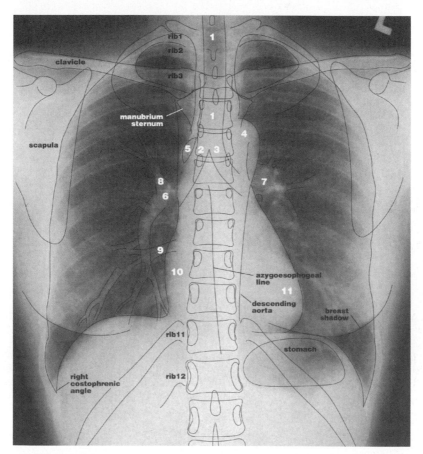

● **Figure 5-6 Posteroanterior (PA) Chest Radiograph.** Note the various numbered and labeled structures. Ribs 1 through 8 can generally be traced from their articulation with the vertebral column to the union of the rib with the costal cartilage. The liver and right dome of the diaphragm cast a domed water-density shadowed at the base of the right lung. The stomach, spleen, and left dome of the diaphragm cast a domed water-density shadowed at the base of the left lung. Both domes generally lie just below vertebra T10. The left dome is lower than the right dome because of the downward thrust of the heart. The right border of the cardiovascular shadow includes the brachiocephalic artery and right brachiocephalic vein, superior vena cava and ascending aorta, right atrium, and inferior vena cava. The left border of the cardiovascular shadow includes the left subclavian artery and left brachiocephalic vein, aortic arch (or aortic knob), pulmonary trunk, auricle of left atrium, and left ventricle. The angle between the right and left main bronchi at the carina is generally 60° to 75°. The left hilum is generally higher than the right hilum. 1 = trachea, 2 = right main bronchus, 3 = left main bronchus, 4 = aortic knob, 5 = azygos vein/superior vena cava, 6 = right pulmonary artery, 7 = left pulmonary artery, 8 = right upper lobe pulmonary artery, 9 = right inferior pulmonary vein, 10 = right atrium, 11 = left ventricle.

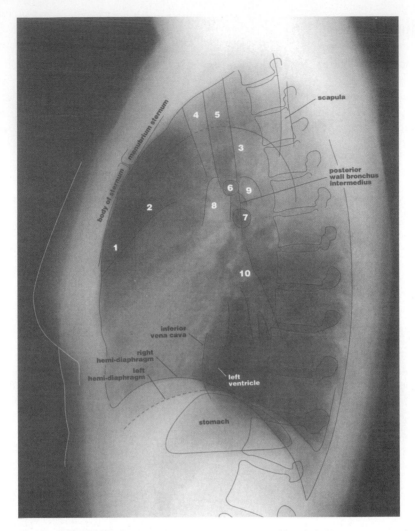

● **Figure 5-7 Lateral Chest Radiograph.** Note the various numbered and labeled structures. 1 = pulmonary outflow tract, 2 = ascending aorta, 3 = aortic arch, 4 = brachiocephalic vessels, 5 = trachea, 6 = right upper lobar bronchus, 7 = left upper lobar bronchus, 8 = right pulmonary artery, 9 = left pulmonary artery, 10 = confluence of pulmonary veins.

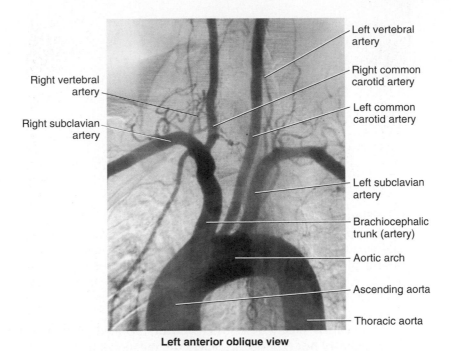

Right vertebral artery

Right subclavian artery

Left vertebral artery

Right common carotid artery

Left common carotid artery

Left subclavian artery

Brachiocephalic trunk (artery)

Aortic arch

Ascending aorta

Thoracic aorta

Left anterior oblique view

● **Figure 5-8 Aortic Angiogram (left anterior oblique view).** Note that injection of contrast dye into the right subclavian artery will visualize the entire circle of Willis because the dye will enter both the right common carotid artery and right vertebral artery (not shown). However, injection of contrast dye into the left subclavian artery will visualize only the posterior part of the circle of Willis because the dye will enter only the left vertebral artery (not shown).

Chapter 6

Pleura, Tracheobronchial Tree, and Lungs

❶ Pleura

A. Types of Pleura
1. **Visceral pleura** adheres to the lung on all its surfaces. The visceral pleura is reflected at the root of the lung and continues as the parietal pleura.
2. **Parietal pleura** adheres to the chest wall, diaphragm, and pericardial sac. The parietal pleura is named according to the anatomic region with which it is associated.
   a. **Costal pleura** is associated with the internal surface of the sternum, costal cartilages, ribs, and sides of the thoracic vertebrae.
   b. **Mediastinal pleura** is associated with the mediastinum and forms the **pulmonary ligament** (located inferior to the root of the lung), which serves to support the lung.
   c. **Diaphragmatic pleura** is associated with the diaphragm.
   d. **Cervical pleura** is associated with the root of the neck.

B. Pleural Recesses
1. **Right and left costodiaphragmatic recesses** are slitlike spaces between the costal and diaphragmatic parietal pleura. During inspiration, the lungs descend into the right and left costodiaphragmatic recesses, causing the recesses to appear radiolucent (dark) on radiographs. During expiration, the lungs ascend so that the costal and diaphragmatic parietal pleura come together and the radiolucency disappears on radiographs. The costodiaphragmatic angle should appear sharp in a posteroanterior (PA) radiograph. If the angle is blunted, pathologic disorder of the pleural space may be suspected such as excess fluid, blood, tumor, or scar tissue. With a patient in the standing position, excess fluid within the pleural cavity will accumulate in the costodiaphragmatic recesses.
2. **Right and left costomediastinal recesses** are slitlike spaces between the costal and mediastinal parietal pleura. During inspiration, the anterior borders of both lungs expand and enter the right and left costomediastinal recesses. In addition, the **lingula of the left lung** expands and enters a portion of the <u>left</u> costomediastinal recess, causing that portion of the recess to appear radiolucent (dark) on radiographs. During expiration, the anterior borders of both lungs recede and exit the right and left costomediastinal recesses.

C. Clinical Considerations
1. **Pleuritis** is inflammation of the pleura. Pleuritis involving only visceral pleura will be associated with **no pain** because the visceral pleura receives no nerves fibers of general sensation. Pleuritis involving the parietal pleura will be associated with **sharp local pain** and **referred pain**. Because parietal pleura is innervated by

intercostal nerves and the phrenic nerve (C3, C4, C5), pain may be referred to the **thoracic wall** and **root of the neck,** respectively.

2. **Inadvertent damage to the pleura** may occur during a:
   a. **Surgical posterior approach to the kidney.** If rib 12 is very short, rib 11 may be mistaken for rib 12. An incision prolonged to the level of rib 11 will damage the pleura.
   b. **Abdominal incision at the right infrasternal angle.** The pleura extends beyond the rib cage in this area.
   c. **Stellate ganglion nerve block**
   d. **Brachial plexus nerve block**
   e. **Knife wounds to the chest wall above the clavicle**
   f. **Fracture of lower ribs**

3. **Chylothorax** occurs when lymph accumulates in the pleural cavity as a result of surgery or trauma that injures the thoracic duct.

4. **Hemothorax** occurs when blood enters the pleura-cavity as a result of trauma or rupture of a blood vessel (e.g. a dissecting aneurysm of the aorta).

5. **Empyema** occurs when a thick pus accumulates in the pleural cavity. Empyema is a variant of **pyothorax** whereby a turbid effusion containing many neutrophils accumulates in the pleural cavity, usually as a result of bacterial pneumonia that extends into the pleural surface.

6. **Open pneumothorax** occurs when the parietal pleura is pierced and the pleural cavity is opened to the outside atmosphere. This causes a loss of the negative intrapleural pressure (P_{IP}) because P_{IP} now equals atmospheric pressure (P_{atm}). This results in an expanded chest wall (its natural tendency) and a collapsed lung (its natural tendency). Upon inspiration, air is sucked into the pleural cavity and results in a **collapsed lung.** Most common causes include chest trauma (e.g., knife wound) and iatrogenic etiology (e.g., thoracocentesis, transthoracic lung biopsy, mechanical ventilation, central line insertion)

7. **Spontaneous pneumothorax (Figure 6-1A)** occurs when air enters the pleural cavity, usually because of a ruptured bleb (bullous) of a diseased lung. The most common site is in the visceral pleura of the upper lobe of the lung. This results in a loss of negative intrapleural pressure and a **collapsed lung.** Clinical findings include chest pain, cough, and mild to severe dyspnea.

8. **Tension pneumothorax (Figure 6-1B)** may occur as a sequela to an open pneumothorax if the inspired air cannot leave the pleural cavity through the wound on expiration (check valve mechanism). This results in a **collapsed lung** on the wounded side and a **compressed lung** on the opposite side because of a deflected mediastinum. Clinical findings include chest pain, shortness of breath, absent breath sounds on the affected side and hypotension because the mediastinal shift compresses the superior vena cava (SVC) and inferior vena cava (IVC), thereby obstructing venous return. It may cause sudden death.

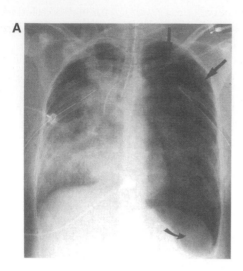
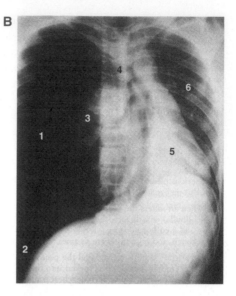

● **Figure 6-1 (A) Pneumothorax.** PA radiograph shows a left apical (straight arrows) and subpulmonic (curved arrow) pneumothorax in a 41-year-old woman with adult respiratory distress syndrome. **(B) Tension Pneumothorax.** AP radiograph shows a tension pneumothorax as a result of a penetrating chest trauma to the right side. 1 = hyperlucent lung field, 2 = hyperexpansion lowers right diaphragm, 3 = collapsed right lung, 4 = deviation of trachea, 5 = mediastinal shift, 6 = compressed left lung.

⓲ Tracheobronchial Tree (Figure 6-2)

A. General Characteristics. The trachea is a tube composed of **16 to 20 U-shaped hyaline cartilages** and the **trachealis** muscle. The trachea begins just inferior to the cricoid cartilage (C6 vertebral level) and ends at the sternal angle (T4 vertebral level), where it bifurcates into the **right and left main bronchi.** At the bifurcation of the trachea, the last tracheal cartilage forms the **carina,** which can be observed by bronchoscopy as a raised ridge of tissue in the sagittal plane. The right main bronchus is shorter and wider and turns to the right at a shallower angle than the left main bronchus. The right main bronchus branches into **3 lobar bronchi** (upper, middle, and lower) and finally into **10 segmental bronchi.** The left main bronchus branches into **2 lobar bronchi** (upper and lower) and finally into **8 to 10 segmental bronchi.** The branching of segmental bronchi corresponds to the **bronchopulmonary segments** of the lung.

B. Clinical Considerations
1. **Compression of the trachea** may be caused by an **enlargement of the thyroid gland** or an **aortic arch aneurysm.** The aortic arch aneurysm may tug on the trachea with each cardiac systole such that it can be felt by palpating the trachea at the sternal notch.
2. **Distortions in the position of the carina** may indicate **metastasis of bronchogenic carcinoma** into the tracheobronchial lymph nodes that surround the tracheal bifurcation or may indicate **enlargement of the left atrium.** The mucous membrane covering the carina is very sensitive in eliciting the cough reflex.
3. **Aspiration of Foreign Objects**
   a. **When a person is sitting or standing.** Aspirated material most commonly enters the **right lower lobar bronchus** and lodges within the **posterior basal bronchopulmonary segment (#10) of the right lower lobe.**

b.   **When a person is supine.** Aspirated material most commonly enters the **right lower lobar bronchus** and lodges within the **superior bronchopulmonary segment (#6) of the right lower lobe.**

c.   **When a person is lying on the right side.** Aspirated material most commonly enters the **right upper lobar bronchus** and lodges within the **posterior bronchopulmonary segment (#2) of the right upper lobe.**

d.   **When a person is lying on the left side.** Aspirated material most commonly enters the **left upper lobar bronchus** and lodges within the **inferior lingular (#5) bronchopulmonary segment of the left upper lobe.**

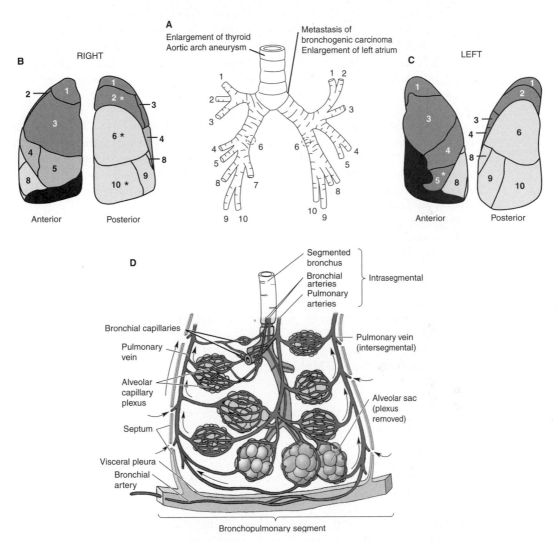

● **Figure 6-2 (A) Diagram of Tracheobronchial Tree. (B) Right Lung.** The bronchopulmonary segments on the anterior and posterior aspects of the right lung are indicated. 1 = apical, 2 = posterior, 3 = anterior, 4 = lateral, 5 = medial, 6 = superior, 8 = anterior basal, 9 = lateral basal, 10 = posterior basal. Note that 7 = medial basal is located on the inner mediastinal surface (not shown). **(C) Left Lung.** The bronchopulmonary segments on the anterior and posterior aspects of the left lung are indicated. 1 = apical, 2 = posterior, 3 = anterior, 4 = superior lingular, 5 = inferior lingular, 6 = superior, 8 = anterior basal, 9 = lateral basal, 10 = posterior basal. Note: There is no 7 segmental bronchus or bronchopulmonary segment in the left lung. * = the bronchopulmonary segments involved in aspiration of foreign objects. **(D) Bronchopulmonary Segment.** Diagram of bronchopulmonary segment 3 shows the centrally located segmental bronchus 3 (SB), branch of the pulmonary artery, and branch of the bronchial artery. Note the location of the pulmonary veins at the periphery of the bronchopulmonary segment.

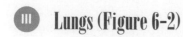 Lungs (Figure 6-2)

A. Right lung consists of **three lobes (upper, middle, and lower)** separated by a **horizontal fissure** and an **oblique fissure.** The right upper lobe lies in a superior–anterior position. The right middle lobe lies in an anterior position between costal cartilages 4 and 6. The right lower lobe lies in an inferior–posterior position. The horizontal fissure runs at the level of costal cartilage 4 and meets the oblique fissure at the midaxillary line. The **diaphragmatic surface** consists of the middle lobe and lower lobe.

B. Left lung consists of **two lobes (upper and lower)** separated by an **oblique fissure.** The left upper lobe lies in a superior–anterior position and contains the **cardiac notch,** where the left ventricle and pericardial sac abut the lung. The **lingula** (which is the embryologic counterpart to the right middle lobe) lies just beneath the cardiac notch. The left lower lobe lies in an inferior–posterior position. The **diaphragmatic surface** consists of the lower lobe.

C. A bronchopulmonary segment contains a **segmental bronchus**, a **branch of the pulmonary artery**, and a **branch of the bronchial artery**, which run together through the **central** part of the segment. It contains **tributaries of the pulmonary vein**, which are found at the **periphery** between two adjacent bronchopulmonary segments. These veins form surgical landmarks during segmental resection of the lung. The bronchopulmonary segments are both named and numbered as indicated below:
   1. Right Lung
      a. Upper lobe: apical (#1), **posterior (#2),** * anterior (#3)
      b. Middle lobe: lateral (#4), medial (#5)
      c. Lower lobe: **superior (#6),** medial basal (#7), anterior basal (#8), lateral basal (#9), **posterior basal (#10)**
   2. Left Lung
      a. Upper lobe: apical (#1), posterior (#2), anterior (#3), superior lingular (#4), **inferior lingular (#5)**
      b. Lower lobe: superior (#6), anterior basal (#8), lateral basal (#9), posterior basal (#10). Note #7 is absent.

D. Breath Sounds
   1. Breath sounds from the upper lobe of each lung can be auscultated on the anterior–superior aspect of the thorax.
   2. Breath sounds from the lower lobe of each lung can be auscultated on the posterior–inferior aspect of the back.
   3. Breath sounds from the middle lobe of the right lung can be auscultated on the anterior thorax near the sternum just inferior to intercostal space 4.

E. Vasculature of the Lung. The adult lung is supplied by two arterial systems and drained by two venous systems.
   1. The **pulmonary trunk** is anterior to the ascending aorta and travels in a superior–posterior direction to the left side for about 5 cm and then bifurcates into the **right pulmonary artery** and **left pulmonary artery**, which carry deoxygenated blood to the lung for aeration. The **right pulmonary** artery runs horizontally toward the hilus beneath the arch of the aorta, posterior to the ascending aorta and superior vena cava, and anterior to the right main bronchus. The **left pulmonary artery**

---

*Bronchopulmonary segments in bold are most frequently involved in aspiration of foreign objects.

PLEURA, TRACHEOBRONCHIAL TREE, AND LUNGS

is shorter and narrower than the right pulmonary artery and is connected to the arch of the aorta by the **ligamentum arteriosum**. The pulmonary arteries branch to follow the airways to the level of the terminal bronchioles, at which point they form a pulmonary capillary plexus.

2. The **bronchial arteries** carry oxygenated blood to the parenchyma of the lung. The **right bronchial artery** is a branch of a posterior intercostal artery. The two **left bronchial arteries** are branches of the thoracic aorta. The bronchial arteries branch to follow the airways to the level of the terminal bronchioles, at which point they drain into the **pulmonary capillary plexus** (i.e. 70% of bronchial blood drains into the pulmonary capillary plexus). Bronchial arteries that supply large bronchi drain into **bronchial veins** (i.e. 30% of bronchial blood drains into the bronchial veins).

3. The **pulmonary veins** carry oxygenated blood from the pulmonary capillary plexus and deoxygenated bronchial blood to the left atrium. There are five pulmonary veins that each drain a lobe of the lungs. However, the pulmonary veins from the right upper and middle lobes generally join so that only **four pulmonary veins** open into the posterior aspect of the **left atrium**. Within the lung, small branches of the pulmonary veins run **solo** (i.e. do not run with the airways, pulmonary arteries, or bronchial arteries). Larger branches of the pulmonary veins are found at the periphery of the bronchopulmonary segments (i.e. **intersegmental location**).

4. The **bronchial veins** carry deoxygenated blood from the bronchial arteries that supply large bronchi. **Right bronchial veins** drain into the **azygos vein**. **Left bronchial veins** drain into the **accessory hemiazygos vein**.

F. **Innervation of the Lung.** The lungs are innervated by the **anterior pulmonary plexus** and **posterior pulmonary plexus**, which are located anterior and posterior to the root of the lung at the hilus, respectively. These plexuses contain both **parasympathetic (vagus; cranial nerve [CN] X)** and **sympathetic components**.

1. **Parasympathetic.** Preganglionic neuronal cell bodies are located in the **dorsal nucleus of the vagus** and **nucleus ambiguus** of the medulla. Preganglionic axons run in the vagus nerve (CN X). Postganglionic neuronal cell bodies are located in the **pulmonary plexuses** and **within the lung** along the bronchial airways. Postganglionic parasympathetic axons terminate on smooth muscle of the bronchial tree, causing **bronchoconstriction**, and seromucous glands, causing **increased glandular secretion**. Postganglionic parasympathetic axons release **acetylcholine (ACh)** as a neurotransmitter, which binds to muscarinic ACh receptors (a G protein-linked receptor). Afferent (sensory) nerve fibers run with CN X and carry touch and stretch modalities.

2. **Sympathetic.** Preganglionic neuronal cell bodies are located in the **intermediolateral cell column** of the spinal cord. Preganglionic axons enter the **paravertebral ganglion**. Postganglionic neuronal cells bodies are located in the paravertebral ganglion at the cervical (superior, middle, and inferior ganglia) and thoracic (T1 through T4) levels. Postganglionic sympathetic axons terminate on postganglionic parasympathetic neurons and modulate their bronchoconstriction activity (thereby causing **bronchodilation**). Circulating epinephrine from the adrenal medulla acts directly on bronchial smooth muscle to cause bronchodilation. Postganglionic sympathetic axons also terminate on smooth muscle of blood vessels causing **vasoconstriction**. Postganglionic sympathetic axons release **norepinephrine (NE)** as a neurotransmitter, which binds to adrenergic receptors (a G protein-linked receptor).

G. **Lymphatic Drainage of the Lung.** The adult lung has lymphatic plexuses that communicate freely. Lymph from the right lung ultimately drains into the **right bronchomediastinal trunk**, which empties into the junction of the right internal jugular vein and right subclavian vein. Most of the lymph from the left lung ultimately drains into the **left bronchomediastinal trunk**, which empties into the junction of the left internal jugular vein and left subclavian vein. Lymph from the lower lobe of the left lung drains into the right lung pathway.

1. The **superficial plexus** of lymphatic vessels lies just deep to the visceral pleura and drains lymph to the **bronchopulmonary lymph nodes** → **inferior and superior tracheobronchial lymph nodes**→ **paratracheal lymph nodes**→ **bronchomediastinal trunk**.

2. The **deep plexus** of lymphatic vessels lies in the submucosa and connective of bronchi and drains lymph to the **pulmonary lymph nodes**→ **bronchopulmonary lymph nodes**→ **inferior and superior tracheobronchial lymph nodes**→ **paratracheal lymph nodes**→ **bronchomediastinal trunk**.

 IV ## Clinical Considerations

A. **Atelectasis (Figure 6-3A)** is the incomplete expansion of alveoli (in neonates) or collapse of alveoli (in adults). **Microatelectasis** is the generalized inability of the lung to expand caused by the loss of surfactant usually seen in the following conditions:

1. **Neonatal respiratory distress syndrome (NRDS)** is caused by a deficiency of surfactant, which may occur in infants because of prolonged intrauterine asphyxia, in premature infants, or in infants of diabetic mothers. Lung maturation is assessed by the **lecithin-to-sphingomyelin ratio** in amniotic fluid (a ratio > 2:1 = maturity). **Thyroxine** and **cortisol** treatment can increase surfactant production. Pathologic findings include hemorrhagic edema within the lung, atelectasis, and **hyaline membrane disease** characterized by eosinophilic material consisting of proteinaceous fluid (fibrin, plasma) and necrotic cells. A deficiency of surfactant causes the surface tension (or attraction) to increase, and therefore the elastance (or collapsing force) of the lung is increased as described by the Laplace Law. The elastance is increased so much that the newborn cannot inflate the lungs with air. The newborn works harder and harder with each successive breath to try to inflate the lungs, but to no avail. The newborn develops hypoxemia, which causes pulmonary vasoconstriction, pulmonary hypoperfusion, and capillary endothelial damage.

2. **Adult respiratory distress syndrome (ARDS; Figure 6-3B)** is defined as a secondary surfactant deficiency caused by other primary pathologic disorders that damage either alveolar cells or capillary endothelial cells in the lung. ARDS is a clinical term for diffuse alveolar damage leading to respiratory failure. ARDS may be caused by the following: inhalation of toxic gases (e.g. seen in 911 emergency responders), water, or extremely hot air; left ventricular failure resulting in cardiogenic pulmonary edema; illicit drugs (e.g. heroin); metabolic disorders (e.g. uremia, acidosis, acute pancreatitis); severe trauma (e.g. car accident with multiple fractures); and shock (e.g. endotoxins or ischemia can damage cells).

B. **Pulmonary embolism (PE; Figure 6-3C, D)** is the occlusion of the pulmonary artery or its branches by an embolic blood clot originating from a deep vein thrombosis (DVT) in the leg or pelvic area. A **large embolus** may occlude the main pulmonary artery or lodge at the bifurcation as a "**saddle embolus**," which may cause sudden death with symptoms easily confused with myocardial infarction (i.e. chest pain, severe dyspnea, shock, increased serum lactate dehydrogenase [LDH] levels). A **medium-sized embolism** may occlude segmental arteries and may produce a **pulmonary infarction** that is wedge-shaped and usually occurs in the lower lobes. A group of **small emboli** ("**emboli showers**") may occlude smaller peripheral branches of the pulmonary artery and cause pulmonary hypertension with time. Risk factors include obesity, cancer, pregnancy, oral contraceptives, hypercoagulability, multiple bone fractures, burns, and prior DVT. A typical clinical scenario involves a postsurgical, bedridden patient who develops sudden shortness of breath.

C. Bronchiectasis (Figure 6-3E, F) is the abnormal, permanent dilatation of bronchi as a result of chronic necrotizing infection (e.g. *Staphylococcus*, *Streptococcus*, *Haemophilus influenzae*), bronchial obstruction (e.g. foreign body, mucous plugs, or tumors), or congenital conditions (e.g. Kartagener syndrome, cystic fibrosis, immunodeficiency disorders). The **lower lobes** of the lung are predominately affected, and the affected bronchi have a **saccular** appearance. Clinical signs include cough, fever, and expectoration of large amounts of foul-smelling purulent sputum.

D. Obstructive lung diseases (Figure 6-4A) are characterized by an **increase in airway resistance (particularly expiratory airflow). Obstructive ventilatory impairment** is the impairment of airflow during expiration with concomitant air trapping and hyperinflation. The increase in airway resistance (as a result of narrowing of the airway lumen) can be caused by the following conditions: **in the wall of the airway**, smooth muscle hypertrophy may cause airway narrowing (e.g. asthma); **outside the airway**, destruction of lung parenchyma may cause airway narrowing on expiration because of loss of radial traction (e.g. emphysema); and **in the lumen of the airway**, increased mucus production may cause airway narrowing (e.g. chronic bronchitis).

1. **Asthma (Figure 6-4B)**
    a. **General Features.** Asthma is associated with **smooth muscle hyperactivity within bronchi and bronchioles, increased mucus production, and edema of the bronchial wall.** Patients with asthma have the following characteristics: a decreased partial pressure of arterial oxygen (PaO_2; hypoxemia) leads to stimulation of the carotid and aortic bodies and hyperventilation, a decreased partial pressure of arterial carbon dioxide ($PaCO_2$; hypocapnia), and respiratory alkalosis. As the asthma attack worsens, hypoventilation occurs and leads to a further decreased PaO_2, a severely increased $PaCO_2$ (hypercapnia), respiratory acidosis, and death.
    b. **Pathology.** Pathologic findings include inflammatory cell infiltrates containing numerous **eosinophils** within the bronchial wall, hyperplasia of bronchial smooth muscle, hypertrophy of seromucous glands, **Curschmann spirals** (formed from shed epithelium), and **Charcot-Leyden crystals** (formed from eosinophil granules) within the mucous plugs.

2. **Emphysema (Figure 6-4C)** is a type of chronic obstructive pulmonary disease (COPD). In the early stages of emphysema, there is enlargement of air spaces distal to the terminal bronchioles called air trapping. In the later stages of emphysema, further lung tissue and alveolar damage result in additional air trapping, which is now called hyperinflation. Emphysematous patients have much less difficulty inhaling air into the lung ($\uparrow$compliance) than a normal individual. However, emphysematous patients have much more difficulty exhaling air out of the lung, which increases the work of breathing (i.e. respiratory muscles), and is manifested by shortness of breath (dyspnea). Emphysematous patient breathe slower with large tidal volumes.
    a. **General Features.** Patients are referred to as "**pink puffers**" with the following characteristics: a thin, barrel-shaped chest, increased breathing rate (tachypnea), a mildly decreased PaO_2 (mild hypoxemia), a mildly decreased or normal $PaCO_2$ (hypocapnia or normocapnia), and a decreased diffusion-limited carbon monoxide ($DLCO$).

b. **Pathology**
    i.   **Centriacinar emphysema** (related to **smoking**). Pathologic findings include a widening of the air spaces within the **respiratory bronchioles** only while the surrounding alveoli remain fairly well preserved.
    ii. **Panacinar emphysema** (related to α_1-**antitrypsin deficiency**). Pathologic findings include a widening of the air spaces within the **alveolar ducts, alveolar sacs,** and **alveoli** as a result of destruction of the alveolar walls by enzymes.
3. **Chronic bronchitis (Figure 6-4D)** is a type of COPD that is related to smoking.
    a. **General Features.** Patients are referred to as **"blue bloaters"** with the following characteristics: a muscular, barrel-shaped chest, severely decreased Pa_{O_2} (severe hypoxemia with cyanosis), increased Pa_{CO_2} (hypercapnia) that leads to chronic respiratory acidosis, increased HCO_3^- reabsorption by the kidney to buffer the acidemia, right ventricular failure, and systemic edema.
    b. **Pathology.** Pathologic findings include inflammatory cell infiltrates within the bronchial wall; hypertrophy of seromucous glands (increase in Reid index); excessive mucus production leading to copious, purulent sputum production; and recurrent inflammation, infection, and scarring in terminal airways that results in a decrease in average small airway diameter.

E. **Restrictive lung diseases (Figure 6-5A)** are characterized by a **decrease in compliance** (i.e. the distensibility of the lung is restricted). The lungs are said to be **"stiff." Restrictive ventilatory impairment** is the inability to fully expand the lung (**inspiratory airflow**), which results in a decrease in total lung capacity (TLC).
1. **Idiopathic Pulmonary Fibrosis (Figure 6-5B)**
    a. **General Features.** Patients with idiopathic pulmonary fibrosis have the following characteristics: a decreased Pa_{O_2} (hypoxemia) and a mildly decreased or normal Pa_{CO_2} (hypocapnia or normocapnia). **During exercise, the hypoxemia worsens without hypercapnia.** As the condition worsens, hypoventilation leads to a further decreased Pa_{O_2}, a severely increased Pa_{CO_2} (hypercapnia), respiratory acidosis, and death, and decreased diffusion limited carbon monoxide (D_{LCO}).
    b. **Pathology.** Pathologic findings include inflammatory cell infiltrates, thickening of the blood–air barrier (i.e. alveolar wall) because of collagen production by fibroblasts, and destruction of alveolar architecture leading to formation of air-filled cystic spaces surrounded by thickened scar tissue (i.e. **"honeycomb lung"**).
2. **Coal worker pneumoconiosis (CWP; "black lung disease"; Figure 6-5C, D)** results from the inhalation of **coal dust** and is generally benign, with little if any reduction in lung function. The appearance of large nodular lesions suggests a change caused by silica in the inhaled dust such that the disease is now called **anthracosilicosis. Anthracosis** is the most innocuous lesion observed whereby carbon pigment is phagocytosed by alveolar macrophages that accumulate along the lymphatics. Simple CWP occurs when carbon pigment is phagocytosed by alveolar macrophages that organize into coal nodules usually found adjacent to respiratory bronchioles. Complicated CWP or progressive massive fibrosis (PMF) occurs when there is a confluent, fibrosing reaction in the lung. PMF occurs on a background of simple CWP and consists of multiple, large scars made up of dense collagen and carbon pigment. Caplan syndrome is the coexistence of rheumatoid arthritis and CWP whereby distinctive pulmonary nodular lesions (similar to rheumatoid nodules) develop rapidly.
3. **Silicosis (Figure 6-5E)** results from the inhalation of **silicon dioxide** (silica; SiO_2) and is associated with an increased disposition to **tuberculosis** (i.e. silicotubercu-

losis). Silicosis is characterized by small, dense, collagenous nodules that contain birefringent silica crystals.

4. **Asbestosis (Figure 6-5F)** results from the inhalation of asbestos fibers. There are two geometric forms of asbestos: a **serpentine form** (curly, flexible fibers) and an **amphibole form** (straight, stiff fibers). The amphibole form is more pathogenic. Asbestosis is characterized by **diffuse pulmonary interstitial fibrosis** and **asbestos bodies.** Asbestos bodies are golden-brown, beaded rods that consist of asbestos fibers coated with iron-containing protein material. These bodies arise when alveolar macrophages attempt to phagocytose asbestos fibers.

   Malignant mesothelioma is the most serious pleural neoplasm and is associated with a history of asbestos exposure.

5. **Sarcoidosis (Figure 6-5G)** is a **type IV hypersensitivity** reaction to an unknown antigen. Sarcoidosis is characterized by a **noncaseating granuloma** distributed along the lymphatics in the lung. The noncaseating granuloma is an aggregation of epithelioid cells with Langerhans cells and foreign body-type giant cells, **asteroid bodies**, which are stellate inclusion bodies found within giant cells, **Schaumann bodies**, which are laminated concretions of calcium, and proteins. Sarcoidosis is common in the southeastern United States and in young black women.

F. **Cystic fibrosis (CF; Figure 6-6A, B)** is caused by production of abnormally thick mucus by epithelial cells lining the respiratory tract (and gastrointestinal tract). This results clinically in obstruction of airways and recurrent bacterial infections (e.g. *Staphylococcus aureus, Pseudomonas aeruginosa*). CF is caused by autosomal recessive mutations of the *CF* gene, which is located on the long arm of chromosome 7 (q7). The *CF* gene encodes for a protein called **CFTR (cystic fibrosis transporter)**, which functions as a Cl^- ion channel. In North America, 70% of CF cases are caused by a three-base deletion that codes for the amino acid **phenylalanine at position 508** such that phenylalanine is missing from CFTR. Clinical signs include meconium ileus (i.e. obstruction of the bowel) in the neonate, steatorrhea (fatty stool) or obstruction of the bowel in childhood, and **cor pulmonale** (manifesting as right-side heart failure) developing secondary to pulmonary hypertension.

G. **Bronchogenic carcinoma (Figure 6-6C, D)** begins as hyperplasia of the bronchial epithelium with continued progression occurring through intraluminal growth, infiltrative peribronchial growth, and intraparenchymal growth. Intrathoracic spread of bronchogenic carcinoma may lead to **Horner syndrome** (miosis, ptosis, hemianhidrosis, and apparent enophthalmos) as a result of cervical sympathetic chain involvement; **SVC syndrome**, causing dilatation of head and neck veins, facial swelling, and cyanosis; **dysphagia** caused by esophageal obstruction; **hoarseness of voice** as a result of recurrent laryngeal nerve involvement; **paralysis of diaphragm** caused by phrenic nerve involvement; and **Pancoast syndrome**, causing ulnar nerve pain and Horner syndrome. Tracheobronchial, parasternal, and supraclavicular lymph nodes are involved in the lymphatic metastasis of bronchogenic carcinoma. Enlargement of the tracheobronchial nodes may **indent the esophagus**, which can be observed radiologically during a barium swallow, or **distort the position of the carina.** Metastasis to the brain via arterial blood may occur by the following route: cancer cells enter a lung capillary → pulmonary vein → left atrium and ventricle → aorta → internal carotid and vertebral arteries. Metastasis to the brain via venous blood may occur by the following route: cancer cells enter a bronchial vein → azygos vein → external and internal vertebral venous plexuses → cranial dural sinuses. Because about 25% of primary lung cancers do not have an obvious bronchial origin, the term "bronchogenic" may not be entirely appropriate. The most important issue in primary lung cancer is the histologic subclassifications, which include the following:

1. **Adenocarcinoma (AD)** has a 35% incidence and is the most common lung cancer in nonsmokers. AD is peripherally located within the lung as it arises from distal airways and alveoli and forms a well-circumscribed gray-white mass. There are four major histologic subtypes of AD although it is common to find mixtures of subtypes.

2. **Squamous cell carcinoma (SQ)** has a 35% incidence and is most closely associated with **smoking history**. SQ is centrally located as it arises from larger bronchi because of injury of the bronchial epithelium followed by regeneration from the basal layer in the form of squamous metaplasia. SQ begins as a small red granular plaque and progresses to a large intrabronchial mass. Cavitation of the lung may occur distal to the mass. SQ may secrete **parathyroid hormone (PTH)**, causing hypercalcemia.

3. **Small cell carcinoma (SC)** has a 20% incidence and is associated with a **smoking history**. SC is centrally located as it arises from larger bronchi. SC forms large, soft, gray-white masses and contains small, oval-shaped cells ("oat cells") derived from **Kulchitsky cells** (neural crest origin) that may produce **adrenocorticotropic hormone (ACTH)** or **antidiuretic hormone (ADH)**, causing Cushing syndrome or syndrome of inappropriate secretion of ADH (SIADH), respectively. SC is a highly malignant and aggressive tumor (median survival time less than 3 months); however, it does respond favorably to chemotherapy. Consequently, from the viewpoint of an oncologist, there are two types of lung carcinomas: small cell carcinomas (chemotherapy sensitive) and non–small cell carcinomas (chemotherapy insensitive).

4. **Undifferentiated large cell carcinoma (LC)** has a 10% incidence. LC is a diagnosis of exclusion in a poorly differentiated non–small cell carcinoma that does not show clear histologic signs of either adenocarcinoma or squamous cell carcinoma.

5. **Carcinoid tumor (CT)** has a 2% incidence and is not associated with a smoking history. CT is a neuroendocrine neoplasm similar to Kulchitsky cells derived from the pluripotential basal layer of the respiratory epithelium. CT is generally endocrinologically silent. CT may be located centrally, peripherally, or in the midportion of the lung. Centrally located CT has a large endobronchial component with a smooth, fleshy mass protruding into the lumen of the bronchus. Patients with CT may develop **carcinoid syndrome**, which is characterized by facial flushing (because of vasomotor disturbances), diarrhea (because of intestinal hypermotility), or wheezing (because of bronchoconstriction).

V Cross-Sectional Anatomy

A. **CT Scan at the Level of Origin of the Three Branches of the Aortic Arch (about vertebral level T2 through T3; Figure 6-7)**

B. **CT Scan and MRI at the Level of the Aortic Arch (Figure 6-8)**

C. **CT scan and MRI at the Level of the Aortic-Pulmonary Window (at about vertebral level T4; Figure 6-9)**

D. **CT Scan at the Level of Origin of the Left Main Pulmonary Artery (Figure 6-10)**

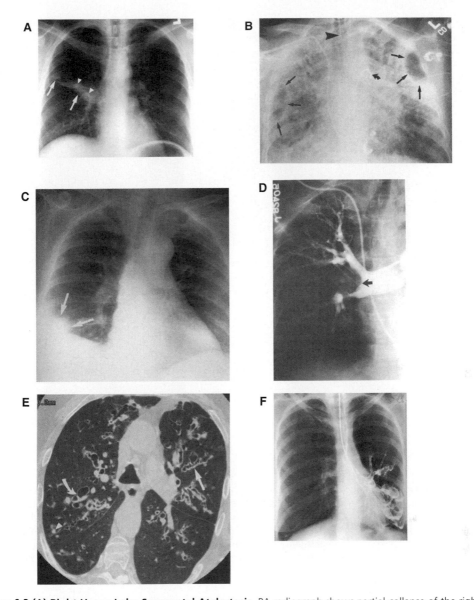

● **Figure 6-3 (A) Right Upper Lobe Segmental Atelectasis.** PA radiograph shows partial collapse of the right upper lobe. The minor fissure is mildly elevated (arrows), outlining the lower border of the atelectatic lung. Note the calcified densities (arrowheads). **(B) Adult Respiratory Distress Syndrome (ARDS).** AP recumbent radiograph shows an endo-tracheal tube (arrowhead), oval collections of air at the periphery of the lung representing pneumatoceles (arrows), and right subclavian Swan-Ganz catheter (curved arrow). **(C) Pulmonary Infarct.** PA radiograph shows a pleural-based, rounded area at the right costophrenic angle (Hampton hump) indicating an acute pulmonary infarct (arrows). **(D) Pulmonary Embolism.** A pulmonary arteriogram shows a large saddle embolus (arrow). Note the poor perfusion of the right middle and lower lobes compared with the upper lobe. **(E, F) Bronchiectasis. (E)** High-resolution CT scan shows a beaded appearance of some airways called varicose bronchiectasis (straight arrow) and a cluster-of-grapes appearance of some airways called cystic bronchiectasis (curved arrow). The bronchial and bronchiolar walls are thickened, and some are filled with mucus-forming nodular opacities (arrowhead). **(F) Bronchogram.** The dilated bronchi have a saccular ap-pearance and are clearly seen within the left lower lobe.

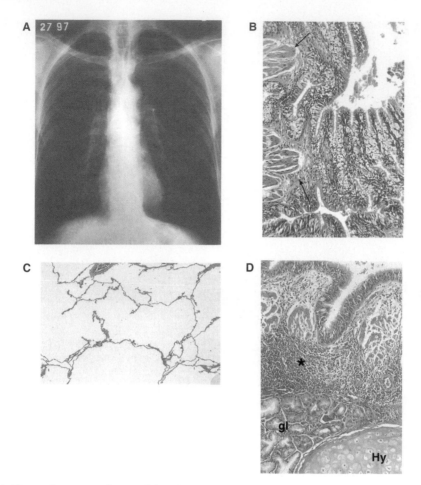

● **Figure 6-4 Obstructive Lung Disease. (A)** Radiograph shows key features of obstructive lung disease. Note the hyperinflation of the lung and destruction of the lung interstitium (i.e. bulla formation), causing the lung to appear hyperlucent. Note that the diaphragm is flat and depressed (i.e. lower than rib 11). **(B) Asthma.** LM shows the respiratory epithelium that lines the bronchus forms invaginations and contains enlarged goblet cells that secrete mucus. Note the hyperplasia of bronchial smooth muscle (arrows). **(C) Emphysema.** LM shows the histologic appearance of panacinar emphysema with large, irregular airspaces and reduced number of alveolar walls. **(D) Chronic Bronchitis.** LM shows the wall of the bronchus contains a large number of inflammatory cells (*) and hypertrophy of seromucous glands (gl). Hy = hyaline cartilage.

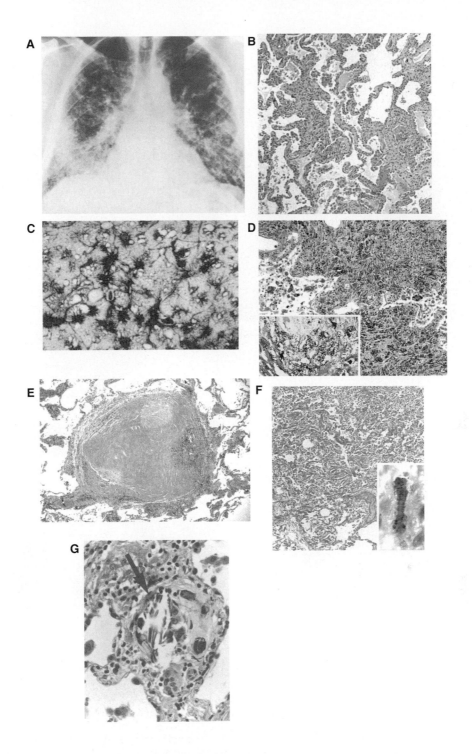

● **Figure 6-5 Restrictive Lung Disease. (A)** Radiograph shows key features of restrictive lung disease. Note a reticular pattern of lung opacities caused by an abnormal lung interstitium that are interspersed between clear areas (lung cysts or "honeycomb lung"); small, contracted lung; and raised diaphragm. **(B) Idiopathic Pulmonary Fibrosis (IPF).** LM shows the appearance of **usual interstitial pneumonia,** which is the most common form of IPF. Note the inflammatory cell infiltrates with the interalveolar septae, thickened interalveolar septae owing to fibrosis, and fibrin in the alveolar spaces. **(C, D) Coal Worker Pneumoconiosis (CWP). (C)** Photograph of a gross specimen of a coal miner's lung showing scattered, irregular, carbon-pigmented nodules throughout the lung parenchyma. **(D)** LM shows fibrotic carbon-pigmented nodules. Inset shows numerous silica particles that appear as birefringent crystals under polarized light. **(E) Silicosis.** LM of a silicotic nodule shows whorls of dense collagen fibers. **(F) Asbestosis.** LM shows prominent diffuse pulmonary interstitial fibrosis and an asbestos body (inset). **(G) Sarcoidosis.** LM shows a laminated concretion of calcium and proteins (arrow) called a Schaumann body.

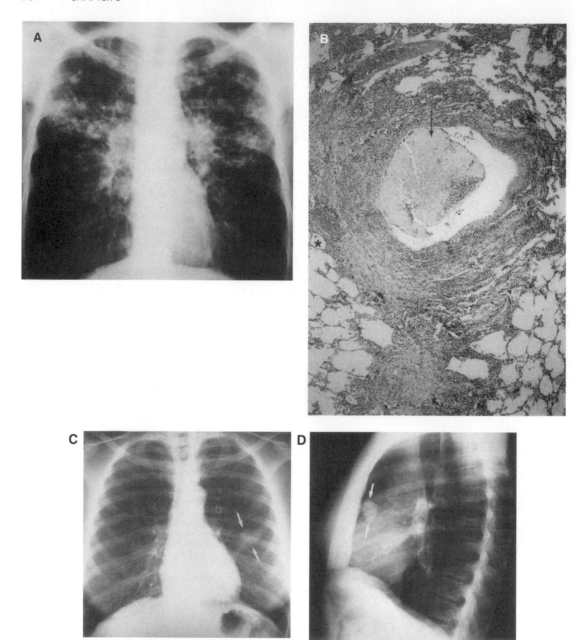

● **Figure 6-6 Cystic Fibrosis and Bronchogenic Carcinoma. (A, B) Cystic Fibrosis. (A)** PA radiograph of cystic fibrosis shows hyperinflation of both lungs, reduced size of the heart because of pulmonary compression, cyst formation, and atelectasis (collapse of alveoli) in both lungs. **(B)** LM of cystic fibrosis shows a bronchus that is filled with a thick mucus and inflammatory cells (arrow). Smaller bronchi may be completely plugged by this material. In addition, surrounding the bronchus there is a heavy lymphocyte infiltration (*). **(C, D) Bronchogenic Carcinoma. (C)** PA radiograph shows a 3-cm nodule in the left lung (arrows). **(D)** Lateral radiograph shows the nodule (arrows) anterior within the left upper lobe.

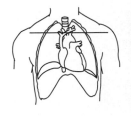
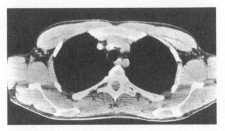

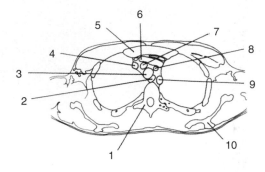

1 - Thoracic vertebra	6 - Left brachiocephalic vein
2 - Esophagus	7 - Brachiocephalic trunk
3 - Trachea	8 - Left common carotid artery
4 - Right brachiocephalic vein	9 - Left subclavian vein
5 - Sternum	10 - Scapula

● **Figure 6-7 CT Scan at Level of Origin of the Three Branches of the Aortic Arch (about vertebral level T2 through T3).** The esophagus is anterior and to the left of the body of the thoracic vertebra. The trachea is anterior and to the right of the esophagus. The brachiocephalic trunk is anterior and to the right of the trachea. The left common carotid artery is anterior and to the left of the trachea. The left subclavian artery is to the left of the posterior border of the trachea. The right brachiocephalic vein is to the right of the brachiocephalic trunk. The left brachiocephalic vein appears in oblique section as it travels to the right side.

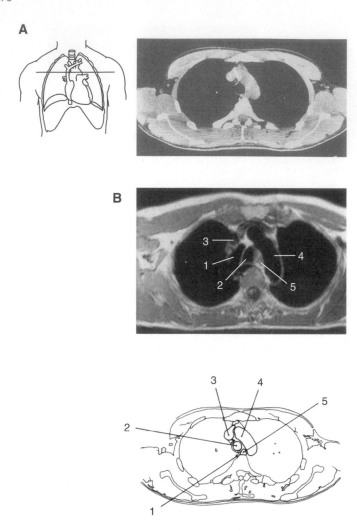

1 - Azygos vein
2 - Trachea
3 - Superior vena cava
4 - Aortic arch
5 - Esophagus

● **Figure 6-8 CT Scan (A) and MRI (B) at the Level of the Aortic Arch.** The esophagus is anterior and to the left of the body of the thoracic vertebra. The trachea is anterior and to the right of the esophagus. The azygos vein is posterior to the trachea and to the right of the esophagus. The aortic arch is a curved image that begins to the left of the superior vena cava (or right brachiocephalic vein), curves around the trachea, and ends to the left of the esophagus. The left brachiocephalic vein appears in oblique section at its union with the right brachiocephalic vein emptying into the superior vena cava.

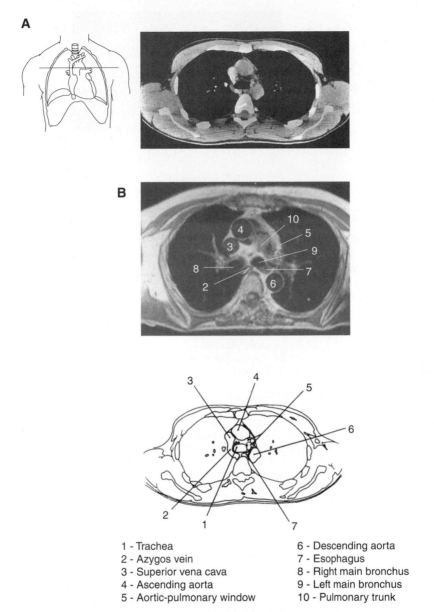

1 - Trachea
2 - Azygos vein
3 - Superior vena cava
4 - Ascending aorta
5 - Aortic-pulmonary window

6 - Descending aorta
7 - Esophagus
8 - Right main bronchus
9 - Left main bronchus
10 - Pulmonary trunk

● **Figure 6-9 CT Scan (A) and MRI (B) at the Level of the Aortic–Pulmonary Window (at about vertebral level T4).** The aortic–pulmonary window is the space in the superior mediastinum from the bifurcation of the pulmonary trunk to the undersurface of the aortic arch. The esophagus is anterior and to the left of the body of the thoracic vertebra. At this level, the trachea bifurcates into the right main bronchus and left main bronchus. The azygos vein appears in longitudinal section as it arches over the right main bronchus and empties into the superior vena cava. The ascending aorta is anterior to the right main bronchus and anterior and to the left of the superior vena cava.

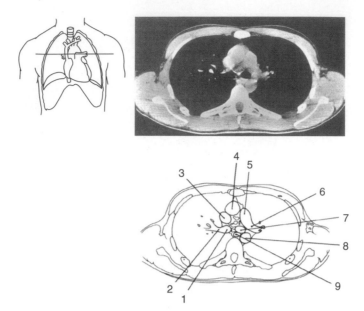

1 - Right main bronchus
2 - Branching of right
    main bronchus
3 - Superior vena cava
4 - Ascending aorta

5 - Pulmonary trunk
6 - Left pulmonary artery
7 - Left main bronchus
8 - Descending aorta
9 - Esophagus

● **Figure 6-10 CT Scan at the Level of the Origin of the Left Pulmonary Artery.** The left main bronchus appears in cross-section anterior to the esophagus and descending aorta. The right main bronchus branches into the right upper lobar bronchus and right middle lobar bronchus. The pulmonary trunk is anterior and to the left of the left main bronchus. The left pulmonary artery appears in longitudinal section as it curves posterolateral toward the hilum of the left lung. The superior vena cava is anterior to the right main bronchus. The ascending aorta is anterior and between the right main bronchus and left main bronchus.

Case Study

A 57-year-old woman who smoked for 38 years was admitted to the hospital because of recurrent nosebleed, chronic cough, and progressive shortness of breath. The nosebleed started 3.5 months ago and required two admissions to the hospital. Dyspnea began 3 years before admission and was particularly noticeable during exercise. The chronic cough has gradually worsened. For the past 24 years, there have been signs of cyanosis of the face and neck, which has gradually worsened over the years. The patient describes distended torturous veins over the front of her chest and neck, and she has also noticed increased dizziness, especially when rising and bending. Although she has not gained weight, her collar size has increased. The patient remarks that just before the development of these veins she had many carbuncles on the trunk and axilla and severe acne on her face that resolved slowly but not completely.

Examination

Cyanosis of the face and neck with deepening of cyanosis when in supine position. Eyes are prominent and eyelids appear swollen. Numerous tortuous superficial veins over the neck and upper chest. Numerous veins cross the anterior costal margins and continue toward the pubic area. The entire trunk is covered with acnelike carbuncles.

Radiographs

Radiographs show widening of the mediastinal shadow in the region of the right upper mediastinum and a group of heavily calcified lymph nodes lying against the right side of the trachea down to the level of the carina. Radiographs of the chest after injection of contrast medium into the cubital vein reveal that the widening of the upper mediastinum is caused by abnormal veins. The termination of the right subclavian vein appears constricted and has collateral channels. No contrast medium entered the heart during the filming. The medium enters an enlarged internal thoracic vein and descends toward the abdomen. Venous pressure shows three times normal in the upper extremity, whereas pressure in the lower extremity is normal.

Explanation

The swelling of the face, bleeding from the nose, cyanosis, and increased venous pressure in the veins in the upper extremity, as well as the distension and tortuosity of the veins in the neck, arms, and upper trunk, are caused by an obstruction of the venous channels that drain the upper body. Because the obstruction is longstanding, there are many collateral venous channels complicating the picture. Because radiographs and other clinical findings do not prove otherwise, one must assume and treat a benign cause. In view of the history of a severe skin infection of the chest wall for many years, the obstruction can reasonably be ascribed to thrombosis in the mediastinal vein originating from inflammation of these veins related to her skin infection. Note that this is not the most common reason for these symptoms.

More than likely, the shortness of breath is caused by pulmonary emphysema, resulting from chronic bronchitis and degenerative changes in the lungs. These symptoms are apparently not connected to the other findings. This is an exception, not the rule.

The calcification of mediastinal lymph nodes in the area of the obstructed veins further suggests the presence of inflammatory changes in these nodes caused by infection of the area. Thus, the combination of chronic inflammation of the mediastinal lymph nodes with scarring, compression of the veins of the mediastinum, and clotting inside these veins resulted in obstruction of the right brachiocephalic vein and the superior vena cava. Further clinical tests and radiographs might also indicate obstruction of the azygos vein at the site of its termination.

Chapter 7

Heart

I   The Pericardium

A. General Features. The pericardium consists of three layers: visceral layer of serous pericardium, parietal layer of serous pericardium, and fibrous pericardium.

1. **Visceral layer of serous pericardium** (known histologically as the **epicardium**) consists of a layer of simple squamous epithelium (called **mesothelium**). Beneath the mesothelium, coronary arteries, coronary veins, and nerves travel along the surface of the heart in a thin collagen bed; adipose tissue is also present.

2. **Parietal layer of serous pericardium.** At the base of the aorta and pulmonary trunk, the mesothelium of the visceral layer of serous pericardium is reflected and becomes continuous with the parietal layer of serous pericardium such that the parietal layer of serous pericardium also consists of a layer of simple squamous epithelium (called **mesothelium**).

3. The **pericardial cavity** lies between the visceral layer and parietal layer of serous pericardium and normally contains a small amount of pericardial fluid (20 mL) that allows friction-free movement of the heart during diastole and systole. The **transverse sinus** is a recess of the pericardial cavity. After the pericardial sac is opened, a surgeon can pass a finger or ligature (posterior to the aorta and pulmonary trunk and anterior to the superior vena cava) from one side of the heart to the other through the transverse sinus. The **oblique sinus** is a recess of the pericardial cavity that ends in a cul-de-sac surrounded by the pulmonary veins.

4. **Fibrous pericardium** is a thick (approximately 1 mm) **collagen layer** (no elastic fibers) with **little ability to distend acutely.** The fibrous pericardium fuses superiorly to the tunica adventitia of the great vessels, inferiorly to the central tendon of the diaphragm, and anteriorly to the sternum. The **phrenic nerve** and **pericardiacophrenic artery** descend through the mediastinum lateral to the fibrous pericardium and are in jeopardy during surgery to the heart.

5. The **thoracic portion of the inferior vena cava (IVC)** lies within the pericardium so that to expose this portion of the IVC the pericardium must be opened.

6. The arterial supply of the pericardium is from the **pericardiacophrenic artery** (a branch of the **internal thoracic artery**) that often accompanies the phrenic nerve. The venous drainage of the pericardium is to the **pericardiacophrenic veins,** which drain into the **brachiocephalic veins.** The innervation of the pericardium is supplied by the phrenic nerve (C3 through C5). Pain sensation carried by the **phrenic nerves** is often referred to the skin (C3 through C5 dermatomes) of the ipsilateral supraclavicular region.

B. Clinical Considerations

1. **Cardiac tamponade (heart compression)** is the accumulation of fluid within the pericardial cavity resulting in compression of the heart because the fibrous

pericardium is inelastic. Clinical findings include hypotension (blood pressure [BP] 90/40 mm Hg) that does not respond to rehydration; compression of the superior vena cava (SVC), which may cause the veins of the face and neck to engorge with blood; a distension of veins of the neck on inspiration (**Kussmaul sign**); paradoxical pulse (inspiratory lowering of BP by greater than 10 mm Hg); spontaneous filling of a syringe when blood is drawn because of increased venous pressure; and distant heart sounds.

2. **Pericardiocentesis** is the removal of fluid from the pericardial cavity, which can be approached in two ways.

   a. **Sternal Approach.** A needle is inserted at intercostal space 5 or 6 on the left side near the sternum. The cardiac notch of the left lung leaves the fibrous pericardium exposed at this site. The needle penetrates the following structures: skin → superficial fascia → pectoralis major muscle → external intercostal membrane → internal intercostal muscle → transverse thoracic muscle → fibrous pericardium → parietal layer of serous pericardium. The internal thoracic artery, coronary arteries, and pleura may be damaged during this approach.

   b. **Subxiphoid Approach.** A needle is inserted at the left infrasternal angle angled in a superior and posterior direction. The needle will penetrate the following structures: skin → superficial fascia → anterior rectus sheath → rectus abdominus muscle → transverse abdominus muscle → fibrous pericardium → parietal layer of serous pericardium. The diaphragm and liver may be damaged during this approach.

II ⬤ Heart Surfaces (Figure 7-1A, B). The heart has six surfaces.

A. Posterior surface (base) consists mainly of the **left atrium**, which receives the pulmonary veins and is related to vertebral bodies T6 through T9.

B. Apex consists of the inferior lateral portion of the **left ventricle** at intercostal space 5 along the midclavicular line. The maximal pulsation of the heart (apex beat) occurs at the apex.

C. Anterior surface (sternocostal surface) consists mainly of the **right ventricle**.

D. Inferior surface (diaphragmatic surface) consists mainly of the **left ventricle** and is related to the central tendon of the diaphragm.

E. Left surface (pulmonary surface) consists mainly of the left ventricle and occupies the cardiac impression of the left lung.

F. Right surface consists mainly of the right atrium located between the SVC and the IVC.

III ⬤ Heart Borders (Figure 7-1A, B). The heart has four borders.

A. Right border consists of the **right atrium, SVC, and IVC.**

B. Left border consists of the **left ventricle, left atrium, pulmonary trunk, and aortic arch.**

C. Inferior border consists of the **right ventricle.**

D. Superior border consists of the **right atrium, left atrium, SVC, ascending aorta, and pulmonary trunk.**

Fibrous Skeleton of the Heart. The fibrous skeleton is a dense framework of collagen within the heart that keeps the orifices of the atrioventricular valves and semilunar valve patent, provides an attachment site of the valve leaflets and cusps, serves as the origin and insertion sites of cardiac myocytes, and forms an electrical "barrier" between the atria and ventricles so that they contract independently. The fibrous skeleton consists of the:

A. **Tricuspid annulus, mitral annulus, pulmonary annulus, and aortic annulus,** which are four fibrous rings (also called **annuli fibrosi**) that surround the orifices of the tricuspid valve, mitral valve, pulmonary semilunar valve, and aortic semilunar valve, respectively.

B. **Right fibrous trigone** (largest and strongest component of the skeleton), **left fibrous trigone, and intervalvular trigone** formed by the collagen connecting all the fibrous rings.

C. **Conus ligament (ligament of Krehl),** which is a small collagenous connection between the pulmonary and aortic valves.

D. **Tendon of Todaro,** which extends from the tricuspid annulus.

E. **Membranous septum,** which consists of an interventricular and atrioventricular portion.

Valves and Auscultation Sites (Figure 7-1C)

A. **Tricuspid (right atrioventricular) Valve.** The tricuspid valve is located between the right atrium and right ventricle and is composed of **three leaflets (anterior, posterior, and septal),** all of which are tethered to **papillary muscles (anterior, posterior, and medial)** by **chorda tendineae.** The auscultation site is **over the sternum at intercostal space 5.**

B. **Bicuspid (mitral; left atrioventricular) Valve.** The bicuspid valve is located between the left atrium and left ventricle and is composed of **two leaflets (anterior and posterior),** both of which are tethered to **papillary muscles (anterolateral and posteromedial)** by **chorda tendineae.** The auscultation site is at the **cardiac apex at left intercostal space 5.**

C. **Pulmonary Semilunar Valve (pulmonic valve).** The pulmonary semilunar valve is the outflow valve of the right ventricle and is composed of **three cusps (anterior, right, and left)** that fit closely together when closed. The orifice of the pulmonary semilunar valve is directed to the left shoulder. The auscultation site is just **lateral to the sternum at left intercostal space 2.** A secondary pulmonic auscultation site is **over the sternum at about intercostal space 4.**

D. **Aortic Semilunar Valve.** The aortic semilunar valve is the outflow valve of the left ventricle and is composed of **three cusps (posterior, right, and left)** that fit closely together when closed. The orifice of the aortic semilunar valve is directed to the right shoulder. The auscultation site is just **lateral to the sternum at right intercostal space 2.**

A
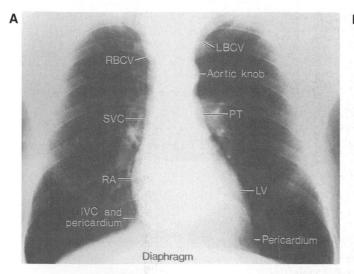

B
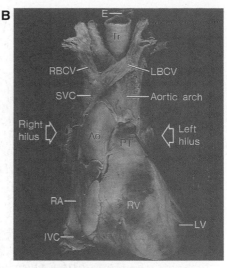

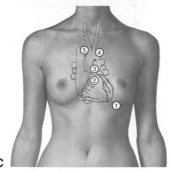

C

● **Figure 7-1 (A)** Radiograph shows the various components of the heart and great vessels. **(B)** Photograph of the anatomic heart and great vessels for comparison to the radiograph in A. RV = right ventricle, Ao = aorta, Tr = trachea, E = esophagus, RBCV = right brachiocephalic vein, LBCV = left brachiocephalic vein, SVC = superior vena cava, RA = right atrium, IVC = inferior vena cava, PT = pulmonary trunk, LV = left ventricle. **(C) Auscultatory Areas of the Chest.** The positions of the auscultatory areas are indicated on the surface of a woman. 1 = mitral valve area at the 5th left intercostal space, 2 = tricuspid valve area at the 4th left intercostal space, 3 = secondary pulmonic valve area at the 3rd left intercostal space, 4 = pulmonic valve area at the left upper sternal border, 5 = aortic valve area at the right upper sternal border.

VI   Vasculature of the Heart

A. Arterial Supply. The right coronary artery and left coronary artery supply oxygenated arterial blood to the heart. The coronary arteries fill with blood during diastole. The coronary arteries have maximal blood flow during diastole and minimal blood flow during systole.

1. **Right Coronary Artery (RCA).** The RCA arises from the right aortic sinus (of Valsalva) of the ascending aorta and courses in the coronary sulcus. The blood supply of the heart is considered **right-side dominant** (most common) if the posterior interventricular artery arises from the RCA. The RCA branches into the **sinoatrial (SA) nodal artery, conus branch, right marginal artery, atrioventricular (AV) nodal artery, terminal branches, posterior interventricular artery,** and **septal branches.**

2. **Left Main Coronary Artery (LMCA).** The LMCA arises from the left aortic sinus (of Valsalva) of the ascending aorta. The blood supply of the heart is considered **left-side dominant** (less common) if the posterior interventricular artery arises from the LMCA. The LMCA branches into the following:

    a. **Left circumflex artery (LCx)** which further branches into the **anterior marginal artery, obtuse marginal artery, atrial branches,** and **posterior marginal artery.**

    b. **Intermediate ramus** (a variable branch).

c. **Anterior interventricular artery** (also called left anterior descending artery [LAD]), which further branches into the **anterior diagonal artery** and **septal branches.**

B. Venous Drainage

1. **Coronary sinus** is the largest vein draining the heart and drains directly into the right atrium. At the opening of the coronary sinus, a crescent-shaped valve remnant (called the **thebesian valve**) is present.
2. **Great cardiac vein** follows the **anterior interventricular artery** and drains into the coronary sinus.
3. **Middle cardiac vein** follows the **posterior interventricular artery** and drains into the coronary sinus.
4. **Small cardiac vein** follows the **right marginal artery** and drains into the coronary sinus.
5. **Oblique vein of the left atrium** is a remnant of the embryonic left superior vena cava and drains into the coronary sinus.
6. **Left posterior ventricular vein** drains into the coronary sinus.
7. **Left marginal vein** drains into the coronary sinus.
8. **Anterior cardiac veins** are found on the anterior aspect of the right ventricle and drain directly into the right atrium.
9. **Smallest cardiac veins** begin within the wall of the heart and drain directly into the nearest heart chamber.

VII   The Conduction System (Figure 7-2)

A. Sinoatrial (SA) node is the **pacemaker** of the heart and is located at the junction of the superior vena cava and right atrium just beneath the epicardium. From the SA node, the impulse spreads throughout the right atrium and to the AV node via the **anterior, middle, and posterior internodal tracts** and to the left atrium via the **Bachmann bundle.** If all SA node activity is destroyed, the AV node will assume the pacemaker role.

B. Atrioventricular (AV) node is located on the right side of the AV portion of the atrial septum near the ostium of the coronary sinus in the subendocardial space. The AV septum corresponds to the **triangle of Koch**, an important anatomic landmark because it contains the AV node and the proximal penetrated portion of the Bundle of His.

C. Bundle of His, Bundle Branches, Purkinje Myocytes. The **bundle of His** travels in the subendocardial space on the right side of the interventricular septum and divides into the **right and left bundle branches.** The left bundle branch is thicker than the right bundle branch. A portion of the right bundle branch enters the septomarginal trabeculae (moderator band) to supply the anterior papillary muscle. The left bundle branch further divides into an **anterior segment** and **posterior segment.** The right and left bundle branches both terminate in a complex network of intramural **Purkinje myocytes.**

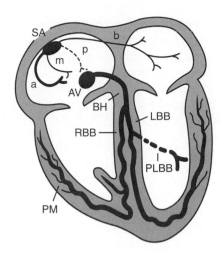

● **Figure 7-2 Diagram of Conduction System of Heart.** SA = sinoatrial node, AV = atrioventricular node, BH = bundle of His, RBB = right bundle branch, LBB = left bundle branch, PLBB = posterior segment of the left bundle branch, PM = Purkinje myocytes, a = anterior internodal tract, m = middle internodal tract, p = posterior internodal tract, b = Bachman bundle.

(VIII) **Innervation of the Heart.** The heart is innervated by the **superficial cardiac plexus**, which is located inferior to the aortic arch and anterior to the right pulmonary artery, and the **deep cardiac plexus**, which is located posterior to the aortic arch and anterior to the tracheal bifurcation. These plexuses contain **both parasympathetic (vagus; cranial nerve [CN] X) and sympathetic components**.

A. **Parasympathetic.** Preganglionic neuronal cell bodies are located in the **dorsal nucleus of the vagus** and **nucleus ambiguus** of the medulla. Preganglionic axons run in the **vagus (CN X) nerve**. Postganglionic neuronal cell bodies are located in the cardiac plexus and atrial wall. Postganglionic axons are distributed to the **SA node, AV node, atrial myocytes (not ventricular myocytes), and smooth muscle of coronary arteries** causing a **decrease in heart rate, decrease in conduction velocity through the AV node,** and **decrease in contractility of atrial myocytes.** Postganglionic axons release **acetylcholine (ACh)** as a neurotransmitter. ACh binds to the **M_2 muscarinic ACh receptor (mAChR)**, which is a G-protein-linked receptor that inhibits adenylate cyclase and decreases cyclic adenosine monophosphate (cAMP) levels. The SA node and AV node contain high levels of **acetylcholinesterase** (degrades ACh rapidly), such that any given vagal stimulation is **short-lived. Vasovagal syncope** is a brief period of lightheadedness or loss of consciousness caused by an intense burst of CN X activity. Afferent (sensory) neurons of CN X whose cell bodies are located in the nodose ganglion innervate **baroreceptors** in the great veins, atria, and aortic arch and relay **changes in blood pressure** to the solitary nucleus within the central nervous system (CNS). Afferent (sensory) neurons of CN X whose cell bodies are located in the nodose ganglion innervate **chemoreceptors** (specifically the **aortic bodies**) and relay **changes in arterial partial pressure of oxygen (Pao_2)** to the solitary nucleus within the CNS.

B. **Sympathetic.** Preganglionic neuronal cell bodies are located in the **intermediolateral columns** of the spinal cord. Preganglionic axons enter the paravertebral ganglion and travel to the stellate or middle cervical ganglia. Postganglionic neuronal cell bodies are located in the **stellate and middle cervical ganglia.** Postganglionic axons are distributed to the **SA node, AV node, atrial myocytes, ventricular myocytes,** and **smooth muscle of coronary arteries** causing an **increase in heart rate, increase in conduction velocity through the AV node,** and **increase in contractility of atrial and ventricular myocytes.** Postganglionic axons release **norepinephrine (NE)** as a neurotransmitter. NE binds to the β_1-**adrenergic receptor**, which is a G-protein-linked receptor that stimulates adenylate cyclase and increases cAMP levels. Released NE is either carried away by the bloodstream or taken up by the nerve terminals so that sympathetic stimulation is relatively **long-lived**. Afferent (sensory) neurons whose cell bodies are located in the dorsal root ganglion run with the sympathetic nerves and relay **pain** information to T1 through T5 spinal cord segments within the CNS. The pain associated with angina pectoris or a "heart attack" may be referred over the T1 through T5 dermatomes (i.e. the classic referred pain down the left arm).

IX   Gross Anatomy of the Heart

A. Right Atrium. The right atrium receives venous blood from the SVC, IVC, and coronary sinus. The right atrium consists of the **right auricle**, which is a conical, muscular pouch; **pectinate muscles**, which form the trabeculated part of the right atrium (2 to 4 mm thick) and develop embryologically from the primitive atrium; **sinus venarum**, which is the smooth part of the right atrium and develops embryologically from the sinus venous; **crista terminalis** (an internal muscular ridge 3 to 6 mm thick), which marks the junction between the trabeculated part and smooth part of the right atrium; **sulcus terminalis** (an external shallow groove), which also marks the junction between the trabeculated part and smooth part of the right atrium; **openings of the SVC, IVC, coronary sinus, and the anterior cardiac vein; atrial septum**, which consists of an interatrial portion and an AV portion; and **fossa ovalis**, which is an oval depression on the interatrial portion consisting of the **valve of the fossa ovalis** (a central sheet of thin fibrous tissue), which is a remnant of septum primum, and the **limbus of the fossa ovalis** (a horseshoe-shaped muscular rim), which is a remnant of the septum secundum. The wall of the right atrium between the pectinate muscles is less than 1 mm thick and can easily be perforated by a catheter or pacemaker lead.

B. Right Ventricle. The trabeculated inflow tract of the right ventricle receives venous blood from the right atrium posteriorly through the tricuspid valve while the smooth outflow tract of the right ventricle expels blood superiorly and to the left into the pulmonary trunk. The right ventricle consists of the **trabeculae carneae** (irregular muscular ridges), which form the trabeculated part of the right ventricle (inflow tract) and develop embryologically from the primitive ventricle; **conus arteriosus (infundibulum)**, which is the smooth part of the right ventricle (outflow tract) and develops embryologically from the bulbus cordis; **supraventricular crest** (a C-shaped internal muscular ridge), which marks the junction between the trabeculated part and smooth part of the right ventricle; **tricuspid valve (anterior, posterior, and septal cusps)**, which attach at their base to the fibrous skeleton; **chordae tendineae** (or cords), which extend from the free edge of the tricuspid valve to the papillary muscles and prevent eversion of the tricuspid valve into the right atrium, thereby preventing regurgitation of ventricular blood into the right atrium during systole; **papillary muscles (anterior, posterior, and septal)**, which are conical muscular projections from the ventricular wall and are attached to the chordae tendineae; **interventricular (IV) septum**, consisting of a **membranous part** (located in a superior posterior position and continuous with the fibrous skeleton) and a **muscular part; septomarginal trabeculae (moderator band)**, which is a curved muscular bundle that extends from the IV septum to the anterior papillary muscle and contains part of the right bundle branch of the Bundle of His to the anterior papillary muscle; **right AV orifice; opening of the pulmonary trunk;** and **pulmonary semilunar valve (anterior, right, and left cusps)**, which lies at the apex of the conus arteriosus and prevents blood from returning to the right ventricle. In fetal and neonatal life, the thickness of the right ventricular wall is similar to the thickness of the left ventricular wall because of the equalization of pulmonary and aortic pressures by the ductus arteriosus. By 3 months of age, the infant heart shows regression of the right ventricular wall thickness.

C. **Left Atrium.** The left atrium receives oxygenated blood from the lungs through the pulmonary veins. The left atrium consists of the **left auricle**, which is a tubular muscular pouch; **pectinate muscles**, which form the trabeculated part of the left atrium and develop embryologically from the primitive atrium; **smooth part of the left atrium**, which develops embryologically by incorporation of the transient common pulmonary vein into its wall; **openings of the valveless pulmonary veins**; **atrial septum**, which consists only of an interatrial portion; and **semilunar depression**, which indicates the valve of the fossa ovalis. The limbus of the fossa ovalis and the AV septum are not visible from the left atrium.

D. **Left Ventricle.** The trabeculate inflow tract of the left ventricle receives oxygenated blood from the left atrium through the mitral valve while the smooth outflow tract of the left ventricle expels blood superoanteriorly into the ascending aorta. The left ventricle consists of the **trabeculae carneae** (irregular muscular ridges), which form the trabeculated part of the left ventricle (inflow tract) and develop embryologically from the primitive ventricle; **aortic vestibule**, which is the smooth part of the left ventricle (outflow tract) and develops embryologically from the bulbus cordis; **mitral valve (anterior and posterior cusps)**, which attach at their base to the fibrous skeleton; **chordae tendineae**, which are cords that extend from the free edge of the mitral valve to the papillary muscles and prevent eversion of the mitral valve into the left atrium, thereby preventing regurgitation of ventricular blood into the left atrium during systole; **papillary muscles (anterior and posterior)**, which are conical muscular projections from the ventricular wall and are attached to the chordae tendineae; **left atrioventricular (AV) orifice**; **opening of the ascending aorta**; and **aortic semilunar valve (posterior, right, and left cusps)**, which lies at the apex of the aortic vestibule and prevents blood from returning to the left ventricle.

Ⓧ Clinical Considerations

A. **Atherosclerosis.** The characteristic lesion of atherosclerosis is an **atheromatous plaque (fibrofatty plaque; atheroma)** within the **tunica intima** of blood vessels. An early stage in the formation of an atheromatous plaque is the subendothelial **fatty streak**. Fatty streaks are elevated, pale yellow, smooth-surfaced, focal in distribution, and irregular in shape with well-defined borders. An atheromatous plaque may undergo many histologic changes to form **complicated plaques**.

1. **Plaque calcification** results in brittle arteries ("brittle pipes").
2. **Plaque hemorrhage** results from tearing of the fibrous cap or rupture of newly formed blood vessels within the plaque.
3. **Plaque rupture** results in **thrombus formation**, whereby the thrombus may partially or completely occlude the lumen (i.e. an **occlusive thrombus**), leading to unstable (crescendo) angina and approximately 90% of all myocardial infarctions. In this situation, thrombus formation is initiated by platelet aggregation induced by **thromboxane A_2 (TXA_2)**. TXA_2 is synthesized from arachidonic acid using the enzyme cyclooxygenase. **Aspirin** covalently inhibits cyclooxygenase, and **nonsteroidal anti-inflammatory drugs (NSAIDs)** such as ibuprofen and acetaminophen reversibly inhibit cyclooxygenase and thereby block the synthesis of TXA_2. Consequently, low doses of aspirin and NSAIDs are effective in prevention of myocardial infarction. Thrombolysis is stimulated by **tissue plasminogen activator**

(TPA) treatment, which successfully decreases the extent of ischemic damage caused by myocardial infarction. TPA stimulates the **conversion of plasminogen to plasmin**. Plasmin is a protease that digests fibrin within the thrombus.

B. **Ischemic Heart Disease (IHD; Figure 7-3).** Coronary artery atherosclerosis leads to three major clinical conditions.

1. **Angina pectoris** is the sudden onset of precordial (anterior surface of the body over the heart and stomach) pain. There are three types of angina pectoris:

   a. **Prinzmetal (variant) angina** is caused by coronary artery spasms. Attacks occur during rest.

   b. **Stable angina** is caused by atherosclerotic narrowing of coronary arteries. Attacks occur during strenuous or excessive activity. This is the most common type of angina.

   c. **Unstable (crescendo) angina** is caused by the formation of a thrombus that occludes the arterial lumen (i.e. occlusive thrombus). Myocardial infarction is imminent.

2. **Myocardial Infarction (MI).** An MI is the ischemic necrosis of the myocardium of the heart. Complications of an MI include **hemopericardium** caused by rupture of the free ventricular wall; **arterial emboli**; **pericarditis** (only in transmural infarcts); **ventricular aneurysm**; which is a bulge in the heart during systole at the postinfarction scar; and **postmyocardial infarction syndrome (Dressler syndrome)**, which is an autoimmune pericarditis. There are two types of infarcts.

   a. **Transmural infarct** is unifocal and solid and follows the distribution of a specific coronary artery; pericarditis is common, often causes shock, and is caused by an occlusive thrombus. The volume of **collateral arterial blood flow** is the chief factor that affects the progression of a transmural infarct. In chronic cardiac ischemia, extensive collateral blood vessels that supply the subepicardial portion of the myocardium develop with time and thereby limit the infarct to the subendocardial portion of the myocardium.

   b. **Subendocardial infarct** is multifocal and patchy and follows a circumferential distribution; pericarditis is uncommon and is caused by hypoperfusion of the heart (e.g. aortic stenosis, hemorrhagic shock, or hypoperfusion during cardiopulmonary bypass).

3. **Congestive Heart Failure (CHF).** CHF is the inability of the heart to pump blood at a rate commensurate with the requirements of the body tissues or can do so only from elevated filling pressures. Most instances of CHF are caused by the progressive deterioration of myocardial contractile function (i.e. systolic dysfunction) as occurs in IHD or hypertension (i.e. the hypertensive left heart). CHF is characterized by the reduced cardiac output (i.e. forward failure), damming back of blood into the venous system (i.e. backward failure), or both.

C. **Right Ventricle (RV) Failure (Figure 7-4A, B)**

1. **General Features.** The RV is susceptible to failure in situations that cause an increase in afterload on the RV. Pure RV failure most often occurs with **cor pulmonale**, which can be induced by intrinsic diseases of the lung or **pulmonary arterial hypertension (PAH)**. **Acute cor pulmonale** is RV dilation caused by a large **pulmonary thromboembolism**. **Chronic cor pulmonale** is RV hypertrophy followed by RV enlargement and RV failure caused by PAH. PAH is defined as pulmonary artery pressures above the normal systolic value of 30 mm Hg. There are numerous causes of PAH, which include vasculitis, idiopathic ("primary PAH), chronic

pulmonary emboli, chronic lung disease, emphysema, Eisenmenger syndrome (mnemonic: "VICE").

2. **Clinical findings include** right hypogastric quadrant discomfort as a result of hepatomegaly, a cut section of the liver that demonstrates a "nutmeg" pattern of chronic passive congestion, peripheral edema (e.g. a hallmark of RV failure is ankle swelling), pulmonary edema absent, jugular vein and portal vein distension, enlarged spleen, peritoneal cavity ascites, pleural effusion, palpable parasternal "heave," presence of S4 heart sound ("atrial gallop"), and tricuspid valve murmur; ascent to high altitudes is contraindicated because of hypoxic pulmonary vasoconstriction, which will exacerbate the condition.

D. Left Ventricle (LV) Failure (Figure 7-4C, D)

1. **General Features.** LV failure most often occurs as a result of impaired LV function caused by an MI. The LV is usually hypertrophied and quite massively dilated. In LV failure, there is progressive damming of blood within the pulmonary circulation such that pulmonary vein pressure mounts and pulmonary edema with wet, heavy lungs is apparent. Coughing is a common feature of LV failure. Transferrin and hemoglobin, which leak from the congested capillaries, are phagocytosed by macrophages in the alveoli (called heart failure cells). In LV failure, the decreased cardiac output causes a reduction in kidney perfusion, which may lead to acute tubular necrosis and also activates the renin-angiotensin system.

2. **Clinical findings include** being overweight, following a poor diet, and having occasional episodes of angina; also may experience crushing pressure on the chest with pain radiating down the left arm ("referred pain"), nausea, profuse sweating and cold, clammy skin because of stress-induced release of catecholamines (epinephrine and norepinephrine) from adrenal medulla that stimulate sweat glands and cause peripheral vasoconstriction, dyspnea, orthopnea, auscultation of pulmonary rales as a result of "popping open" of small airways that were closed off because of pulmonary edema, noisy breathing ("cardiac asthma"), pulmonary wedge pressure (indicator of left atrial pressure) increased versus normal (30 versus 5 mm Hg, respectively), ejection fraction decreased versus normal (0.35 versus 0.55, respectively).

3. **Treatment includes** sublingual nitroglycerin; β-adrenergic antagonist (e.g. propranolol "β-blocker") to relieve tachycardia and hypertension, although there is a risk because β-blockers will further decrease an already compromised cardiac output; streptokinase IV or TPA to reduce amount of infarcted tissue if administered within 6 hours of MI; atropine to relieve bradycardia; and heparinization and warfarin therapy to prevent ventricular aneurysms, pulmonary thromboembolisms, and deep vein thrombosis.

E. Pericarditis is inflammation of the visceral layer of serous pericardium (known histologically as the epicardium) and the parietal layer of serous pericardium usually secondary to a variety of cardiac disease, systemic disorders, or neoplastic metastases from remote areas. Pericarditis is recognized clinically by a **pericardial friction rub** that results from external compression of the heart.

A

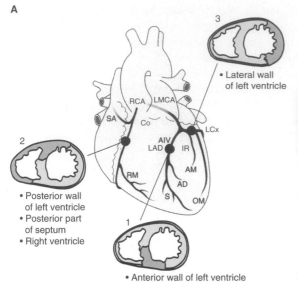

3
• Lateral wall
  of left ventricle

RCA LMCA
SA   Co
          AIV
     LAD IR
  RM   AM
       S AD
          OM
LCx

2
• Posterior wall
  of left ventricle
• Posterior part
  of septum
• Right ventricle

1
• Anterior wall of left ventricle
• Anterior part of septum

B

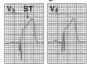

Troponin I

CK-MB

LDH$_1$

[serum]

1   2

↑
MI pain

C Early Anterior MI (2-24 hours)
       • ST segment elevated in V$_3$ and V$_4$

V$_3$ ST V$_4$

Recent Anterior MI (24-72 hours)
  • Q waves in V$_3$ and V$_4$
  • T waves inverted in V$_3$ and V$_4$

V$_3$ V$_4$
Q   T

Old Anterior MI
  • Q waves persist in V$_3$ and V$_4$
  • No T-wave inversion

V$_3$ V$_4$
Q

D   Day 1

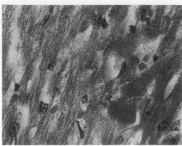

• Coagulation necrosis
• Wavy myocytes
• Pyknotic nuclei
• Eosinophilic cytoplasm
• Contraction bands

Days 2–4

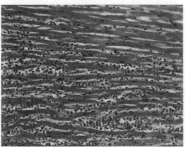

• Total coagulation
  necrosis
• Loss of nuclei
• Loss of striations
• Dilated vessels
  (hyperemia)
• Neutrophil infiltration

Days 5–10

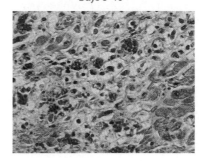

• Macrophage infiltration
• Phagocytosis of
  necrotic myocytes

Week 7

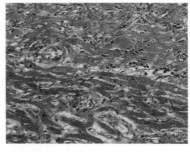

• Collagenous scar

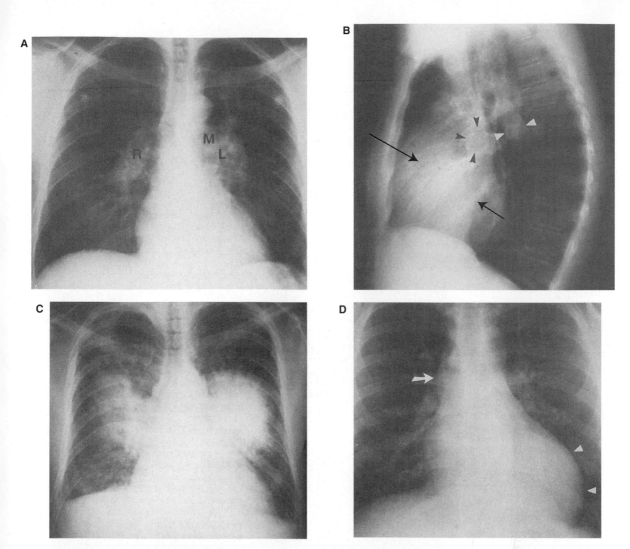

● **Figure 7-4 (A, B) Right Ventricle Failure. (A)** PA radiograph of pulmonary arterial hypertension (PAH) shows enormously dilated pulmonary trunk (M) and right (R) and left (L) pulmonary arteries with diminutive peripheral pulmonary vessels. **(B)** Lateral radiograph of PAH shows the enlarged right ventricle (RV hypertrophy) and atrium extending anteriorly into the anterior mediastinum (arrow). Note that the posterior border of the heart (left ventricle) is flat (double arrows). Fine curvilinear calcifications can be seen outlining the enlarged right and left pulmonary arteries (arrowheads). **(C, D) Left Ventricle Failure. (C)** AP radiograph shows alveolar (airspace) pulmonary edema at the central, parahilar regions of the lung in the classic "bat's wing" appearance. **(D)** AP radiograph shows left ventricle enlargement. Note the prominence of the LV with rounding along the inferior heart border and a downward pointing apex (arrowheads).

←

● **Figure 7-3 Myocardial Infarction (MI). (A)** Transmural MIs are caused by thrombotic occlusion of a coronary artery. Infarction is localized to the anatomic area supplied by the occluded artery. Coronary artery occlusion occurs most commonly in the anterior interventricular artery ([AIV]; also called the left anterior descending artery [LAD]), followed by the right coronary artery (RCA), and then the left circumflex artery (LCx). This is indicated by the numbers 1, 2, and 3. LMCA = left main coronary artery, SA = sinoatrial artery, RM = right marginal artery, S = septal branches, OM = obtuse marginal artery, AM = anterior marginal artery, AD = anterior diagonal artery, IR = intermediate ramus. **(B)** Serum markers of MI. Troponin I is a highly specific cardiac marker that can be detected within 4 hours and up to 7 to 10 days after MI pain. Creatine kinase (CK) consists of M and B subunits. CK-MM is found in skeletal muscle and cardiac muscle. CK-MB is found mainly in cardiac muscle. CK-MB is the test of choice in the first 24 hours after MI pain. CK-MB begins to rise 4 to 8 hours after MI pain, peaks at 24 hours, and returns to normal within 48 to 72 hours. This sequence is important because skeletal muscle injury or non-MI conditions may raise serum CK-MB but do not show this pattern. It is common to calculate the ratio of CK-MB to total CK. A CK-MB/total CK > 2.5% indicates MI. Lactate dehydrogenase (LDH) consists of H and M subunits. LDH-HHHH (or LDH_1) and LDH-HHHM (or LDH_2) are found in cardiac muscle. LDH_1 is the test of choice 2 to 3 days after MI pain because CK-MB levels have already returned to normal by this time. It is common to calculate the ratio LDH_1/LDH_2. An LDH_1/LDH_2 > 1.0 indicates MI. **(C) Electrocardiograms (ECGs).** An acute MI is associated with ST segment elevation. A recent MI (within 1 to 2 days) is associated with deep Q waves and inverted T waves. An old MI (weeks later) is associated with persistence of deep Q waves but no T-wave inversion. **(D) Evolution of a Myocardial Infarction (MI).** The histologic changes of an MI are indicated.

XI Radiology

A. **Angiograms of Coronary Arteries (Figure 7-5)**

B. **MRIs at Six Different Levels (Figures 7-6, 7-7, and 7-8)**

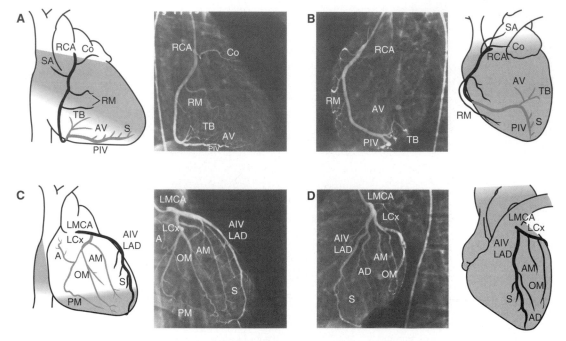

● **Figure 7-5 Angiograms of Right and Left Main Coronary Arteries. (A, B) Right Coronary Artery (RCA).** **(A)** Right anterior oblique (RAO) angiogram shows the various branches of the RCA that can be observed in this view. **(B)** Left anterior oblique (LAO) angiogram shows the various branches of the RCA that can be observed in this view. **(C, D) Left Main Coronary Artery (LMCA). (C)** Right anterior oblique (RAO) angiogram shows the various branches of the LMCA that can be observed in this view. **(D)** Left anterior oblique (LAO) angiogram shows the various branches of the LMCA that can be observed in this view. LCx = left circumflex artery, Co = conus branch, AIV = anterior interventricular artery, LAD = left anterior descending artery, AD = anterior diagonal artery, S = septal branches, RM = right marginal artery, AM = anterior marginal, SA = sinoatrial nodal artery, A = atrial branches, OM = obtuse marginal artery, PM = posterior marginal artery, AV = atrioventricular nodal artery, TB = terminal branches, PIV = posterior interventricular artery.

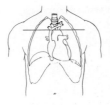
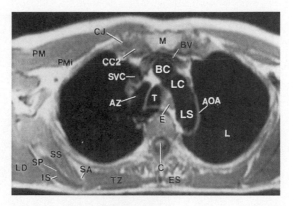

● **Figure 7-6 MRI scan at About T2 Through T3.** The line diagram shows the level of the cross-section. AOA = aortic arch, AZ = azygos vein, BC = brachiocephalic artery, BV = left brachiocephalic vein, C = spinal cord, CC2 = second costal cartilage, CJ = costochondral junction, E = esophagus, ES = erector spinae, IS = infraspinatus, L = lung, LC = left common carotid artery, LS = left subclavian artery, M = manubrium, PM = pectoralis major, PMi = pectoralis minor, SA = serratus anterior, SP = scapula, SS = subscapularis, SVC = superior vena cava, T = trachea, TZ = trapezius.

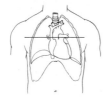
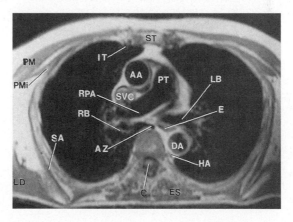

● **Figure 7-7 MRI scan at About T5 Through T6.** The line diagram shows the level of cross-section. AA = ascending aorta, AZ = azygos vein, C = spinal cord, DA = descending aorta, E = esophagus, ES = erector spinae, HA = hemi-azygos vein, IT = internal thoracic artery, LB = left main bronchus, LD = latissimus dorsi, PM = pectoralis major, PMi = pectoralis minor, PT = pulmonary trunk, RB = right main bronchus, RPA = right pulmonary artery, SA = serratus anterior, ST = sternum, SVC = superior vena cava.

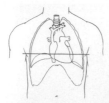

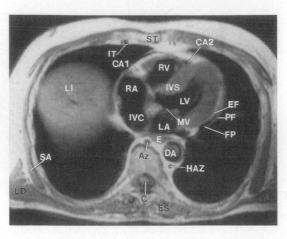

● **Figure 7-8 MRI Scan at About T7 Through T8.** The line diagram shows the level of the cross-section. It is important to know the arrangement of the heart chambers in the anteroposterior direction. A typical clinical vignette question may ask about a patient who is shot through the sternum. In what order would the bullet pass through the chambers of the heart before it exits the back? Az = azygos vein, C = spinal cord, CA1 = right coronary artery, CA2 = left anterior descending artery, DA = descending aorta, E = esophagus, EF = epicardial artery, ES = erector spinae, FP = fibrous pericardium, HAZ = hemiazygos vein, IT = internal thoracic artery, IVC = inferior vena cava, IVS = interventricular septum, LA = left atrium, LD = latissimus dorsi, LI = liver, LV = left ventricle, MV = mitral valve, PF = pericardial fat, RA = right atrium, RV = right ventricle, SA = serratus anterior, ST = sternum.

Case Study

Karen, a 33-year-old fashion buyer, presents complaining of chest pain. The pain is retrosternal with some radiation to the left shoulder and jaw. The pain characteristically comes on with exertion and is rapidly relieved by rest. She first noticed the pain a month ago, and it has progressively worsened to the point where she now has to stop after climbing one flight of stairs. She remarked that the pain was particularly bad after a business dinner in a very cold dining room. She is a nonsmoker, does not take oral contraceptives, and has a 7-year-old daughter.

Family history: Father died at age 40 of a myocardial infarction. Her elder 36-year-old brother has just undergone coronary artery bypass grafting surgery.

Examination

Blood pressure is 125/82 mm hg; pulse 70 beats/min and regular. There is a soft systolic murmur in the aortic area. There is no evidence of left ventricular hypertrophy. Carotid pulses are normal. Of note are prominent corneal arcus, swellings in the tendons of the hands, and thickening of both Achilles tendons.

Resting 12-lead electrocardiogram (ECG) is normal. Her exercise ECG was equivocal.

Explanation

Karen presents with the classic picture of angina, which is characterized by substernal chest pain and referred pain in the left arm and jaw. This type of pain pattern may occur with aortic stenosis, hypertrophic cardiomyopathy, or coronary artery disease (CAD); however, these are not likely in a woman her age. With her family history and evidence of hypercholesteremia (note the prominent corneal arcus), Karen is a likely candidate for future ischemic heart disease or CAD. Angina can be precipitated by exercise, cold, and stress, and relieved by rest.

Coronary artery occlusion occurs most commonly in the anterior interventricular artery. In clinical literature, it is referred to as the left anterior descending coronary artery (LAD). The LAD supplies the anterior wall of the left ventricle and the anterior part of the interventricular septum.

Cardiac referred pain is a phenomenon whereby pain originating in the heart is sensed by the person as originating from a superficial part of the body, e.g. upper left limb. The afferent (sensory) pain fibers from the heart run centrally in the thoracic cardiac branches of the sympathetic trunk and enter spinal cord segments T1 through T5 (dermatomes T1 through T5) especially on the left side. On entering the spinal cord, afferent neurons travel to higher brain centers in the CNS, and some afferent neurons synapse on interneurons that cross to the contralateral side. Classically, precordial pain (deep visceral retrosternal pain) is not specific for cardiac disease. Precordial pain is the prime symptom for the region supplied by dermatomes T1 through T6. Usually such pain is maximal in the retrosternal region and often extends into the neck, to either the right or left hemithorax, and down the anteromedial aspects of one or both arms or forearms. If the patient sustains an inferior wall or anterior inferior wall infarct with subsequent irritation of the diaphragm, the phrenic nerve, which innervates the diaphragm, may contribute to the pain pattern.

Karen's familial history of premature coronary artery disease suggests familial hyperlipidemia (FH). The findings of prominent corneal arcus, swellings in the tendons of the hands, and thickening of both Achilles tendons suggest that a lipid disorder is present in this patient. It is unlikely that diet therapy alone will correct the problem. Desirable therapeutic goals for this patient would be a low-density lipoprotein (LDL) cholesterol of approximately 100 mg/dL. Studies have demonstrated regression of atherosclerotic lesions 2 years after attaining these goals. Given the unstable nature of the angina, she is a likely candidate for angioplasty or coronary artery bypass grafting surgery. Her daughter should be referred for cholesterol testing.

Chapter 8

Abdominal Wall

I **Abdominal Regions (Figure 8-1).** The abdomen can be topographically divided into nine regions, namely the **right hypochondriac, epigastric, left hypochondriac, right lumbar, umbilical, left lumbar, right inguinal, hypogastric,** and **left inguinal.**

II **Muscles** include the rectus abdominis, transverse abdominis, internal oblique, and external oblique.

III **Arterial Supply**

A. **Musculophrenic artery** arises from the internal thoracic artery and descends along the costal margin.

B. **Superior epigastric artery** arises from the internal thoracic artery, enters the rectus sheath, and descends on the posterior surface of the rectus abdominis. The superior epigastric artery anastomoses with the inferior epigastric artery, thereby providing a collateral circulation between the subclavian artery and the external iliac artery.

C. **Tenth and eleventh posterior intercostal arteries** arise from the aorta and continue beyond the ribs to descend between the transverse abdominis muscle and the internal oblique muscle.

D. **Subcostal artery** arises from the aorta and continues beyond the ribs to descend between the transverse abdominis muscle and the internal oblique muscle.

E. **Inferior epigastric artery** arises from the external iliac artery above the inguinal ligament, enters the rectus sheath, and ascends between the rectus abdominis and the posterior layer of the rectus sheath. The inferior epigastric artery anastomoses with the superior epigastric artery, thereby providing a collateral circulation between the subclavian artery and the external iliac artery.

F. **Deep circumflex iliac artery** arises from the external iliac artery and runs laterally along the inguinal ligament and the iliac crest between the transverse abdominis muscle and the internal oblique muscle.

G. **Superficial circumflex iliac artery** arises from the femoral artery and runs laterally upward and parallel to the inguinal ligament.

H. **Superficial epigastric artery** arises from the femoral artery and runs superiorly toward the umbilicus over the inguinal ligament.

Ⅳ Venous Drainage

A. **Superficial Veins.** The skin and subcutaneous tissue of the abdominal wall contain an intricate subcutaneous venous plexus that drains into larger veins as follows.

1. **Internal thoracic vein** empties into the subclavian vein.
2. **Lateral thoracic vein** empties into the axillary vein.
3. **Superficial epigastric vein** empties into the femoral vein.
4. **Inferior epigastric vein** empties into the external iliac vein.
5. **Thoracoepigastric vein** may develop (because of altered venous flow) between the superficial epigastric vein and the lateral thoracic vein, providing a superficial venous collateral circulation between the femoral vein and the axillary vein.
6. **Paraumbilical veins** are small tributaries of the portal vein.

B. **Deep Veins.** The deep veins accompany the arteries bearing the same name. The inferior epigastric vein may anastomose with the superior epigastric vein or internal thoracic vein, providing a deep venous collateral circulation between the external iliac vein and the subclavian vein.

C. **Clinical Consideration. Varicose superficial epigastric veins** are caused by obstruction of either the inferior vena cava (IVC) or the hepatic portal vein, both of which drain structures below the diaphragm.

Ⅴ Nerves

A. **Thoracoabdominal nerves** arise as a continuation of intercostal nerves 7 through 11 distal to the costal margin and innervate the muscles of the abdominal wall and overlying skin.

B. **Lateral cutaneous branches** arise from intercostal nerves 7 through 9 and innervate the skin of the right and left hypochondriac regions.

C. **Subcostal nerve** arises from spinal nerve T12 and innervates the muscles of the abdominal wall and the skin superior to the iliac crest and inferior to the umbilicus.

D. **Iliohypogastric nerve** arises from spinal nerve L1 and innervates the internal oblique muscle, the transverse abdominis muscle, and the skin of the iliac crest, upper inguinal, and hypogastric regions.

E. **Ilioinguinal nerve** arises from spinal nerve L1 and innervates the internal oblique muscle, the transverse abdominis muscle, and the skin of the lower inguinal region, mons pubis, anterior scrotum or labium majus, and adjacent medial thigh.

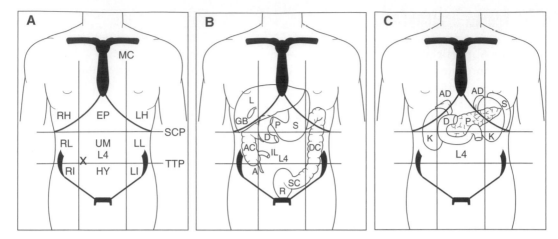

● **Figure 8-1 Abdominal Regions. (A)** A commonly used clinical method for subdividing the abdomen into specific regions using the subcostal plane (SCP), transtubercular plane (TTP; joining the tubercles of the iliac crests), and the midclavicular lines (MC). RH = right hypochondriac, EP = epigastric, LH = left hypochondriac, RL = right lumbar, UM = umbilical, LL = left lumbar, RI = right inguinal, HY = hypogastric, LI = left inguinal, L4 = vertebral level lumbar 4. **(B)** Surface projection of the stomach (S), pylorus (P), duodenum (D), liver (L), gallbladder (GB), ascending colon (AC), appendix(A), ileum (IL), descending colon (DC), sigmoid colon (SC), and rectum (R). **(C)** Surface projection of the duodenum (D), pancreas (P), kidneys (K), suprarenal gland (AD), and spleen (S). Many clinical vignette questions will describe pain associated with a particular region of the abdomen. Knowing what viscera are associated with each region will help in deciphering the clinical vignette (e.g. pain in the right lumbar region may be associated with appendicitis). X = McBurney's point.

VI **Clinical Procedure. Paracentesis (Figure 8-2)** is a procedure in which a needle is inserted through the layers of the abdominal wall to withdraw excess peritoneal fluid. Knife wounds to the abdomen will also penetrate the layers of the abdominal wall.

A. Midline Approach. The needle or knife will pass through the following structures in succession: skin → superficial fascia (Camper's and Scarpa's) → linea alba → transversalis fascia → extraperitoneal fat → parietal peritoneum.

B. Flank Approach. The needle or knife will pass through the following structures in succession: skin → superficial fascia (Camper's and Scarpa's) → external oblique muscle → internal oblique muscle → transverse abdominis muscle → transversalis fascia → extraperitoneal fat → parietal peritoneum.

VII **Inguinal region** is an area of weakness of the anterior abdominal wall owing to the penetration of the testes and spermatic cord (in males) or the round ligament of the uterus (in females) during embryologic development.

A. Inguinal ligament is the coiled lower border of the **external oblique muscle** and extends from the anterior–superior iliac spine to the pubic tubercle.

B. Deep inguinal ring is an oval opening in the **transversalis fascia** located lateral to the inferior epigastric artery.

C. Superficial inguinal ring is a triangular defect of the **external oblique muscle** located lateral to the pubic tubercle.

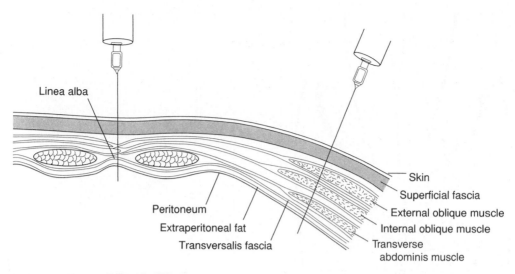

Linea alba

Skin
Superficial fascia
External oblique muscle
Internal oblique muscle
Transverse
abdominis muscle

Peritoneum
Extraperitoneal fat
Transversalis fascia

● **Figure 8-2 Anterior Abdominal Wall.** A transverse section through the anterior abdominal wall demonstrating the various layers that would be penetrated by a needle during paracentesis or a knife wound.

D. Inguinal canal begins at the deep inguinal ring and ends at the superficial inguinal ring and transmits the **spermatic cord** (in males) or **round ligament of the uterus** (in females).

E. Types of Hernias (Figure 8-3)
  1. Direct Inguinal Hernia
  2. Indirect Inguinal Hernia
  3. Femoral Hernia
  4. Surgical Repair
    a. Bassini repair: the transversalis fascia and **conjoint tendon** (combined tendinous insertion of the transverse abdominis muscle and internal oblique muscle) are sutured to the shelving edge of the inguinal ligament (Poupart's ligament).
    b. Cooper's ligament repair (McVay's method): the transversalis fascia and conjoint tendon are sutured to the periosteum of the pubic ramus (**Cooper's ligament or pectineal ligament**).
    c. Surgical hernia repair may damage the **iliohypogastric nerve**, causing anesthesia of the ipsilateral abdominal wall and inguinal region, or the **ilioinguinal nerve**, causing anesthesia of the ipsilateral penis, scrotum, and medial thigh.

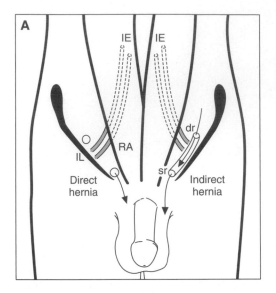 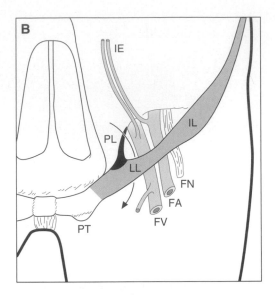

HERNIA CHARACTERISTICS

Type of Hernia	Characteristics
Direct inguinal	Protrudes directly through the anterior abdominal wall within Hesselbach's triangle[a] Protrudes *medial* to the inferior epigastric artery and vein[b] Common in *older* men; rare in women Clinical signs include mass in inguinal region that protrudes on straining and disappears at rest (i.e. easily reduced), constipation, prostate enlargement, and felt with pulp of finger
Indirect inguinal	Protrudes through the deep inguinal ring to enter the inguinal canal and may exit through the superficial inguinal ring into the scrotum Protrudes *lateral* to the inferior epigastric artery and vein[b] Protrudes *above* and *medial* to the pubic tubercle[c] Common in *young* men More common than a direct inguinal hernia Clinical signs include tender painful mass in the inguinal region that continues into the scrotum, and felt with the tip of the finger
Femoral	Protrudes through the femoral canal below the inguinal ligament Protrudes *below* and *lateral* to the pubic tubercle[c] Protrudes medial to the femoral vein More common in women on the right side Prone to early strangulation

[a]Hesselbach's (inguinal) triangle is bounded laterally by the inferior epigastric artery and vein, medially by the rectus abdominus muscle, and inferiorly by the inguinal ligament.

[b]Distinguishing feature of a direct hernia versus an indirect hernia.

[c]Distinguishing feature of an indirect hernia versus a femoral hernia.

● **Figure 8-3 Inguinal Hernias. (A)** A schematic demonstrating the anatomy associated with a direct and indirect inguinal hernia. **(B)** A schematic demonstrating the anatomy associated with a femoral hernia. IE = inferior epigastric artery and vein, IL = inguinal ligament, PL = pectineal (Cooper's) ligament, LL = lacunar ligament, FV = femoral vein, FA = femoral artery, FN = femoral nerve, PT = pubic tubercle, RA = rectus abdominis muscle, dr = deep inguinal ring, sr = superficial inguinal ring.

VIII The Scrotum (Figure 8-4)

A. **General Features.** The scrotum is an outpouching of the lower abdominal wall in which layers of the abdominal wall continue into the scrotal area to cover the spermatic cord and testes.

B. **Clinical Considerations**
   1. **Cancer of the scrotum** will metastasize to **superficial inguinal nodes**.
   2. **Cancer of the testes** will metastasize to **deep lumbar nodes** because of the embryologic development of the testes within the abdominal cavity and subsequent descent into the scrotum.
   3. **Extravasated urine** from a straddle injury will be found within the **superficial perineal space** located between Colles' fascia and dartos muscle (layer 2) and the external spermatic fascia (layer 3).
   4. In a **vasectomy**, the scalpel will cut through the following layers in succession: skin → Colles' fascia and dartos muscle → external spermatic fascia → cremasteric fascia and muscle → internal spermatic fascia → extraperitoneal fat. The tunica vaginalis is not cut, as it is present only over the anterior aspect of the testes.
   5. **Cremasteric Reflex.** Stroking the skin of the superior and medial thigh stimulates sensory fibers that run with the **ilioinguinal nerve** and serve as the afferent limb of the cremasteric reflex. Motor fibers that run with the **genital branch of the genitofemoral nerve** are distributed to the cremasteric muscle where they cause contraction of the cremasteric muscle, thereby elevating the testis (i.e. the efferent limb of the cremasteric reflex).

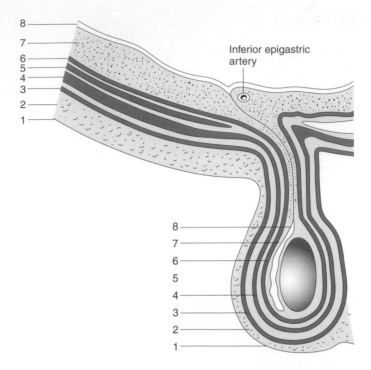

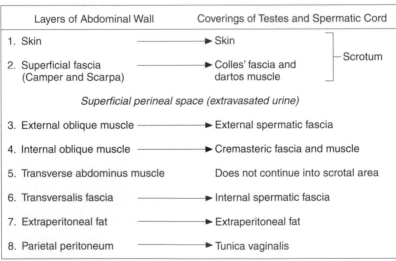

Layers of Abdominal Wall	Coverings of Testes and Spermatic Cord
1. Skin	► Skin
2. Superficial fascia (Camper and Scarpa)	► Colles' fascia and dartos muscle
Superficial perineal space (extravasated urine)	
3. External oblique muscle	► External spermatic fascia
4. Internal oblique muscle	► Cremasteric fascia and muscle
5. Transverse abdominus muscle	Does not continue into scrotal area
6. Transversalis fascia	► Internal spermatic fascia
7. Extraperitoneal fat	► Extraperitoneal fat
8. Parietal peritoneum	► Tunica vaginalis

● **Figure 8-4 The Scrotum.** A schematic showing the layers of the abdominal wall continuing into the scrotal area as the coverings of the spermatic cord and testes. Note that the transverse abdominis muscle does not continue into the scrotal area but instead joins with the tendon of the internal oblique muscle to form the conjoint tendon. Extravasated urine as a result of a straddle injury will leak between layers 2 and 3.

Chapter 9

Peritoneal Cavity

I **Peritoneal Cavity (Figure 9-1)** is a potential space between the visceral and parietal peritoneum. It is divided into the lesser peritoneal sac and greater peritoneal sac.

A. **Lesser peritoneal sac (omental bursa)** is an irregular-shaped sac that communicates with the greater peritoneal sac via the **omental (Winslow) foramen.** The lesser peritoneal sac forms because of the 90-degree clockwise rotation of the stomach during embryologic development. The boundaries of the lesser peritoneal sac are:
1. **Anterior**—liver, stomach, and lesser omentum
2. **Posterior**—diaphragm
3. **Right side**—liver
4. **Left side**—gastrosplenic and splenorenal ligaments

B. **Greater peritoneal sac** is the remainder of the peritoneal cavity and extends from the diaphragm to the pelvis. The greater peritoneal sac contains a number of pouches, recesses, and paracolic gutters through which peritoneal fluid circulates.
1. **Paracolic gutters** are channels that run along the ascending and descending colon. Normally, peritoneal fluid flows **upward** through the paracolic gutters to the **subphrenic recess,** where it enters the lymphatics associated with the diaphragm.
2. **Excess peritoneal fluid** as a result of peritonitis or ascites flows downward through the paracolic gutters to the **rectovesical pouch** (in males) or the **rectouterine pouch** (in females) when the patient is in a **sitting** or **standing position.**
3. **Excess peritoneal fluid** as a result of peritonitis or ascites flows upward through the paracolic gutters to the **subphrenic recess** and the **hepatorenal recess** when the patient is in the **supine position.** The patient may complain of shoulder pain (referred pain) caused by irritation of the phrenic nerve (C3, C4, and C5 nerve roots). The hepatorenal recess is the **lowest** part of the peritoneal cavity when the patient is in the supine position.

C. **Omental (Winslow) foramen** is the opening (or connection) between the lesser peritoneal sac and greater peritoneal sac. If a surgeon places his or her finger in the omental foramen, the inferior vena cava (IVC) will lie posterior and the portal vein will lie anterior.

II **Omentum**

A. **Lesser omentum** is a fold of peritoneum that extends from the porta hepatis of the liver to the lesser curvature of the stomach. It consists of the **hepatoduodenal ligament** and **hepatogastric ligament.** The **portal triad** lies in the free margin of the hepatoduo-denal ligament and consists of the:

1. **Portal vein** lying posterior
2. **Common bile duct** lying anterior and to the right
3. **Hepatic artery** lying anterior and to the left

B. **Greater omentum** is a fold of peritoneum that hangs down from the greater curvature of the stomach. It is known as the "abdominal policeman" because it adheres to areas of inflammation.

III Intraperitoneal and Retroperitoneal Viscera (Figure 9-1)

IV Clinical Considerations

A. **Ascites** is an accumulation of fluid in the peritoneal cavity caused by peritonitis or congestion of the venous drainage of the abdomen.

B. **Inflammation of the parietal peritoneum** occurs when there is an enlarged visceral organ or escape of fluid from a visceral organ and results in a sharp, localized pain over the inflamed area. Patients exhibit rebound tenderness and guarding over the site of inflammation. **Rebound tenderness** is pain that is elicited after the pressure of palpation over the inflamed area is removed. **Guarding** is the reflex spasms of the abdominal muscles in response to palpation over the inflamed area.

C. **Peritonitis** is inflammation and infection of the peritoneum and commonly occurs as a result of a burst appendix, a penetrating abdominal wound, a perforated ulcer, or poor sterile technique during surgery. Peritonitis is treated by rinsing the peritoneal cavity with large amounts of sterile saline and administering antibiotics.

D. **Peritoneal adhesions** occur after abdominal surgery, when scar tissue forms and limits the normal movement of the viscera. This tethering may cause chronic pain or emergency complications such as volvulus (i.e. twisting of the intestines).

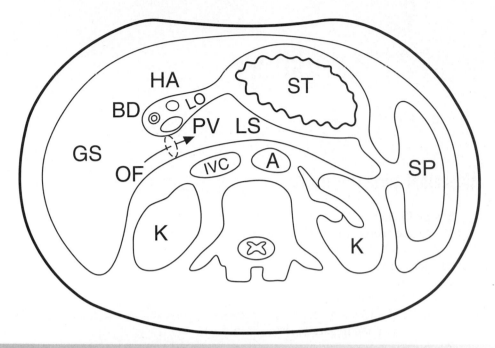

INTRAPERITONEAL AND RETROPERITONEAL VISCERA

Intraperitoneal	Retroperitoneal
Stomach	
First 2 cm of the superior part of the duodenum (duodenal cap)	Distal 3 cm of the superior part of the duodenum Descending part of the duodenum Horizontal part of the duodenum Ascending part of the duodenum
Jejunum	Ascending colon
Ileum	Descending colon
Cecum	Rectum
Appendix	Head, neck, body of pancreas
Transverse colon	Kidneys
Sigmoid colon	Ureters
Liver	Suprarenal gland
Gall bladder	Abdominal aorta
Tail of pancreas	Inferior vena cava
Spleen	

● **Figure 9-1 Cross-Section of the Abdomen Demonstrating the Peritoneal Cavity.** Note the greater peritoneal sac (GS) and lesser peritoneal sac (LS) connected by the omental foramen (OF; arrow). The portal triad is shown at the free margin of the hepatoduodenal ligament of the lesser omentum (LO). ST = stomach, SP = spleen, K = kidney, IVC = inferior vena cava, A = aorta, BD = common bile duct, PV = portal vein, HA = hepatic artery.

Chapter 10

Abdominal Vasculature

Abdominal Aorta (Figure 10-1)

A. Major Branches

1. **Celiac trunk** is located at the **T12** vertebral level and supplies viscera that derive embryologically from the **foregut** (i.e. intra-abdominal portion of esophagus, stomach, upper part of duodenum, liver, gallbladder, and pancreas). It further branches into the:
   a. Left gastric artery
   b. Splenic artery
   c. Common hepatic artery
2. **Superior mesenteric artery** is located at the **L1** vertebral level and supplies viscera that derive embryologically from the **midgut** (i.e. lower part of duodenum, jejunum, ileum, cecum, appendix, ascending colon, proximal two thirds of transverse colon).
3. **Renal arteries** supply the kidneys.
4. **Gonadal arteries** supply the testes or ovaries.
5. **Inferior mesenteric artery** is located at the **L3** vertebral level and supplies viscera that derive embryologically from the **hindgut** (i.e. distal one-third of transverse colon, descending colon, sigmoid colon, upper portion of rectum).
6. **Common iliac arteries** are the terminal branches of the abdominal aorta.

B. Clinical Considerations

1. **Abdominal aortic aneurysm (AAA)** is most commonly seen in atherosclerotic elderly men below the L1 vertebral level (i.e. below the renal arteries and superior mesenteric artery). The most common site of a ruptured AAA is below the renal arteries in the **left posterolateral wall (i.e. retroperitoneal)**. In a patient with a ruptured AAA, the first step is immediate compression of the aorta against the vertebral bodies **above the celiac trunk.** During a transabdominal surgical approach to correct a ruptured AAA, the **left renal vein** is put in jeopardy. The **inferior mesenteric artery** generally lies in the middle of an AAA. Clinical findings include sudden onset of severe, central abdominal pain, which may radiate to the back, and a pulsatile tender abdominal mass; if rupture occurs, hypotension and delirium may occur. Surgical complications include **ischemic colitis** caused by ligation of the inferior mesenteric artery or **spinal cord ischemia** as a result of ligation of the great radicular artery (Adamkiewicz; see Chapter 2 III.C.).
2. **Acute mesenteric ischemia** is most commonly caused by an embolism within the **superior mesenteric artery.** Clinical signs include severe abdominal pain out of proportion to physical findings and no evidence of peritonitis; it usually occurs in elderly patients with a history of heart disease taking digoxin (a potent splanchnic vasoconstrictor).

3. **Gradual occlusion** is most commonly seen in atherosclerotic patients at the bifurcation of the abdominal aorta. It may result in **claudication** (i.e. pain in the legs when walking) and **impotence** as a result of the lack of blood to the internal iliac arteries.

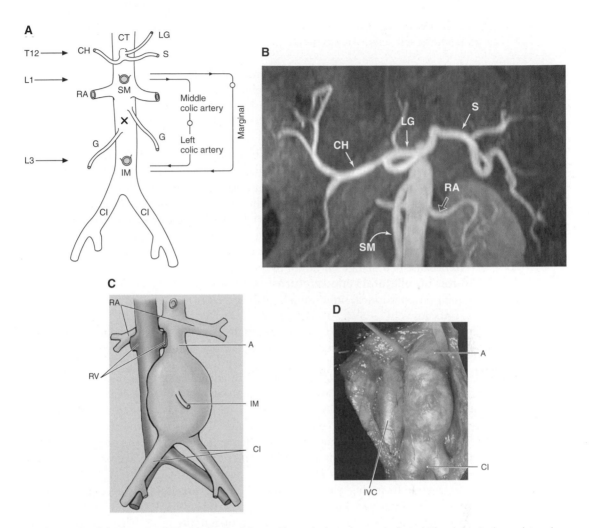

● **Figure 10-1 (A) Diagram of the Abdominal Aorta.** The major branches are indicated. The abdominal vasculature has a fairly robust collateral circulation. Any blockage (see X) between the superior mesenteric artery (SM; at L1 vertebral level) and inferior mesenteric artery (IM; at L3 vertebral level) will cause blood to be diverted along two routes of collateral circulation. The first route uses the middle colic artery (a branch of the SM), which anastomoses with the left colic artery (a branch of the IM). The second route uses the marginal artery. Circles (○) indicate a site of anastomosis. **(B) Arteriogram Showing the Branches of the Celiac Trunk and Other Arteries in the Vicinity. (C,D) Abdominal Aortic Aneurysm.** (C) Diagram of an abdominal aortic aneurysm. (D) Photograph of an abdominal aortic aneurysm. A = aorta, CH = common hepatic artery, CI = common iliac artery, CT = celiac trunk, G = gonadal artery, IM = inferior mesenteric artery, IVC = inferior vena cava, LG = left gastric artery, RA = renal artery, RV = renal vein, S = splenic artery, SM = superior mesenteric artery, T12, L1, and L3 = vertebral level of the various branches.

II   Venous Drainage of Abdomen (Figure 10-2A)

A. Azygos Venous System. The azygos vein ascends on the right side of the vertebral column and drains blood from the inferior vena cava (IVC) to the superior vena cava (SVC). The **hemiazygos vein** ascends on the left side of the vertebral column and drains blood from the left renal vein to the azygos vein.

B. Inferior vena cava (IVC) is formed by the union of the right and left common iliac veins at vertebral level L5. The IVC drains all the blood from below the diaphragm (even portal blood from the gastrointestinal tract after it percolates through the liver) to the right atrium. It is in jeopardy during surgical repair of a herniated intervertebral disk. The IVC above the kidneys (suprarenal) should never be ligated (there is a 100% mortality rate); the IVC below the kidneys (infrarenal) may be ligated (there is a 50% mortality rate).

1. The **right gonadal vein** drains directly into the IVC, whereas the **left gonadal vein** drains into the left renal vein. This is important in women in whom the appearance of a **right-side hydronephrosis** may indicate thrombosis of the right ovarian vein, which constricts the ureter because the right ovarian vein crosses the ureter to drain into the IVC. This is also important in men, in whom the appearance of a **left-side testicular varicocele** may indicate occlusion of the **left testicular vein** or **left renal vein** because of a malignant tumor of the kidney.

2. **Routes of collateral venous return** exist in case the IVC is blocked by either a malignant retroperitoneal tumor or a large blood clot (thrombus). These include:
   a. Azygos vein → SVC → right atrium
   b. Lumbar veins → external and internal vertebral venous plexuses → cranial dural sinuses → internal jugular vein → right atrium

III   Hepatic Portal System (Figure 10-2B, C).

In general, the term "portal" refers to a vein interposed between two capillary beds, i.e. capillary bed → vein → capillary bed. The hepatic portal system consists specifically of the following vascular structures: capillaries of gastrointestinal tract → portal vein → hepatic sinusoids. The **portal vein** is formed posterior to the neck of the pancreas by the union of the **splenic vein** and **superior mesenteric vein**. The **inferior mesenteric vein** usually ends by joining the splenic vein. The blood within the portal vein carries high levels of nutrients from the gastrointestinal tract and products of red blood cell destruction from the spleen. **Portal–IVC (caval) anastomosis** becomes clinically relevant when **portal hypertension** occurs. Portal hypertension will cause blood within the portal vein to reverse its flow and enter the IVC to return to the heart. There are three main sites of portal–IVC anastomosis: esophagus, umbilicus, and rectum. Clinical signs of portal hypertension include vomiting copious amounts of blood, alcoholism, liver cirrhosis, schistosomiasis, enlarged abdomen because of ascites fluid, and splenomegaly.

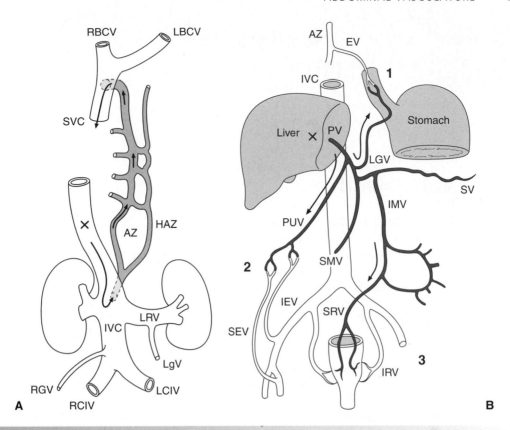

Site of Anastomosis	Clinical Sign	Veins Involved in Portal ↔ Inferior Venal Caval Anastomosis
Esophagus (site 1)	Esophageal varices	Left gastric vein ↔ esophageal vein
Umbilicus (site 2)	Caput medusa	Paraumbilical vein ↔ superficial and inferior epigastric veins
Rectum (site 3)	Hemorrhoids	Superior rectal vein ↔ middle and inferior rectal veins

C

● **Figure 10-2 (A) Diagram of the Azygos Venous System and the Inferior Vena Cava (IVC).** Note that the left go-nadal vein (LGV) drains into the left renal vein (LRV), which has clinical implications in the case of men (e.g. left testicu-lar varicocele). Note how the azygos vein (AZ) provides a route of collateral venous (arrows) return in cases in which the IVC is blocked (X). **(B, C) Hepatic Portal System. (B)** Diagram of the hepatic portal system. Note the three main sites (1, 2, 3) of portal–IVC (caval) anastomosis. In case of portal hypertension in which blood flow through the liver is severely reduced (X), these anastomoses provide collateral circulation (arrows) through the IVC back to the heart. **(C)** Table showing the clinical signs of portal hypertension. EV = esophageal vein, HAZ = hemiazygos vein, IEV = inferior epigas-tric vein, IMV = inferior mesenteric vein, IRV = inferior rectal vein, LBCV = left brachiocephalic vein, LCIV = left com-mon iliac vein, LGV = left gastric vein, PUV = paraumbilical vein, PV = portal vein, RBCV = right brachiocephalic vein, RCIV = right common iliac vein, RGV = right gonadal vein, SEV = superior epigastric vein, SMV = superior mesenteric vein, SRV = superior rectal vein, SV = splenic vein, SVC = superior vena cava, LgV = left gonadal vein.

Chapter 11

Abdominal Viscera

① Esophagus (Figure 11-1)

A. **General Features.** The esophagus is a muscular tube that is continuous with the pharynx and runs in the thorax through the superior and posterior mediastinum. The esophagus begins at the **cricoid cartilage** (at vertebral level C6) and ends at the **gastroesophageal (GE) junction**. The esophagus pierces the diaphragm to form the esophageal hiatus (at vertebral level T10).

The muscular wall of the esophagus (i.e. the muscularis externa histologically) changes from cephalad to caudad. The **upper 5%** of the esophagus (some authors say the upper 33% but on close inspection this does not seem to be the case) consists of skeletal muscle only. The **middle 45%** of the esophagus consists of both **skeletal muscle and smooth muscle** interwoven together. The **distal 50%** of the esophagus consists of smooth muscle only.

The overall length of the esophagus obviously varies with trunk length, but the average adult length of the esophagus is **23 to 25 cm**. In clinical practice, endoscopic distances are measured from the incisor teeth, and in the average man the GE junction is 38 to 43 cm away from the incisor teeth. For purposes of classification, staging, and reporting of esophageal malignancies, the esophagus is divided into four segments based on the distance from the incisor teeth: cervical segment, upper thoracic segment, midthoracic segment, and lower thoracic segment.

B. **Constrictions.** Along the course of the esophagus, there are five main sites where the esophagus is constricted: (1) at the junction of the pharynx and esophagus (cricoid origin), (2) at the aortic arch, (3) at the tracheal bifurcation (vertebral level T4) where the left main bronchus crosses the esophagus, (4) at the left atrium, and (5) at the esophageal hiatus.

C. **Sphincters**
   1. The **upper esophageal sphincter** (UES) separates the pharynx from the esophagus. The UES is composed of **opening muscles** (i.e. thyrohyoid and geniohyoid muscles) and **closing muscles** (i.e. inferior pharyngeal constrictor and **cricopharyngeus** [main player]). The UES is skeletal muscle. The UES relaxes (opens) during swallowing (deglutition), belching, and vomiting. The UES maintains closure of the upper end of the esophagus, prevents air from entering the esophagus, and with severe gastric acid reflux prevents refluxed material from entering the pharynx.
   2. The **lower esophageal sphincter** (LES) separates the esophagus from the stomach. The LES is composed of smooth muscle and is difficult to identify anatomically. Human autopsies have found an asymmetric, thickened, ringlike area in the area of the GE junction that may aid the muscularis externa in the physiologic role as a

sphincter. The LES **relaxes** during swallowing. LES relaxation occurs within 2 seconds after swallowing at a time when peristaltic waves are observed in the middle portion of the esophagus. When the ingested bolus reaches the LES, the LES is relaxed but closed. The ingested bolus with the aid of peristalsis forces the LES open. The LES is tonically contracted and can increase the force of contraction in response to increased stomach contents (postprandial). The LES **prevents gastroesophageal reflux.**

D. Clinical Considerations

1. **Enlarged left atrium** may constrict the esophagus as a result of their close anatomic relationship.

2. **Bronchogenic carcinoma** may indent the esophagus as a result of the enlargement of mediastinal lymph nodes. This indentation can be observed radiologically during a barium swallow.

3. **Malignant tumors of the esophagus** most commonly occur in the lower one third of the esophagus and metastasize below the diaphragm to the **celiac lymph nodes.**

4. **Forceful vomiting,** which is commonly seen in alcoholism, bulimia, and pregnancy, may tear the posterior wall of the esophagus. Clinical findings include severe retrosternal pain after vomiting and extravasated contrast medium. **Mallory-Weiss tears** involve only the mucosal and submucosal layers. **Boerhaave syndrome** involves tears through all layers of the esophagus.

5. **Sliding hiatal hernia** occurs when the stomach along with the GE junction herniate through the diaphragm into the thorax. Clinical findings include deep, burning, retrosternal pain and reflux of gastric contents into the mouth (i.e. heartburn), which are accentuated in the supine position.

6. **Paraesophageal hiatal hernia** occurs when only the stomach herniates through the diaphragm into the thorax. Clinical findings include no reflux of gastric contents, but strangulation or obstruction may occur.

7. **Achalasia** is failure of the LES to relax during swallowing probably because of the absence of the myenteric plexus. Clinical findings include progressive dysphagia (difficulty in swallowing), barium swallow shows dilated esophagus above the LES and distal stenosis at the LES ("bird beak"). **Chagas disease** (caused by *Trypanosoma cruzi*) may lead to achalasia.

8. **Esophageal reflux** is caused by LES dysfunction that allows gastric acid reflux into the lower esophagus. Clinical findings include substernal pain and heartburn, which may worsen with bending or lying down. **Scleroderma** may be a systemic cause of esophageal reflux.

9. **Esophageal Strictures (narrowing). Caustic strictures** are caused by ingestion of caustic agents (e.g. drain openers, oven cleaners). **Other strictures** are caused by recurrent mucosal destruction as a result of gastric acid reflux. These strictures most often occur at the GE junction.

10. **Esophageal varices** refer to the dilated subepithelial and submucosal venous plexuses of the esophagus that drain into the **left gastric (coronary) vein.** The left gastric vein empties into the portal vein from the distal esophagus and proximal stomach. Esophageal varices are caused by **portal hypertension** as a result of cirrhosis of the liver.

11. **Barrett's Esophagus.** The GE junction in gross anatomy is fairly easy to demarcate. However, the histologic GE junction does NOT correspond to the gross anatomic GE junction. The mucosal lining of the cardiac portion of the stomach **extends about 2 cm into the esophagus** such that the distal 2 cm of the esophagus is lined by a simple columnar epithelium instead of stratified squamous epithelium. The

junction where stratified squamous epithelium changes to simple columnar epithelium (or the mucosal GE junction) can be seen macroscopically as a **zigzag line** (called the **Z-line**). This distinction is clinically very important, especially when dealing with Barrett's esophagus. Barrett's esophagus can be defined as the replacement of esophageal stratified squamous epithelium with metaplastic "intestinalized" simple columnar (with goblet cells) epithelium extending **at least 3 cm** into the esophagus. The clinical importance of this metaplastic invasion is that virtually all lower esophageal adenocarcinomas occur as a sequela.

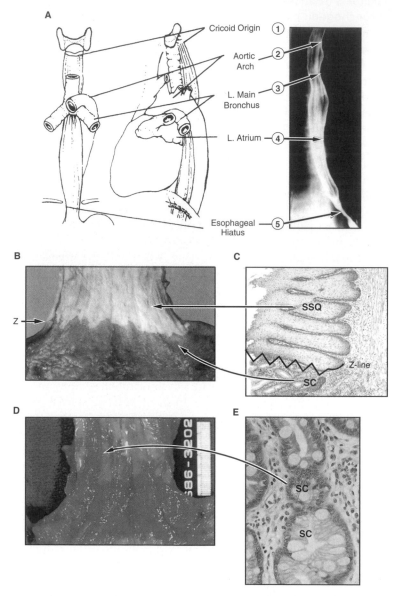

● **Figure 11-1 Esophagus. (A)** This diagram shows the normal constrictions of the esophagus. **(B, C) The Mucosal Gastroesophageal (GE) Junction. (B)** Photograph of a formalin-fixed esophagus shows the Z-line where the stratified squamous epithelium (white portion) changes to a simple columnar epithelium (dark portion). **(C)** LM shows the Z-line where stratified squamous epithelium (SSQ) changes to a simple columnar epithelium (SC). **(D, E) Barrett's Esophagus. (D)** Photograph of Barrett's esophagus shows the cephalad extension of simple columnar epithelium above the Z-line. **(E)** LM shows the cephalad extension of simple columnar epithelium (SC) above the Z-line.

Stomach (Figure 11-2)

A. **General Features.** The stomach is a muscular organ that macerates, homogenizes, and partially digests the swallowed food into a semisolid paste called **chyme**. The stomach is divided into four parts:
   1. **Cardia** is near the GE junction.
   2. **Fundus** is above the GE junction.
   3. **Body** is between the fundus and antrum.
   4. **Pylorus** is the distal part of the stomach and is divided into the **pyloric antrum** (wide part) and the **pyloric canal** (narrow part). The pyloric orifice is surrounded by the **pyloric sphincter**, which is a well-defined muscular sphincter that controls movement of food out of the stomach and prevents reflux of duodenal contents into the stomach.

B. **Clinical Considerations**
   1. **Gastric ulcers (Figure 11-3A)** most often occur within the **body of the stomach** along the **lesser curvature** above the **incisura angularis** at a histologic transition zone where the gastric glands change from predominately parietal cells (HCl-producing) to G cells (gastrin-producing). They are caused by **damage to the mucosal barrier** (resulting in decreased mucus and bicarbonate production) as a result of smoking, salicylate or nonsteroid anti-inflammatory drug (NSAID) ingestion, type B chronic atrophic gastritis, mucosal ischemia because of reduced prostaglandin E (PGE) production, or bile reflux. About 80% of patients with gastric ulcers have associated *Helicobacter pylori* infection. Clinical findings include burning epigastric pain **soon after eating;** pain increases with food intake; pain is relieved by antacids; patient is afraid to eat and loses weight. Treatment is the same as that for duodenal ulcers (see Section III.B.1.).
   2. **Hypertrophic pyloric stenosis** is a congenital condition that presents within weeks after birth. Clinical findings include projectile vomiting containing no bile, visible peristalsis from the left hypochondriac to the right hypochondriac region, and a hard, mobile mass palpated in the epigastric region.
   3. **Dumping syndrome** refers to the abnormally rapid emptying of **hyperosmotic** stomach contents (especially high-carbohydrate foods) into the jejunum within 30 minutes after a meal ("early dumping") or 1 to 3 hours later ("late dumping"). The dumping syndrome usually occurs after a partial gastrectomy or vagotomy for treatment of an ulcer or obesity. Clinical findings include epigastric discomfort, borborygmi (rumbling sounds caused by gas movement), palpitations, dizziness, diarrhea, and hypoglycemia.
   4. **Carcinomas of the stomach** are most commonly found in the **pylorus** of the stomach and may metastasize to **supraclavicular lymph nodes (Virchow's nodes)** on the left side, which can be palpated within the posterior triangle of the neck. Carcinoma of the stomach may also metastasize to the ovaries, where it is called a **Krukenberg tumor.**

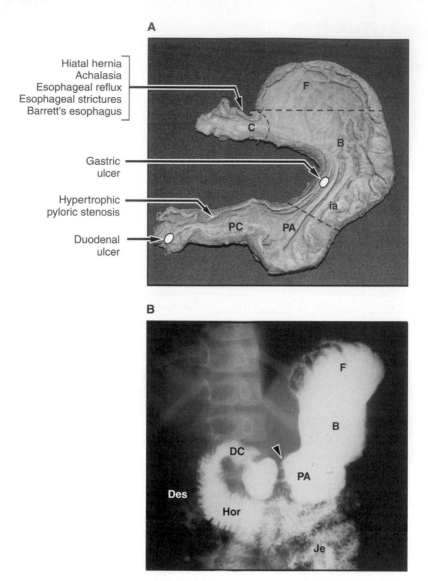

● **Figure 11-2 (A) Photograph of the Stomach.** Note the various parts of the stomach. High-yield clinical considerations associated with the esophagus, stomach, and duodenum are indicated. **(B) Radiograph after Barium Swallow.** Note the parts of the stomach and duodenum. B = body, C = cardia, DC = duodenal cap or superior part of duodenum, Des = descending part of duodenum, F = fundus, Hor = horizontal part of duodenum, ia = incisura angularis, Je = jejunum, PA = pyloric antrum, PC = pyloric canal, arrowhead = peristaltic wave.

Ⅲ Duodenum

A. General Features. The duodenum pursues a C-shaped course around the head of the pancreas. The duodenum is divided into four parts:

1. **Superior Part (first part).** The first 2 cm of the superior part is intraperitoneal and therefore has a mesentery and is mobile; the remaining distal 3 cm of the superior part is retroperitoneal. Radiologists refer to the first 2 cm of the superior part of the duodenum as the **duodenal cap** or **bulb**. The superior part begins at the pylorus of the stomach (**gastroduodenal junction**), which is marked by the **prepyloric vein**. Posterior relationships include the **common bile duct** and **gastroduodenal artery**.

The **hepatoduodenal ligament** attaches superiorly and the **greater omentum** attaches inferiorly.

2. **Descending part (second part)** is retroperitoneal and receives the **common bile duct** and **main pancreatic duct** on its posterior/medial wall at the **hepatopancreatic ampulla (ampulla of Vater)**.

3. **Horizontal part (third part)** is retroperitoneal and runs horizontally across the L3 vertebra between the superior mesenteric artery anteriorly and the aorta and inferior vena cava (IVC) posteriorly. In severe abdominal injuries, this part of the duodenum may be crushed against the L3 vertebra.

4. **Ascending part (fourth part)** is retroperitoneal and ascends to meet the jejunum at the **duodenojejunal junction**, which occurs approximately at the L2 vertebral level about 2 to 3 cm to the left of the midline. This junction usually forms an acute angle that is called the **duodenojejunal flexure**, which is supported by the **ligament of Treitz** (also called the suspensory muscle of the duodenum).

B. Clinical Considerations

1. **Duodenal ulcers (Figure 11-3B)** most often occur on the anterior wall of the first part of the duodenum (i.e. at the **duodenal cap**) followed by the posterior wall (danger of perforation into the pancreas). They are caused by **damage to the mucosal barrier** (resulting in decreased mucus and bicarbonate production) and **gastric acid hypersecretion** as a result of increased parietal cell mass, increased secretion to stimuli, increased nocturnal secretion, or rapid gastric emptying. About 95% of patients have associated *H. pylori* infection. Clinical findings include burning epigastric pain **1 to 3 hours after eating**; pain decreases with food intake; pain is relieved by antacids; patient does not lose weight; patient wakes at night because of pain. Treatment includes:

    a. **Sucralfate (Carafate or Sulcrate)** is a drug that forms a polymer in an acidic environment and protects ulcers from further irritation and damage.

    b. The antibiotic regimens of **bismuth subsalicylate (Pepto-Bismol), tetracycline, and metronidazole** or **amoxicillin and clarithromycin** are effective in eradication of *H. pylori*.

    c. **Omeprazole (Prilosec), esomeprazole (Nexium), lansoprazole (Prevacid)** are irreversible H^+-K^+ ATPase inhibitors that inhibit HCl secretion from parietal cells.

    d. **Atropine** is a muscarinic acetylcholine receptor (mAChR) antagonist that blocks the stimulatory effects of acetylcholine (Ach) released from postganglionic parasympathetic neurons (cranial nerve [CN] X) on HCl secretion.

    e. **Cimetidine (Tagamet), ranitidine (Zantac), nizatidine (Axid), and famotidine (Pepcid)** are histamine-2 (H_2) receptor antagonists that block the stimulatory effects of histamine released from inflammatory cells or mast cells on HCl secretion. The H_2 receptor is a G-protein–linked receptor that increases cyclic adenosine monophosphate (cAMP) levels.

    f. **Misoprostol (Cytotec)** is a PGE_1 analog that inhibits HCl secretion and stimulates secretion of mucus and HCO_3^- from surface mucous cells of the stomach.

    g. **Proximal Gastric Vagotomy (PGV).** A PGV transects the vagus nerve (CN X) fibers only to the distal esophagus and fundus of the stomach and results in decreased gastric acid secretion.

2. **Perforations of the duodenum** occur most often with ulcers on the **anterior** wall of the duodenum. Perforations occur less often with ulcers on the **posterior** wall; however, these may erode the **gastroduodenal artery**, causing severe hemorrhage, and perforate into the pancreas. Clinical findings include air under the diaphragm and pain that radiates to the left shoulder.

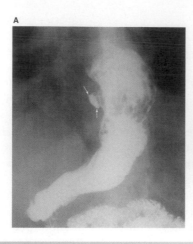
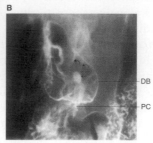

COMPARISON OF GASTRIC AND DUODENAL ULCERS

	Gastric Ulcer	Duodenal Ulcer
% of ulcer cases	25%	75%
Epidemiology	Male to female ratio = 1:1	Male to female ratio = 2:1
	Increased risk with blood type A	Increased risk with blood type O
	No association with MEN I or II	Associated with Zollinger-Ellison syndrome (MEN I)
	COPD	Liver cirrhosis or alcoholism
	Renal failure	COPD
		Renal failure
		Hyperparathyroidism
		Family history with an autosomal dominant pattern
Pathogenesis	*H. pylori* infection in 80% of cases	*H. pylori* infection in 95% of cases
	Damage to mucosal barrier caused by smoking, salicylate or NSAID ingestion, type B chronic atrophic gastritis, mucosal ischemia because of reduced PGE production, or bile reflux	Damage to mucosal barrier
		Gastric acid hypersecretion caused by increased parietal cell mass, increased secretion to stimuli, increased nocturnal secretion, or rapid gastric emptying
Location	Single ulcer within the body of the stomach along the lesser curvature above the incisura angularis	Single ulcer on the anterior wall of the first part of the duodenum (i.e. at the **duodenal cap**) most common
		Single ulcer on the posterior wall (danger of perforation into the pancreas)
Malignant Potential	No malignant potential	No malignant potential
	Cancer may be associated with a benign ulcer in 1–3% of cases (biopsy necessary)	
Complications	Bleeding from left gastric artery	Bleeding from gastroduodenal artery
	Perforation	Perforation (air under diaphragm, pain radiates to left shoulder)
	Both are less common than seen in duodenal ulcers	Gastric outlet obstruction
		Pancreatitis
Clinical Findings	Burning epigastric pain **soon after eating**	Burning epigastric pain **1–3 hours after eating**
	Pain increases with food intake	Pain decreases with food intake
	Pain is relieved by antacids	Pain is relieved by antacids
	Patient is afraid to eat and loses weight	Patient does not lose weight
		Patient wakes at night because of pain

COPD = chronic obstructive pulmonary disease, MEN = multiple endocrine neoplasia, NSAID = nonsteroidal anti-inflammatory drug, PGE = prostaglandin E.

● **Figure 11-3 (A) Gastric Ulcer.** Radiograph shows a gastric ulcer (arrows) along the lesser curvature of the stomach. **(B) Duodenal Ulcer.** Radiograph shows a duodenal ulcer (straight arrow) located in the duodenal bulb (DB). The duodenal mucosal folds (curved arrows) radiate toward the ulcer crater. PC = pyloric canal.

Ⓘ Jejunum, Ileum, and Large Intestine

A. General features are indicated in Table 11-1.

TABLE 11-1	CHARACTERISTICS OF JEJUNUM, ILEUM, AND LARGE INTESTINE	
Jejunum	**Ileum**	**Large Intestine**
Villi present (long, finger-shaped)	Villi present (short, club-shaped)	Villi absent
Intestinal glands (crypts) present	Intestinal glands (crypts) present	Intestinal glands (crypts) present
>3 cm in diameter	<3 cm in diameter	~6–9 cm in diameter
Large, numerous, and palpable circular folds[a]	Small and few circular folds that disappear distally	No circular folds; inner luminal surface is smooth
Initial 2/5 of small intestine	Terminal 3/5 of small intestine	———
Located in the umbilical region on left side of abdomen	Located in the hypogastric and inguinal regions on the right side of abdomen	———
Long vasa recta	Short vasa recta	———
Main site of nutrient absorption Often empty (no fecal contents)	Site of vitamin B_{12} and H_2O and electrolyte absorption Site of bile recirculation	Site of H_2O and electrolyte absorption Site of sedatives, anesthetics, and steroid absorption when medications cannot be delivered orally
Thicker wall, more vascular, and redder in the living person than ileum	Terminal ileum ends several centimeters above the cecal tip	**Taeniae coli** (three longitudinal bands of smooth muscle) are present **Appendices epiploicae** (fatty tags) are present **Haustra** (sacculations of the wall) are present

[a]Folds of the mucosa and submucosa (also called **plicae circularis**).

B. Clinical Considerations

1. **Celiac disease** is a hypersensitivity to **gluten** and **gliadin** protein found in wheat and other grains. On ingestion of gluten-containing foods, a large number of lymphocytes, plasma cells, macrophages, and eosinophils accumulate within the lamina propria of the intestinal mucosa. Gliadin antibodies are generally detectable in the blood. These factors may contribute to the immunologic damage of the mucosa. Clinical findings include chronic diarrhea, flatulence, weight loss, and fatigue.

2. **Appendicitis** begins with the obstruction of the appendix lumen with a fecal concretion (fecalith) and lymphoid hyperplasia followed by distension of the appendix. Clinical findings include initial pain in the umbilical or epigastric region, later pain that localizes to the right lumbar region, nausea, vomiting, anorexia, and tenderness to palpation and percussion in the right lumbar region. Complications may include peritonitis as a result of rupture of the appendix. **McBurney's point** is located by drawing a line from the right anterior superior iliac spine to the umbilicus. The midpoint of this line locates the root of the appendix at the junctions of the right inguinal region and the umbilical region of the abdominal wall. The appendix is suspended by the **mesoappendix** (i.e. intraperitoneal) and is generally found in the **retrocecal fossa** (although its position is variable).

3. **Toxic megacolon** is most commonly a dilatation of the transverse colon that results in perforation of the colonic wall. Clinical signs include abdominal pain, fever, and leukocytosis.

4. **Ogilvie syndrome** is most commonly a dilatation of the cecum that is often seen in critically ill or bedridden patients.

5. **Crohn disease (CR; Figure 11-4A, B)** is a chronic inflammatory bowel disease that most commonly affects the **ileum** and involves an abundant accumulation of lymphocytes forming a **granuloma** (a typical feature of CR) within the submucosa that may further extend into the muscularis externa. Neutrophils infiltrate the intestinal glands and ultimately destroy them, leading to ulcers. With progression of CR, the ulcers coalesce into long, **serpentine ulcers** ("**linear ulcers**") oriented along the long axis of the bowel. A classic feature of CR is the clear demarcation between diseased bowel segments located directly next to uninvolved normal bowel and a cobblestone appearance that can be seen grossly and radiographically. The cause of CR is unknown. Clinical findings include intermittent bouts of diarrhea, weight loss, and weakness. Complications include strictures of the intestinal lumen, formation of fistulas, and perforation.

6. **Ulcerative colitis (Figure 11-4 C, D)** is a type of idiopathic inflammatory bowel disease. It always involves the rectum and extends proximally for varying distances. The inflammation is continuous, i.e. there are no "skip areas" as in Crohn disease. The cause of ulcerative colitis is unknown. Clinical signs include bloody diarrhea with mucus and pus, malaise, fever, weight loss, and anemia, and it may lead to toxic megacolon.

7. **Familial adenomatous polyposis (FAP)** is the archetype of adenomatous polyposis syndromes in which patients develop 500 to 2,000 polyps that most commonly carpet the mucosal surface of the **rectosigmoid colon** (60% of all cases) and invariably become malignant. Malignant polyps are irregular in shape, sessile, greater than 2 cm in diameter, and exhibit sudden growth, and their base is broader than their height. FAP is an autosomal dominant disease and involves a mutation in the **adenomatous polyposis coli (APC) anti-oncogene**. The progression from a small polyp to a large polyp is associated with a mutation in the *ras* proto-oncogene. The progression from a large polyp to metastatic carcinoma is associated with mutations in the **DCC anti-oncogene** (deleted in colon carcinoma) and the **p53 anti-oncogene**. **Gardner syndrome** is a variation of FAP in which patients demonstrate adenomatous polyps and multiple osteomas. **Turcot syndrome** is a variation of FAP in which patients demonstrate adenomatous polyps and gliomas.

8. **Adenocarcinoma of the colon** will invariably develop in patients with FAP and accounts for 98% of all cancers in the large intestine. Mutations in the *HNPCC* **gene** (hereditary nonpolyposis colorectal cancer gene), which codes for a DNA repair enzyme, have been implicated in some cases. Clinical findings include fatigue, weakness, change in bowel habits, and weight loss. Right-sided tumors are associated with iron deficiency anemia. Left-sided tumors are associated with obstruction and bloody stools. It is a clinical maxim that iron-deficiency anemia in an older man means adenocarcinoma of the colon until shown otherwise. Metastasis occurs most commonly to the **liver** because the sigmoid veins and superior rectal veins drain into the hepatic portal system. A posterior metastasis may involve the **sacral nerve plexus**, causing sciatica.

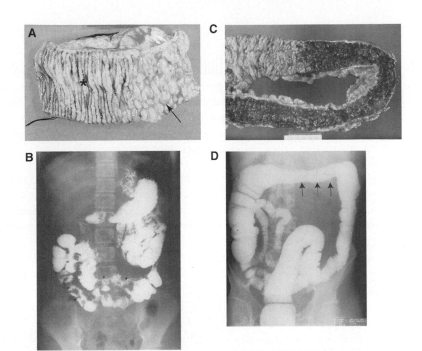

COMPARISON OF CROHN DISEASE AND ULCERATIVE COLITIS

	Crohn Disease	Ulcerative Colitis
Epidemiology	More common in whites vs. blacks More common in Jews vs. non-Jews More common in women Affects young adults	More common in whites vs. blacks No sex predilection Affects young adults
Extent	Transmural	Mucosal and submucosal
Location	Terminal ileum alone (30%) Ileum and colon (50%) Colon alone (20%) Involves other areas of GI tract (mouth to anus)	Mainly the rectum May extend into descending colon May involve entire colon Does not involve other areas of GI tract
Gross Features	Thick bowel wall and narrow lumen (leads to obstruction) Aphthous ulcers (early sign) Skip lesions, strictures, and fistulas Deep linear ulcers with cobblestone pattern Fat creeping around the serosa	Inflammatory pseudopolyps Areas of friable, bloody residual mucosa Ulceration and hemorrhage
Microscopic Findings	Noncaseating granulomas Lymphoid aggregates Dysplasia or cancer less likely	Ulcers and intestinal gland abscesses with neutrophils Dysplasia or cancer may be present
Clinical Findings	Recurrent right lower quadrant colicky pain with diarrhea Bleeding occurs with colon or anal involvement	Recurrent left-sided abdominal cramping with bloody diarrhea and mucus
Radiography	"String" sign in terminal ileum because of luminal narrowing	"Lead pipe" appearance in chronic state
Complications	Fistulas, obstruction Calcium oxalate renal calculi Malabsorption because of bile deficiency Macrocytic anemia because of vitamin B_{12} deficiency	Toxic megacolon Primary sclerosing cholangitis Adenocarcinoma

GI = gastrointestinal.

● **Figure 11-4 (A, B) Crohn Disease. (A)** Photograph of a gross specimen of the ileum shows prominent cobblestoning (arrow) as a result of multiple transverse and linear ulcers. The other portion of the ileum is normal (*). **(B)** Radiograph shows the luminal narrowing ("string sign") and cobblestone pattern of the affected small intestines. **(C, D) Ulcerative Colitis. (C)** Photograph of a gross specimen of the colon shows inflammatory pseudopolyps and ulceration. **(D)** Radiograph shows the "lead pipe" appearance of the affected transverse and descending colon. Note the small ulcerations extending from the colon lumen (arrows).

Innervation of the Gastrointestinal (GI) Tract. The GI tract is innervated by the **celiac plexus, superior mesenteric plexus, inferior mesenteric plexus, and superior hypogastric plexus**, which are located around the abdominal aorta and its major branches. These plexuses contain both **parasympathetic (vagus nerve [CN X] and pelvic splanchnic nerves)** and **sympathetic components**. In addition, the GI tract is innervated by an entirely separate nervous system called the **enteric nervous system**.

A. Enteric Nervous System. The phylogenetically primitive enteric nervous system is an entirely separate nervous system in the body because most functions of the GI tract are controlled by the enteric nervous system even in the absence of parasympathetic or sympathetic innervation. The enteric nervous system is composed of two distinct interconnected neuronal circuits as indicated below:

   1. Submucosal Plexus of Meissner. The neuronal cell bodies of the submucosal plexus are found in the submucosa. This plexus extends from the small intestine to the upper anal canal.

   a. **Motor Component.** The motor component of this plexus controls primarily **mucosal and submucosal gland secretion and blood flow.**

   b. **Sensory Component.** The sensory component of this plexus consists of **mucosal mechanosensitive neurons.**

   2. Myenteric Plexus of Auerbach. The neuronal cell bodies of the myenteric plexus are found between the inner circular and outer longitudinal layer of the muscularis externa. This plexus extends from the esophagus to the upper anal canal.

   a. **Motor Component.** The motor component of this plexus controls primarily **GI motility (contraction and relaxation of GI smooth muscle).**

   b. **Sensory Component.** The sensory component of this plexus consists of **tension-sensitive neurons** and **chemosensitive neurons.**

B. Parasympathetic Nervous System

   1. Motor Component. Preganglionic neuronal cell bodies are located in the **dorsal nucleus of the vagus** and the **nucleus ambiguus** in the medulla or in the **gray matter of the S2 through S4 spinal cord.** Preganglionic axons travel in CN X (vagus nerve) and **pelvic splanchnic nerves (S2 through S4)** and synapse in the complex neuronal circuitry of the enteric nervous system. Hence, it is difficult to detail specific parasympathetic motor functions, although they are usually considered excitatory in nature.

   2. Sensory Component. The neuronal cell bodies are located in the **nodose (inferior) ganglion** of CN X and the **dorsal root ganglion of S2 through S4 spinal nerves.** These neurons send a peripheral process to the viscera and a central process to either the solitary nucleus in the brainstem or the spinal cord, respectively. These neurons transmit the sensations of **visceral pressure, visceral movement, visceral stretch, visceral osmolarity, and visceral temperature.** Reflexes in which the motor and sensory components travel in CN X are called **vagovagal reflexes.**

C. Sympathetic Nervous System

   1. Motor Component. Preganglionic neuronal cell bodies are located in the **intermediolateral cell column** of the T5 through L2 or L3 spinal cord. Preganglionic axons travel in the **greater splanchnic nerve, lesser splanchnic nerve, least splanchnic nerve,** and **lumbar splanchnic nerves** and synapse in the **celiac ganglion, superior mesenteric ganglion, inferior mesenteric ganglion** (also called prevertebral ganglia), and **superior hypogastric plexus.** Postganglionic neurons synapse in the complex neuronal circuitry of the enteric nervous system. Hence, it is difficult to detail specific sympathetic motor functions, although they are usually considered inhibitory in nature. However, one motor function that is fairly well established is the **regulation of GI blood flow.**

2. **Sensory Component.** The neuronal cell bodies are located in the dorsal root ganglia at T5 through L2 or L3 spinal cord levels. These neurons send a peripheral process to the viscera via splanchnic nerves and a central process to the spinal cord. These neurons transmit the sensation of **visceral pain.**

VI Gallbladder, Extrahepatic Biliary Ducts, and Bile (Figure 11-5)

A. General Features

1. **Gallbladder** is divided into the **fundus** (anterior portion), **body**, and **neck** (posterior portion). A small pouch (**Hartmann's pouch**) may extend from the neck as a sequela to pathologic changes and is a common site for gallstones to lodge. **Rokitansky-Aschoff sinuses** occur when the mucosa of the gallbladder penetrates deep into the muscularis externa. They are an early indicator of pathologic changes (e.g. acute cholecystitis or gangrene). Arterial blood supply is via the **cystic artery** (a branch of the right hepatic artery). Venous drainage is via **cystic veins** that empty into the portal vein or directly into liver sinusoids. Lymphatic drainage is into **hepatic** and **pancreaticoduodenal** lymph nodes. Sensory nerve fibers for pain from the gallbladder travel with the **greater thoracic splanchnic nerve** to the T7 through T10 spinal levels. Motor nerve fibers that stimulate contraction of the gallbladder are the preganglionic and postganglionic parasympathetic neurons of the **vagus (CN X) nerve.** **Cholecystokinin (CCK)** is a hormone (secreted from I cells of the small intestine) that stimulates contraction of the gallbladder. Motor nerve fibers that inhibit contraction of the gallbladder are preganglionic sympathetic neurons of the **greater thoracic splanchnic nerve** and postganglionic sympathetic neurons from the **celiac plexus. Somatostatin** is a hormone that inhibits contraction of the gallbladder. Functions include storage of bile, concentration of bile (about tenfold) through absorption of water and electrolytes, acidification of bile, addition of mucus ("white bile") to bile, and release of bile through the simultaneous contraction of the gallbladder and relaxation of the sphincter of Oddi, predominately controlled by CCK.

2. **Extrahepatic Biliary Ducts.** The **right and left hepatic ducts** join together after leaving the liver to form the **common hepatic duct.** The common hepatic duct is joined at an acute angle by the **cystic duct** to form the **common bile duct.** The cystic duct drains bile from the gallbladder. The mucosa of the cystic duct is arranged in a spiral fold with a core of smooth muscle known as the **spiral valve (valve of Heister).** The spiral valve keeps the cystic duct constantly open so that bile can flow freely in either direction. The common bile duct passes posterior to the pancreas and ends at the **hepatopancreatic ampulla (ampulla of Vater),** where it joins the **pancreatic duct.** The **sphincter of Oddi** is an area of thickened smooth muscle that surrounds the bile duct as it traverses the ampulla. The sphincter of Oddi **controls bile flow** (sympathetic innervation causes contraction of the sphincter).

3. **Bile** is mainly produced by hepatocytes (600 mL/day). Bile is mainly composed of water, electrolytes, bilirubin glucuronide (bile pigment), cholic acid and chenodeoxycholic acid conjugated to glycine or taurine (bile salts), cholesterol and lecithin (lipids), calcium, and secretory IgA. The function of bile is to emulsify fats. **Lactated Ringer's solution** is a good replacement fluid for bile loss.

B. Clinical Considerations. The term **cholelithiasis** refers to the presence or formation of gallstones either in the gallbladder (called **cholecystolithiasis**) or common bile duct (called **choledocholithiasis**).

1. **Gallstones** form when bile salts and lecithin are overwhelmed by cholesterol. Most stones consist of **cholesterol (major component), bilirubin, and calcium.** There are three main types of gallstones:

   a. **Cholesterol stones** are yellow, large, and smooth and are composed mainly of cholesterol. These stones are associated with obesity, Crohn disease, cystic fibrosis, clofibrate, estrogens, rapid weight loss, and the US or Native American population (4 Fs: female, fat, fertile, over forty).

   b. **Pigment (bilirubin) stones** are brown or black, smooth, and composed mainly of bilirubin salts. These stones are associated with chronic red blood cell hemolysis (e.g. sickle cell anemia or spherocytosis), alcoholic cirrhosis, biliary infection, and the Asian population.

   c. **Calcium bilirubinate stones** are associated with infection or inflammation of the biliary tree.

2. **Gallstone Obstruction.** There are three clinically important sites of gallstone obstruction as follows:

   a. **Within the cystic duct.** A stone may transiently lodge within the cystic duct and cause pain (**biliary colic**) within the epigastric region as a result of distension of the duct. If a stone becomes entrapped within the cystic duct, bile flow from the gallbladder will be obstructed, resulting in inflammation of the gallbladder (**acute cholecystitis**), and pain will shift to the right hypochondriac region. Bile becomes concentrated and precipitates in the gallbladder, forming a layer of high-density material called "**milk of calcium**" **bile** as a result of a large amount of calcium carbonate. Bile flow from the liver remains open (i.e. **no jaundice**). This may lead to **Mirizzi syndrome,** in which impaction of a large gallstone in the cystic duct extrinsically obstructs the nearby common hepatic duct.

   b. **Within the common bile duct.** If a stone becomes entrapped within the common bile duct, bile flow from both the gallbladder and liver will be obstructed, resulting in inflammation of the gallbladder and liver. **Jaundice** is frequently present and is first observed clinically **under the tongue.** The jaundice is moderate and fluctuates as a stone rarely causes complete blockage of the lumen.

   c. **At the hepatopancreatic ampulla.** If a stone becomes entrapped at the ampulla, bile flow from both the gallbladder and liver will be obstructed. In addition, the pancreatic duct may be blocked. In this case, **jaundice** and **pancreatitis** are frequently observed.

● **Figure 11-5 Gallbladder and Biliary Tree. (A)** Diagram of the gallbladder and biliary tree. Note the termination of the common bile duct (CBD) at the hepatopancreatic ampulla (HPA) along with the pancreatic duct (PD). Note the three main sites (X) of gallstone obstruction. **(B)** Endoscopic retrograde cholangiograph shows the normal gallbladder and biliary tree. Note that the cystic duct normally lies on the right side of the common hepatic duct and joins it superior to the duodenal cap. **(C)** Photograph shows a solitary cholesterol gallstone. **(D)** Photograph shows a pigment gallstone embedded in a mucous gel. **(E)** Longitudinal decubitus sonogram shows gallstones within the gallbladder (cholelithiasis; curved arrows), which cast acoustic shadows (between the straight arrows) because the sound waves cannot penetrate the dense gallstones. Ultrasonography generally elicits **Murphy's sign,** in which a patient reports pain as the operator presses on the gallbladder. **(F, G) Hepatobiliary iminodiacetic acid (HIDA) scan of a normal patient.** HIDA makes use of the radionuclide technetium 99m attached to bilirubin analogs bound to iminodiacetic acid. This compound is injected intravenously, processed

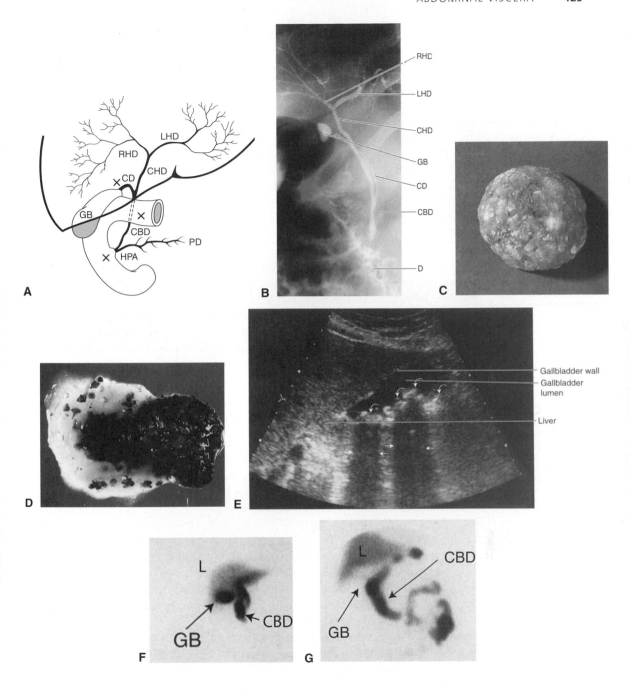

by hepatocytes, and excreted into the bile. In a normal person, filling of the liver, gallbladder, and biliary tract occurs within 60 minutes after injection. Note the filling of the liver (L), gallbladder (GB), and common bile duct (CBD) within 60 minutes after injection. **(G) Hepatobiliary iminodiacetic acid (HIDA) scan of a patient with acute cholecystitis.** Note the absence of filling of the gallbladder minutes after morphine injection that contracts the sphincter of Odi and leads to a rise of biliary system pressure. Even after the morphine injection the gallbladder does not fill, which is diagnostic of a blockage. However, the liver and common bile duct are filled. Because most gallstones are composed of cholesterol (and therefore radiolucent), plain abdominal radiographic films are often of little value. Therefore, ultrasonography and HIDA are the methods of choice for diagnosis. CHD = common hepatic duct, CD = cystic duct, LHD = left hepatic duct, RHD = right hepatic duct, D = duodenum.

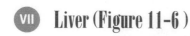

Liver (Figure 11-6)

A. General Features. The liver is the largest internal gland in the body. The **liver parenchyma** consists of radially arranged plates of **hepatocytes**. The **liver stroma** consists of **reticular fibers (type III collagen).** The stroma begins as a thin connective tissue capsule called the **Glisson capsule** that extends into the liver around the portal triads, around the periphery of the hepatic lobules, and into the perisinusoidal space of Disse to surround hepatocytes, and then terminates around the central vein. Gross anatomically, one can identify at the **porta hepatis** components of the (1) **common bile duct**, (2) **portal vein**, (3) **hepatic artery**, and (4) **lymphatics.** The hepatic bile duct, portal vein, and hepatic artery are referred to as the **portal triad** (the lymphatics are forgotten about in this designation). Histologically, branches of these same components can be found within the substance of the liver as they help define a classic hepatic lobule.

B. Lobes of the Liver. The liver is classically divided into the **right lobe** and **left lobe** by the **interlobar fissure** (an invisible line running from the gallbladder to the inferior vena cava), **quadrate lobe**, and **caudate lobe.** The left lobe contains the **falciform ligament** (a derivative of the ventral mesentery), with the **ligamentum teres** (a remnant of the left umbilical vein) along its inferior border. The **bare area** of the liver is located on the diaphragmatic surface and is devoid of peritoneum. The liver is secured in its anatomic location by the attachment of the hepatic veins to the IVC, which allows for very little rotation of the liver during surgery.

C. Segments and Subsegments of the Liver. There are five liver segments, which include the **anterior segment of the right lobe, posterior segment of the right lobe, medial segment of the left lobe, lateral segment of the left lobe**, and **caudate lobe.** The hepatic veins define the boundaries of the liver segments. There are nine liver subsegments, which include the **posterior superior, posterior inferior, anterior superior, anterior inferior, medial superior, medial inferior** (which corresponds to the classic quadrate lobe), **lateral superior, lateral inferior**, and the classic **caudate lobe.**

D. Clinical Considerations

1. **Liver biopsies** are frequently performed by needle puncture through right intercostal space 8, 9, or 10 when the patient has exhaled. The needle will pass through the following structures: skin → superficial fascia → external oblique muscle → intercostal muscles → costal parietal pleura → costodiaphragmatic recess → diaphragmatic parietal pleura → diaphragm → peritoneum.

2. **Congenital biliary atresia** affects the development of the intrahepatic and extrahepatic bile ducts and generally presents within weeks after birth. This is the most common cause of persistent jaundice in infancy. Clinical findings include jaundice (does not start immediately after birth as with physiologic jaundice), dark urine, and clay-colored stool; liver biopsy shows bile duct proliferation with dilatation of bile canaliculi and bile plugs.

3. **Primary sclerosing cholangitis** is caused by inflammation, fibrosis, and segmental dilatation of both **intrahepatic and extrahepatic bile ducts.** It is frequently seen in association with chronic ulcerative colitis of the bowel. Clinical findings include right hypochondriac region pain or painless jaundice, no fever or chills, pruritus, fatigue, and nausea.

4. **Primary biliary cirrhosis** is caused by an autoimmune granulomatous destruction of medium-sized **intrahepatic bile ducts**, with cirrhosis appearing late in the course of the disease, and occurs principally in middle-aged women. It is characterized by

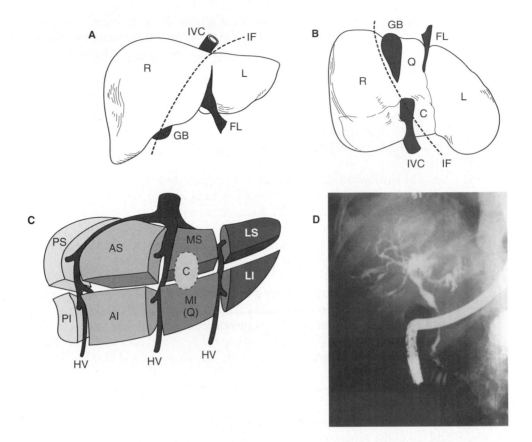

● **Figure 11-6 Liver. (A)** Diagram of the anterior surface of the liver. Note the right lobe (R) and left lobe (L) divided by the interlobar fissure (IF). IVC = inferior vena cava, FL = falciform ligament, GB = gallbladder. **(B)** Diagram of the inferior surface of the liver. Note the quadrate lobe (Q) and caudate lobe (C). **(C)** Diagram of the five liver segments and nine liver subsegments used in liver resectioning. The five liver segments include the posterior segment and anterior segment of the right lobe, the medial segment and lateral segment of the left lobe, and the caudate lobe. Note the hepatic veins (HV) at the periphery of the liver segments. The nine liver subsegments include posterior superior (PS), posterior inferior (PI), anterior superior (AS), anterior inferior (AI), medial superior (MS), medial inferior (MI), which corresponds to the classic quadrate lobe (Q), lateral superior (LS), lateral inferior (LI), and the classic caudate lobe (C). **(D)** Primary sclerosing cholangitis radiograph shows stenosis of both intrahepatic and extrahepatic bile ducts with intervening areas of ductal dilation.

mitochondrial pyruvate dehydrogenase autoantibodies, the role of which is not clear. Primary biliary cirrhosis is often associated with other autoimmune diseases (e.g. Sjögren syndrome, rheumatoid arthritis, CREST syndrome, Hashimoto thyroiditis, and renal tubular acidosis).

5. **Surgical resection of the liver** may be performed by removing one of the **liver segments** (five total segments) or one of the **liver subsegments** (nine total subsegments). **Hepatic veins** form the surgical landmarks that mark the periphery (or border) of a liver segment during segmental resection of the liver. Recall that **pulmonary veins** form the surgical landmarks that mark the periphery of a bronchopulmonary segment during segmental resection of the lung.

VIII   Pancreas (Figure 11-7)

A. General Features. In the adult, the pancreas is a retroperitoneal organ that measures 15 to 20 cm in length and weighs about 85 to 120 g. The normal pancreas is tan-pink to yellow in color and uniformly lobulated. A cut section of the pancreas reveals an extensive branching network of ducts extending into the lobules of the pancreas. The pancreas is both an exocrine gland and an endocrine gland. Gross anatomically, the pancreas consists of four parts as follows:

1. **Head of the Pancreas.** The head is the expanded part of the pancreas that lies in the concavity of the C-shaped curve of the duodenum and is firmly attached to the descending and horizontal parts of the duodenum. The **uncinate process** is a projection from the inferior portion of the pancreatic head. The head of the pancreas is related posteriorly to the IVC, right renal artery, right renal vein, and left renal vein.

2. **Neck of the Pancreas.** The neck is related posteriorly to the confluence of the superior mesenteric vein and splenic vein to form the portal vein.

3. **Body of the Pancreas.** The body is related posteriorly to the aorta, superior mesenteric artery, left suprarenal gland, left kidney, renal artery, and renal vein.

4. **Tail of the Pancreas.** The tail is related to the splenic hilum and the left colic flexure.

B. **Arterial Supply.**

1. **Anterior and posterior superior pancreaticoduodenal arteries** are branches of the gastroduodenal artery and supply the head and neck of the pancreas.

2. **Anterior and posterior inferior pancreaticoduodenal arteries** are branches of the superior mesenteric artery and supply the head and neck of the pancreas.

3. **Dorsal pancreatic artery** is a branch of the splenic artery and supplies the body and tail of the pancreas.

4. **Great pancreatic artery** is a branch of the splenic artery and supplies the body and tail of the pancreas.

5. **Caudal pancreatic arteries** are branches of the splenic artery and supply the body and tail of the pancreas.

C. **Venous Drainage.** The venous drainage of the pancreas is predominately to the **splenic vein** and **superior mesenteric vein**, both of which empty into the **portal vein**, which ultimately empties into the **liver sinusoids**.

D. **Exocrine Pancreas.** The exocrine pancreas is a compound tubuloacinar gland that has histologic features similar to the salivary glands.

1. The functional unit of the exocrine pancreas is the histologic **pancreatic acinus**, which consists of acinar cells that contain rough endoplasmic reticulum (rER), Golgi, and zymogen granules. Acinar cells secrete digestive enzymes, which include trypsinogen, chymotrypsinogen, procarboxypeptidase, lipase, amylase, elastase, ribonuclease, deoxyribonuclease, cholesterol esterase, and phospholipase. The secretion of digestive enzymes is stimulated by cholecystokinin (CCK) released by I-cells of the small intestine.

2. The exocrine pancreas also contains a network of ducts: centroacinar cells of the intercalated duct → intralobular duct → interlobular duct → main pancreatic duct (duct of Wirsung) → joins the common bile duct at the hepatopancreatic ampulla (ampulla of Vater) → duodenum. The sphincter of the pancreatic duct, the sphincter of the common bile duct, and the sphincter of the hepatopancreatic ampulla (sphincter of Oddi) are smooth muscle sphincters that control the flow of bile and pancreatic juice. An **accessory pancreatic duct (duct of Santorini)** opens into the duodenum superior to the opening of the main pancreatic duct. In about 60% of cases, the accessory pancreatic duct communicates with the main pancreatic duct. In other cases, the main pancreatic duct is smaller than the accessory pancreatic

duct and there is no communication between the two; in this situation the accessory pancreatic duct carries the majority of the pancreatic juice. The duct network delivers digestive enzymes to the duodenum and secretes HCO_3^-. Secretion of HCO_3^- by the intercalated and intralobular ducts is stimulated by **secretin**, released by S-cells of the small intestine.

E. Endocrine Pancreas. The endocrine pancreas comprises only 2% of the entire pancreas and consists of the **islets of Langerhans** that are scattered throughout the pancreas. The islets of Langerhans consists mainly of the following cell types: **alpha (α) cells** (20% of the islet) secrete **glucagon** in response to hypoglycemia, which will elevate blood glucose, free fatty acid, and ketone levels; **beta (β) cells** (75% of the islet) secrete **insulin** in response to hyperglycemia, which will lower blood glucose, free fatty acid, and ketone levels; and **delta (δ) cells** (5% of the islet) secrete **somatostatin**, which inhibits hormone secretion from nearby cells in a paracrine manner.

F. Clinical Considerations

1. **Pancreatitis** is the inflammation of the pancreas that is almost always associated with acinar cell injury. **Chronic pancreatitis** is the relapsing inflammation of the pancreas, causing pain and eventually irreversible damage in which **pancreatic calcifications** (pathognomonic) are frequently diagnosed by imaging procedures. **Acute pancreatitis** is an acute condition associated with abdominal pain and raised levels of pancreatic enzymes in the blood and urine. An increased level of amylase in the pleural fluid is pathognomonic of acute pancreatitis. About 80% of acute pancreatitis cases are associated with **biliary tract disease** or **alcoholism.** Its most severe form is known as **acute hemorrhagic pancreatitis.** The ultimate pathologic process is the destructive effect of pancreatic enzymes released from damaged acinar cells, resulting in the **autodigestion** of the pancreas. Clinical findings include pain in the epigastric region that radiates to the back, nausea, vomiting, elevated amylase or lipase levels, and retroperitoneal hemorrhage that may lead to flank ecchymosis (Turner sign) or periumbilical ecchymosis (Cullen sign).

2. **Pancreatic Adenocarcinoma.** About 90% of all tumors of the pancreas involve the pancreatic ducts; the remaining 10% involve the islets. Pancreatic adenocarcinoma is a very aggressive malignant tumor that usually occurs within the head of the pancreas and is more common in men in the 60- to 80-year-old range. Mutations in the p53 tumor suppressor gene and the *ras* oncogene have been clearly implicated. It has a poor prognosis and usually has already metastasized on presentation. Clinical findings include midepigastric pain that radiates to the back and worsens on lying down, weight loss, obstructive jaundice, clay-colored stools, hepatomegaly, glucose intolerance, palpable gallbladder (Courvoisier sign), and elevated CA19-9 (the gold standard marker). A pancreaticoduodenectomy (**Whipple procedure**), which removes the head of the pancreas, duodenum, distal common bile duct, gallbladder, and distal stomach, may be a surgical treatment.

3. **Pancreatic divisum** (4% incidence) occurs when the **distal two-thirds of the dorsal pancreatic duct** and the **entire ventral pancreatic duct** fail to anastomose and the proximal one-third of the dorsal pancreatic duct persists, thereby forming two separate duct systems. The dorsal pancreatic duct drains a **portion of the head, body,** and **tail of the pancreas** by opening into the duodenum through the minor papillae. The ventral pancreatic duct drains the **uncinate process** and a **portion of the head of the pancreas** by opening into the duodenum through the major papillae. Patients with pancreas divisum are prone to pancreatitis, especially if the opening of the dorsal pancreatic duct at the minor papillae is small.

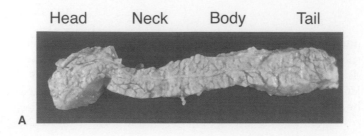

Head   Neck   Body   Tail

A

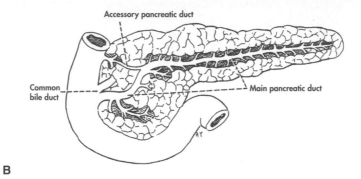

Accessory pancreatic duct

Common bile duct

Main pancreatic duct

B

C

Dorsal pancreatic duct

Common bile duct

Ventral pancreatic duct

D

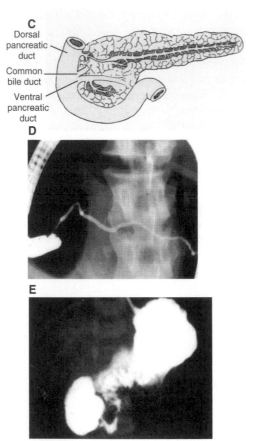

E

● **Figure 11-7 Pancreas. (A)** Photograph of a gross specimen of the pancreas. **(B)** Diagram of the duct system of the pancreas. **(C)** Diagram of the duct system showing pancreatic divisum. Note that distal two thirds of the dorsal pancreatic duct and the ventral pancreatic bud fail to anastomose, thereby forming two separate duct systems. **(D)** An endoscopic retrograde pancreatogram performed through the accessory minor papillae shows the dorsal pancreatic duct in pancreatic divisum. **(E)** Annular pancreas. Barium contrast radiograph showing partial duodenal obstruction is consistent with an annular pancreas.

4. **Annular pancreas** occurs when the ventral pancreatic bud fuses with the dorsal bud both dorsally and ventrally, thereby forming a **ring of pancreatic tissue** around the duodenum, causing severe **duodenal obstruction** noticed shortly after birth. Newborns and infants are intolerant of oral feeding and often have bilious vomiting. Radiographic evidence of an annular pancreas is indicated by a duodenal obstruction in which a "double bubble" sign is often seen because of dilation of the stomach and distal duodenum.

IX Cross-Sectional Anatomy

A. **At About T12 Where the Portal Triad is Located (Figure 11-8)**

B. **At the Level of the Gallbladder (Figure 11-9)**

C. **At the Level of the Hilum of the Kidneys (Figure 11-10)**

X Radiology

A. **Radiograph of the Stomach and Small Intestines After a Barium Meal (Figure 11-11A)**

B. **AP Radiograph of the Large Intestine After a Barium Enema (Figure 11-11B)**

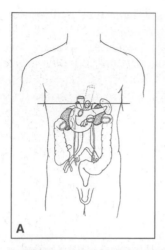

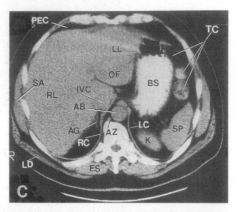

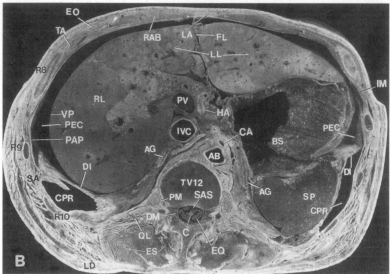

● **Figure 11-8 Cross-Section and CT Scan at About T12, Where the Portal Triad is Located. (A)** A schematic to show where the cross section was taken. **(B)** A cross-section through a cadaver. **(C)** A CT scan. Note the various structures as indicated by the key. In addition, note the psoas major and quadratus lumborum muscles along the sides of the vertebral body. The right and left lobes of the liver are shown in their relationship to the portal vein, common hepatic artery, and IVC. The right adrenal gland lies posterolateral to the IVC. The left adrenal gland lies between the body of the stomach and the abdominal aorta. Abdominal aorta (AB), Adrenal gland (AG), Azygous vein (AZ), Body of stomach (BS), Sacral spinal cord (C), Celiac artery (CA), Posterior costophrenic recess (CPR), Diaphragm (DI), Dura mater (DM), External abdominal oblique (EO), Cauda equina (EQ), Erector spinae (ES), Falciform ligament (FL), Common hepatic artery (HA), Intercostal muscles (IM), Inferior vena cava (IVC), Kidney (K), Linea alba (LA), Left crus of diaphragm (LC), Latissimus dorsi (LD), Left lobe of liver (LL), Oblique fissure (OF), Parietal peritoneum (PAP), Peritoneal cavity (PEC), Psoas major (PM), Portal vein (PV), Quadratus lumborum (QL), Ribs 8–10 (R8-10), Rectus abdominis (RAB), Right crus of diaphragm (RC), Right lobe of liver (RL), Serratus anterior (SA), Subarachnoid space (lumbar cistern) (SAS), Spleen (SP), Transversus abdominis (TA), Transverse colon (TC), Body of thoracic vertebra 12 (TV12), Visceral peritoneum (VP).

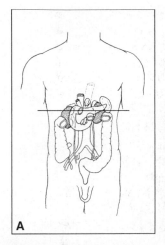

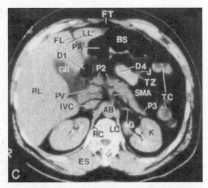

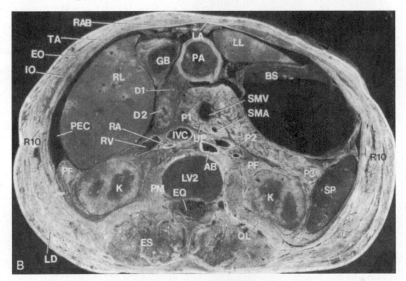

● **Figure 11-9 Cross-Section and CT Scan at the Level of the Gallbladder. (A)** A schematic to show where the cross-section was taken. **(B)** A cross-section through a cadaver. **(C)** A CT scan. Note the various structures as indicated by the key. The second part of the duodenum is adjacent to the head of the pancreas. The body of the pancreas extends to the left, posterior to the stomach. The tail of the pancreas reaches the spleen. The uncinate process of the pancreas lies posterior to the superior mesenteric artery. The gallbladder lies between the right and left lobes of the liver just to the right of the antrum of the stomach. Note the location of the adrenal gland. A large mass in this area is indicative of a pheochromocytoma or neuroblastoma, both of which are associated with the adrenal medulla. Abdominal aorta (AB), Adrenal gland (AG), Body of stomach (BS), First part of duodenum (D1), Second part of duodenum (D2), Fourth part of duodenum (D4), External abdominal oblique (EO), Cauda equina (EQ), Erector spinae (ES), Falciform ligament (FL), Fat (FT), Gallbladder (GB), Internal abdominal oblique (IO), Inferior vena cava (IVC), Jejunum (J), Kidney (K), Linea alba (LA), Left crus of diaphragm (LC), Latissimus dorsi (LD), Left lobe of liver (LL), Body of lumbar vertebra 2 (LV2), Head of pancreas (P1), Body of pancreas (P2), Tail of pancreas (P3), Antrum of stomach (PA), Peritoneal cavity (PEC), Perirenal fat (PF), Psoas major (PM), Portal vein (PV), Quadratus lumborum (QL), Rib 10 (R10), Renal artery (RA), Rectus abdominis (RAB), Right crus of diaphragm (RC), Right lobe of liver (RL), Renal vein (RV), Superior mesenteric artery (SMA), Superior mesenteric vein (SMV), Spleen (SP), Transversus abdominis (TA), Transverse colon (TC), Ligament of Treitz (TZ), Uncinate process of pancreas (UP).

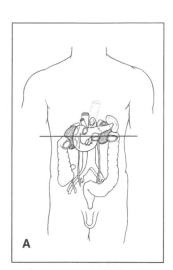

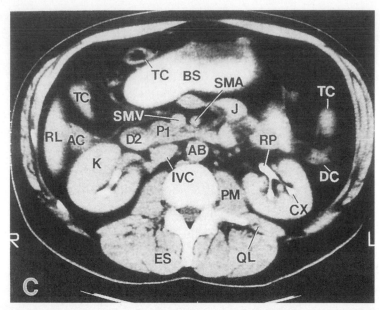

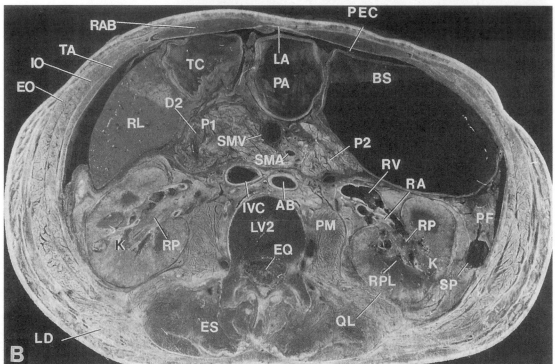

● **Figure 11-10 Cross-Section and CT Scan at the Level of the Hilum of the Kidney. (A)** A schematic to show where the cross-section was taken. **(B)** A cross-section through a cadaver. **(C)** A CT scan. Note the various structures as indicated by the key. The IVC and the abdominal aorta lie side-by-side as both vessels pass posterior to the pancreas. The second part of the duodenum contacts the right kidney and the right lobe of the liver. The left renal vein lies anterior to the renal artery. Abdominal aorta (AB), ascending colon (AC), body of stomach (BS), renal calyx (minor) (CX), second part of duodenum (D2), descending colon (DC), external abdominal oblique (EO), cauda equina (EQ), erector spinae (ES), internal abdominal oblique (IO), inferior vena cava (IVC), jejunum (J), kidney (K), linea alba (LA), latissimus dorsi (LD), body of lumbar vertebra 2 (LV2), head of pancreas (P1), body of pancreas (P2), antrum of stomach (PA), peritoneal cavity (PEC), perirenal fat (PF), psoas major (PM), quadratus lumborum (QL), renal artery (RA), rectus abdominis (RAB), right lobe of liver (RL), renal pelvis (RP), renal papilla (RPL), renal vein (RV), superior mesenteric artery (SMA), superior mesenteric vein (SMV), spleen (lower tip) (SP), transversus abdominis (TA), transverse colon (TC),.

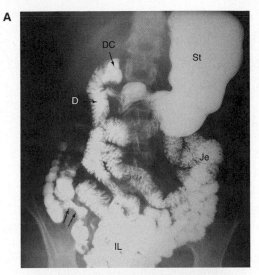

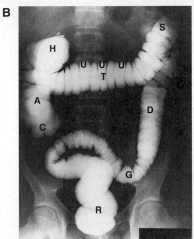

● **Figure 11-11 (A) Radiograph of the Stomach and Small Intestines After a Barium Meal.** Note the structures indicated. Note the barium-filled stomach (St), duodenal cap (DC), duodenal C-loop (D), feathered jejunum in the upper portion and left side of the abdomen (Je), and the relatively formless mucosa of the ileum (Il) in the lower portion and right side of the abdomen. The terminal ileum (arrows) entering the cecum is shown. **(B) Radiograph After a Barium Enema.** A = ascending colon, C = cecum, D = descending colon, G = sigmoid colon, H = hepatic or right colic flexure, R = rectum, S = splenic or left colic flexure, T = transverse colon, U = haustra.

Chapter 12

Sigmoid Colon, Rectum, and Anal Canal

① Sigmoid Colon (Figure 12-1)

A. General Features. The sigmoid colon is a segment of the large intestine between the descending colon and rectum whose primary function is **storage of feces**. It begins at vertebral level S1 (sacral promontory; pelvic inlet) and ends at S3 (**rectosigmoid junction**), where **teniae coli** (longitudinal bands of smooth muscle) are replaced by a complete circular layer of smooth muscle of the rectum. The sigmoid colon is suspended by the **sigmoid mesocolon** (i.e. intraperitoneal). The **left ureter** and **left common iliac artery** lie at the apex of the sigmoid mesocolon. The arterial supply is from the inferior mesenteric artery via the **sigmoid arteries** and **rectosigmoid artery**. The venous drainage is to the sigmoid veins → inferior mesenteric vein → hepatic portal system.

B. Clinical Considerations
1. **Colonic aganglionosis (Hirschsprung disease)** is caused by the arrest of the caudal migration of neural crest cells. The hallmark is the absence of ganglionic cells in the myenteric and submucosal plexuses most commonly in the sigmoid colon and rectum, resulting in a narrow segment of colon (i.e. the colon fails to relax). Although the ganglionic cells are absent, there is a proliferation of hypertrophied nerve fiber bundles. The most characteristic functional finding is the failure of the internal anal sphincter to relax after rectal distention (i.e. abnormal rectoanal reflex). Mutations of the **RET proto-oncogene** (chromosome 10q.11.2) have been associated with Hirschsprung disease. Clinical findings include a distended abdomen, inability to pass meconium, gushing of fecal material on a rectal digital examination, fecal retention, and a loss of peristalsis in the colon segment distal to the normal innervated colon.
2. **Diverticulosis** is the presence of diverticula (abnormal pouches or sacs), most commonly found in the sigmoid colon in patients older than 60 years of age. It is associated with a low-fiber, modern Western diet. Perforation or inflammation of the diverticula results in **diverticulitis**. Clinical findings include pain in the left lumbar region, palpable inflammatory mass in the left lumbar region, fever, leukocytosis, ileus, and peritonitis.
3. **Flexible sigmoidoscopy** permits examination of the sigmoid colon and rectum. During sigmoidoscopy, the large intestine may be punctured if the angle at the rectosigmoid junction is not negotiated properly. At the rectosigmoid junction, the sigmoid colon bends in an **anterior direction and to the left**. During sigmoidoscopy, the transverse rectal folds (Houston's valves) must be negotiated also.
4. **Colostomy.** The sigmoid colon is often used in a **colostomy** because of the mobility rendered by the sigmoid mesocolon (mesentery). An ostomy is an intestinal diversion that brings out a portion of the gastrointestinal tract through the **rectus**

abdominis muscle. A colostomy may ablate the pelvic nerve plexus, which results in loss of ejaculation, loss of erection, urinary bladder retention, and decreased peristalsis in the remaining colon.

Ⅱ Rectum

A. **General Features.** The rectum is a segment of the large intestine between the sigmoid colon and the anal canal. It begins at vertebral level S3 and ends at the tip of the coccyx (**anorectal junction**), where the **puborectalis muscle** forms a U-shaped sling causing a 90-degree **perineal flexure**. The **ampulla of the rectum** lies just above the pelvic diaphragm and generates the **urge to defecate** when feces move into it. The rectum contains three **transverse rectal folds (Houston's valves)** formed by the mucosa, submucosa, and inner circular layer of smooth muscle that permanently extend into the lumen of the rectum.

The arterial supply is chiefly from the inferior mesenteric artery via the **superior rectal artery**; the **middle rectal artery**, **inferior rectal artery**, and **middle sacral artery** also play a role. The venous drainage is chiefly to the superior rectal vein → inferior mesenteric vein → hepatic portal system; the middle rectal vein and inferior rectal vein also play a role and drain into the inferior vena cava (IVC).

B. **Clinical Consideration. Rectal prolapse** is the protrusion of the **full thickness of the rectum** through the anus (should be distinguished from **mucosal prolapse**, which is the protrusion of only the rectal mucosa through the anus). Clinical findings include bowel protruding through anus, bleeding, anal pain, mucous discharge, and anal incontinence cause by stretching of the **internal and external anal sphincters** or stretch injury to the **pudendal nerve.**

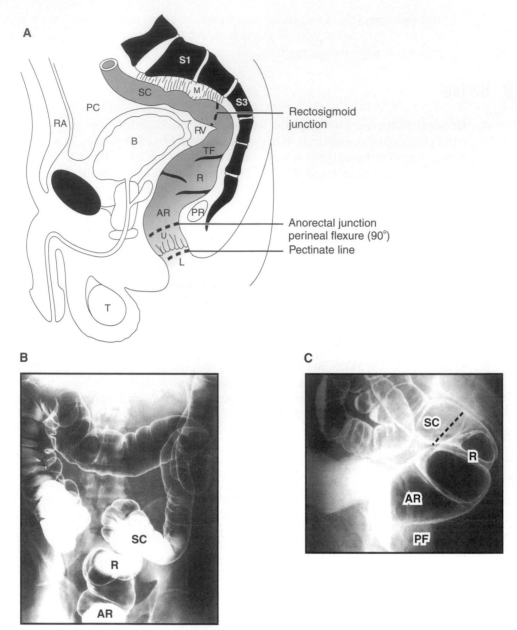

● **Figure 12-1 (A) Sagittal View of the Male Pelvis.** The sigmoid colon (SC) extends from vertebral level S1 to S3 suspended by the sigmoid mesocolon (M) and ends at the rectosigmoid junction (dotted line). The rectum (R) and ampulla of the rectum (AR) are shown along with the transverse rectal folds (TF; Houston's valve). The rectum ends at the anorectal junction (dotted line) at the tip of the coccyx where the puborectalis muscle (PR) maintains a perineal flexure of 90 degrees. The anal canal is divided into the upper anal canal (U) and lower anal canal (L) by the pectinate line. RV = rectovesical pouch, B = urinary bladder, T = testes, PC = peritoneal cavity, RA = rectus abdominis. **(B)** AP barium radiograph shows the sigmoid colon (SC), rectum (R), and ampulla of the rectum (AR). **(C)** A lateral barium radiograph shows the sigmoid colon (SC), rectosigmoid junction (dotted line), rectum (R), ampulla of the rectum (AR), and perineal flexure (PF).

III   **Anal Canal (Figure 12-2)** is divided into the upper and lower anal canal by the **pectinate line**. The anal canal is surrounded by the **internal anal sphincter** (a continuation of smooth muscle from the rectum with involuntary control via autonomic innervation) and the **external anal sphincter** (striated muscle under voluntary control via the pudendal nerve).

A.   Upper anal canal extends from the anorectal junction (perineal flexure) to the pectinate line. The mucosa of the upper anal canal is thrown into longitudinal folds called the **anal columns (of Morgagni)**. The base of the anal columns defines the **pectinate line**. At the base of the anal columns are folds of tissue called the **anal valves**. Behind the anal valves are small, blind pouches called the **anal sinuses** into which the **anal glands** open.

B.   Lower anal canal extends from the pectinate line to the **anal verge** (the point at which perianal skin begins).

C.   Clinical Considerations
1.   **Internal hemorrhoids** are varicosities of the **superior rectal veins**. They are located above the pectinate line and are covered by rectal mucosa. Clinical findings include: bleeding, mucous discharge, prolapse, pruritus, and pain.
2.   **External hemorrhoids** are varicosities of the **inferior rectal veins**. They are located below the pectinate line near the anal verge and are covered by skin. Clinical findings include: bleeding, swelling, and pain.

IV   **Defecation Reflex.** Sensory impulses from **pressure-sensitive receptors** within the ampulla of the rectum travel to sacral spinal cord levels when feces are present. Motor impulses travel with the **pelvic splanchnic nerves (parasympathetics; S2 through S4)**, which increase peristalsis and relax the internal anal sphincter. If the external anal sphincter and puborectalis muscle are also relaxed, defecation takes place with the help of contraction of the anterior abdominal wall muscles and closure of the glottis. If the external anal sphincter and puborectalis muscle are voluntarily contracted via the **pudendal nerve**, defecation is delayed and the feces moves back into the sigmoid colon for storage. The **hypogastric plexus** and **lumbar splanchnic nerves (sympathetics)** decrease peristalsis and maintain tone of the internal anal sphincter.

V   **Radiology**

A.   Hirschsprung Disease and Diverticulosis (Figure 12-3)

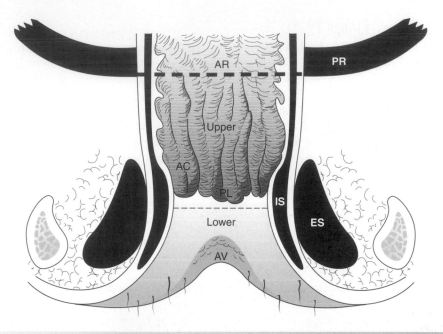

Feature	Upper Anal Canal	Lower Anal Canal
Arterial supply	Superior rectal artery (branch of inferior mesenteric artery)	Inferior rectal artery (branch of internal pudendal artery)
Venous drainage	Superior rectal vein → inferior mesenteric vein → hepatic portal system	Inferior rectal vein → internal pudendal vein → internal iliac vein → IVC
Lymphatic drainage	Deep nodes	Superficial inguinal nodes
Innervation	Motor: autonomic innervation of internal anal sphincter (smooth muscle)	Motor: somatic innervation (pudendal nerve) of external anal sphincter (striated muscle)
	Sensory: stretch sensation; no pain sensation	Sensory: pain, temperature, touch sensation
Embryologic derivation	Endoderm (hindgut)	Ectoderm (proctodeum)
Epithelium	Simple columnar	Stratified squamous
Tumors	Palpable enlarged superficial nodes will not be found	Palpable enlarged superficial nodes will be found
	Patients do not complain of pain	Patients do complain of pain
Hemorrhoids	Internal hemorrhoids (varicosities of superior rectal veins)	External hemorrhoids (varicosities of inferior rectal veins)
	Covered by rectal mucosa	Covered by skin
	Patients do not complain of pain	Patients do complain of pain

IVC = inferior vena cava.

● **Figure 12-2 Diagram of the Anal Canal.** Note the following structures: anal columns (AC), anal verge (AV), pectinate line (PL), internal anal sphincter (IS), and external anal sphincter (ES). AR = ampulla of rectum, PR = puborectalis muscle.

A

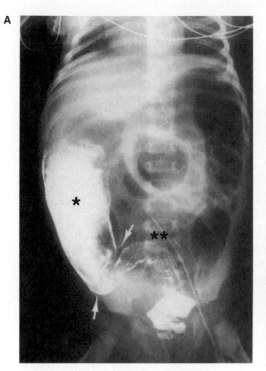

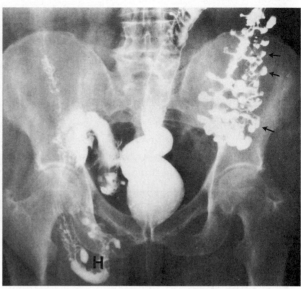

B

● **Figure 12-3 (A) Hirschsprung Disease.** A barium radiograph shows a narrowed rectum and a classic transition zone (arrows). The upper segment (*) of normal colon is distended with fecal material. The distal segment (**) of the colon is narrow and is the portion of the colon where the myenteric plexus of ganglion cells is absent. **(B) Colonic Diverticulosis.** A postevacuation barium radiograph shows numerous small outpouchings or diverticula (arrows) from the colonic lumen. These diverticula are filled with barium and fecal material. Note the hernia (H) on the right.

Chapter 13

Spleen

I **General Features (Figure 13-1).** The spleen is located in the left hypochondriac region anterior to the 9th, 10th, and 11th ribs, which puts the spleen in jeopardy in the case of rib fractures. The spleen does not extend below the costal margin and therefore is not palpable unless splenomegaly is present. It is attached to the stomach by the **gastrosplenic ligament**, which contains the **short gastric arteries and veins** and the **left gastroepiploic artery and vein**. The spleen is attached to the kidney by the **splenorenal ligament**, which contains the **five terminal branches of the splenic artery**, **tributaries of the splenic vein**, and the **tail of the pancreas**. **Accessory spleens** occur in 20% of the population and are commonly located near the hilum or the tail of the pancreas, or within the gastrosplenic ligament.

II **Functions.** The functions of the spleen include removal of old or abnormal red blood cells (RBCs), removal of inclusion bodies from RBCs (e.g. **Howell-Jolly bodies** [nuclear remnants]; **Pappenheimer bodies** [iron granules]; **Heinz bodies** [denatured hemoglobin]), removal of poorly opsonized pathogens, IgM production by plasma cells, storage of platelets, and protection from infection.

III **Arterial Supply.** The arterial supply is from the **splenic artery** (the largest branch of the celiac trunk). The splenic artery gives off the following branches: **dorsal pancreatic artery**, **great pancreatic artery**, **caudal pancreatic arteries**, **short gastric arteries**, and **left gastroepiploic artery**, and ends with **five terminal branches**. The five terminal branches of the splenic artery supply individual segments of the spleen with no anastomoses between them (i.e. **end arteries**), so that obstruction or ligation of any terminal branch will result in **splenic infarction** (i.e. the spleen is very prone to infarction). **Splenic artery aneurysms** show a particularly high incidence of rupture in **pregnant women** such that these aneurysms should be resected in women of childbearing age.

IV **Venous Drainage.** The venous drainage is to the **splenic vein** via tributaries. The splenic vein joins the superior mesenteric vein to form the portal vein. The inferior mesenteric vein usually joins the splenic vein. **Splenic vein thrombosis** is most commonly associated with **pancreatitis** and shows the following clinical signs: gastric varices and upper gastrointestinal bleeding.

V **Clinical Considerations**

A. **Splenectomy** is the surgical removal of the spleen. Nearby anatomic structures, which may be injured during a splenectomy, include the **gastric wall (stomach)** if the short gastric arteries are compromised, the **tail of the pancreas** if the caudal pancreatic arteries are compromised or during manipulation of the splenorenal ligament, and the **left**

kidney during manipulation of the splenorenal ligament. The most common complication of a splenectomy is **atelectasis of the left lower lobe of the lung. Thrombocytosis** (i.e. increased number of platelets within the blood) is common postoperatively such that anticoagulation therapy may be necessary to prevent spontaneous thrombosis. Abnormal RBCs with bizarre shapes, some of which contain **Howell-Jolly bodies** (nuclear remnants), are found in the blood postoperatively.

B. **Overwhelming Postsplenectomy Sepsis.** Postsplenectomy patients (especially children) are at a great risk for **bacterial septicemia** because of decreased opsonic production, decreased IgM levels, and decreased clearance of bacteria from blood. The most commonly involved pathogens are *Streptococcus pneumoniae, Haemophilus influenzae,* and *Neisseria meningitidis.* Patients with **sickle cell anemia** usually undergo "autosplenectomy" as a result of multiple infarcts caused by stagnation of abnormal RBCs and are therefore prime targets for postsplenectomy sepsis. Clinical signs include influenza-like symptoms that progress to high fever, shock, and death.

C. **Hypersplenism** describes a state of increased splenic function (i.e. not to be confused with splenomegaly). Clinical findings include anemia (leading to pallor and fatigue), leukopenia (leading to increased susceptibility to infection), thrombocytopenia (leading to easy bruising and nosebleeds), and a compensatory increase in bone marrow activity. It may be caused by hematopoietic disorders (e.g. hereditary spherocytosis, thalassemia) or immune disorders (i.e. immune thrombocytopenic purpura).

   1. **Hereditary spherocytosis** is a genetic hematopoietic disease characterized by a deficiency in the **spectrin** protein that helps stabilize the RBC membrane and is usually caused by a mutation in the gene for **ankyrin.** This results in anisocytosis (variation in size of RBCs) and spherocytes with no central pallor zone. Clinical signs include anemia, fatigue, jaundice, pigmented gallstones, and splenomegaly. The treatment is splenectomy for all patients.

   2. **Immune thrombocytopenic purpura** is an immune disorder in which circulating antibodies (IgG) directed against **platelet-associated antigen** cause the rapid destruction of platelets. Clinical signs include low platelet count, easy bruising, petechiae, mucosal bleeding, menorrhagia, and increased megakaryocyte count. The treatment is steroid (e.g. prednisone) administration, platelet transfusions, and plasmapheresis. Splenectomy is recommended for patients refractive to steroid administration.

D. **Splenic vein thrombosis** most commonly is associated with pancreatitis. Clinical signs include gastric varices and upper gastrointestinal bleeding.

E. **Splenomegaly.** The causes of splenomegaly include autoimmune disease (e.g. systemic lupus erythematous, rheumatoid arthritis), infectious disease (e.g. mononucleosis, visceral leishmaniasis), infiltrative disease (e.g. lysosomal storage disease, leukemias), extramedullary hematopoiesis (e.g. myeloproliferative diseases such as myelofibrosis and myeloid metaplasia), and vascular congestion (portal hypertension in cirrhosis). In the United States, myeloproliferative disease and lymphoid malignancies (e.g. chronic lymphocytic leukemia) are the most common causes of massive splenomegaly.

F. **Splenic Infarct.** An infarction is a process by which coagulating necrosis develops in an area distal to the occlusion of an end artery. The necrotic tissue or zone is called an infarct.

VI Radiology (Figure 13-2)

A. **CT Scan at the Level of the Liver and Spleen**

B. **Splenomegaly**

C. **Chronic Lymphocytic Leukemia**

D. **CT Scan of Splenic Infarction**

E. **Laceration of the Spleen**

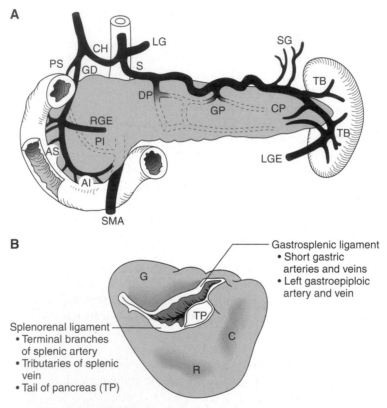

● **Figure 13-1 (A) Diagram of Arterial Supply of the Spleen.** The splenic artery (S) is the largest branch of the celiac trunk. LG = left gastric artery, CH = common hepatic artery, PS = posterior-superior pancreaticoduodenal artery, PI = posterior-inferior pancreaticoduodenal artery, GD = gastroduodenal artery, AS = anterior-superior pancreaticoduodenal artery, AI = anterior-inferior pancreaticoduodenal artery, RGE = right gastroepiploic artery, LGE = left gastroepiploic artery, DP = dorsal pancreatic artery, GP = great pancreatic artery, CP = caudal pancreatic arteries, SG = short gastric arteries, TB = terminal branches of splenic artery, SMA = superior mesenteric artery. **(B) Diagram of Visceral Surface of the Spleen.** The gastrosplenic ligament and splenorenal ligament are shown along with the structures they contain. G = gastric depression, C = colon depression, R = renal depression.

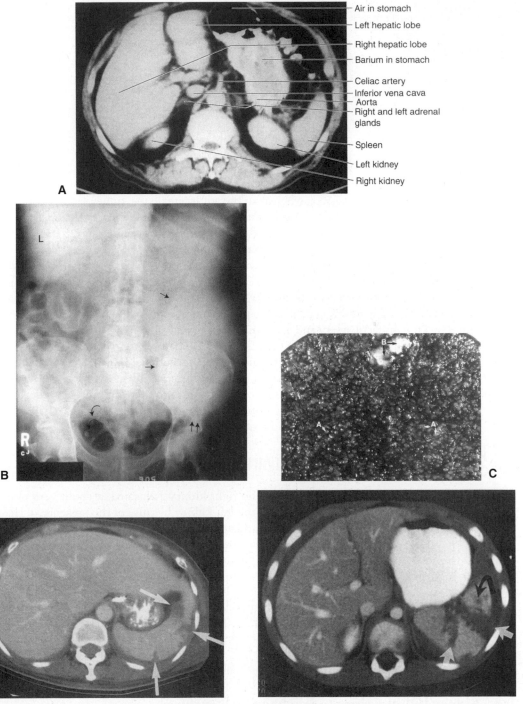

● **Figure 13-2 (A) CT Scan at the Level of the Liver and Spleen. (B) Splenomegaly.** Radiograph shows that the water-density spleen is enlarged (straight arrow) and that the inferior margin projects just above the left hip (double straight arrows). The enlarged spleen has pushed the intestinal gas into the right abdomen. The liver (L) size is normal. Note the small intravenous stones (phleboliths; curved arrows) secondary to calcified thrombi. **(C) Chronic Lymphocytic Leukemia.** Photograph of a gross specimen shows diffuse enlargement of the white pulp (A) with focally prominent tumor nodules (B). **(D) Splenic Infarction.** CT scan shows multiple wedge-shaped areas of diminished contrast enhancement in the spleen representing multiple areas of embolic infarction (arrows). **(E) Laceration of the Spleen.** CT scan shows two lacerations that intersect (straight arrows). Contusion causes heterogeneous enhancement in the anterior fragment of the spleen (curved arrow). Hemoperitoneum is present.

Chapter 14

Kidney

I   **General Features (Figure 14-1A).** A human adult kidney in the fresh state is reddish-brown and is about 11 cm in length, 6 cm in width, and 3 cm in thickness. In adult males, the kidney weighs about 150 g, whereas in the adult female the kidney weighs about 135 g. The kidneys are retroperitoneal organs that lie on the ventral surface of the quadratus lumborum muscle and lateral to the psoas muscle and vertebral column. The kidneys are directly covered by a fibrous capsule called the **renal capsule (or true capsule)**, which can be readily stripped from the surface of the kidney except in some pathologic conditions in which it is strongly adherent because of scarring. The kidneys are further surrounded by the **perirenal fascia of Gerota (or false capsule)**, which is important in staging renal cell carcinoma. The perirenal fascia of Gerota defines the **perirenal space** that contains the **kidney**, **adrenal gland**, **ureter**, **gonadal artery and vein**, and **perirenal fat**. Any fat located outside the perirenal space is called **pararenal fat**, which is most abundant posterolaterally. At the concave medial margin of each kidney is a vertical cleft called the **renal hilum**, where the following anatomic structures are arranged in an anterior to posterior direction: **renal vein (most anterior)** → **renal artery** → **renal pelvis (most posterior)**. The renal hilum is continuous with a space called the **renal sinus** that contains the renal pelvis, major and minor calyces, renal blood vessels, nerves, lymphatics, and a variable amount of fat.

II   **Kidney Surface Projections (Figure 14-1B, C)**

   A. Right Kidney. The upper pole of the right kidney is located at about vertebral level T12. The right kidney is lower than the left kidney because of the presence of the liver on the right side. The right kidney is related to rib 12. The renal hilum of the right kidney lies 5 cm from the median plane just below the transpyloric plane (which passes through vertebral level L1). The renal hilum of the right kidney lies about 5 cm from the median plane at the lower border of the spinous process of vertebra L1.

   B. Left Kidney. The upper pole of the left kidney is located at about vertebral level T11. The left kidney is higher than the right kidney. The left kidney is related to ribs 11 and 12. The renal hilum of the left kidney lies 5 cm from the median plane along the transpyloric plane (which passes through vertebral level L1). The renal hilum of the left kidney lies about 5 cm from the median plane at the lower border of the spinous process of vertebra L1.

III   **Kidney Relationships to Neighboring Structures**

   A. Anterior Surface
     1. Right Kidney. The anterior surface of the right kidney is related to the right suprarenal gland, liver, descending part of the duodenum, right colic flexure of the large intestine, and small intestine.

2. **Left Kidney.** The anterior surface of the left kidney is related to the left suprarenal gland, spleen, pancreas, stomach, left colic flexure of the large intestine, and jejunum.

B. **Posterior Surface**
1. **Right Kidney.** The posterior surface of the right kidney is related to rib 12, the diaphragm, psoas major, quadratus lumborum, tendon of the transversus abdominis muscle, and transverse process of vertebra L1.
2. **Left Kidney.** The posterior surface of the left kidney is related to ribs 11 and 12, the diaphragm, psoas major, quadratus lumborum, tendon of the transversus abdominis muscle, and transverse process of vertebra L1.

IV **Internal Macroscopic Anatomy of the Kidney.** A coronal section through the kidney reveals the following macroscopic structures:

A. **Renal Cortex.** The renal cortex lies under the renal capsule and also extends between the renal pyramids as the **renal columns of Bertin.** The renal cortex may be divided into the **cortical labyrinth** and the **medullary rays.**

B. **Renal Medulla.** The renal medulla is composed of **5 to 11 renal pyramids of Malpighi** whose tips terminate as **5 to 11 renal papillae.** The base of a renal pyramid abuts the renal cortex, whereas the tip of a renal pyramid (i.e. the renal papillae) abuts a minor calyx. The renal medulla may be divided into the **outer medulla** and **inner medulla.** The **papillary ducts of Bellini** open onto the surface of the renal papillae at the **area cribrosa.**

C. **Five to 11 Minor Calyces.** The minor calyces are cup-shaped structures that abut the renal papillae. Each minor calyx may receive one to three renal papillae.

D. **Two to Three Major Calyces.** The major calyces are continuous with the minor calyces.

E. **Renal Pelvis.** The renal pelvis is continuous with the major calyces. The renal pelvis tapers inferomedially as it traverses the renal hilum to become continuous with the ureter at the **ureteropelvic junction,** which is usually found in an extrahilar location adjacent to the lower part of the medial border of the kidney.

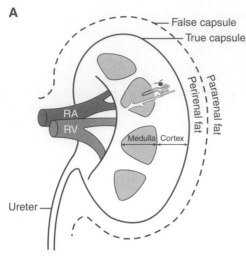

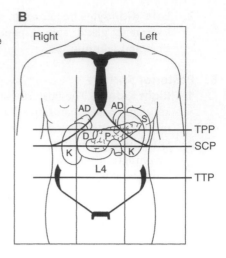

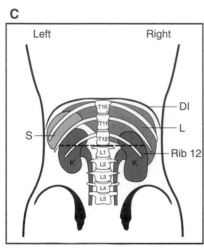

● **Figure 14-1 (A) Diagram of General Features of the Kidney.** Note the true capsule and false capsule. Note the location of the perirenal fat and pararenal fat. **(B) Anterior Kidney Surface Projections.** A commonly used clinical method for subdividing the abdomen into specific regions uses the subcostal plane (SCP), transtubercular plane (TTP; joining the tubercles of the iliac crest), and midclavicular lines (MC) is shown. Note also the transpyloric plane (TTP). **(C) Posterior Kidney Surface Projections.** Note that the pleura extends across rib 12 (dotted line). AD = suprarenal glands, D = duodenum, P = pancreas, L1–L5 = lumbar vertebrae, T10–T12 = thoracic vertebrae, S = spleen, K = kidney, L = liver, D1 = diaphragm.

ⓥ Vasculature of the Kidney (Figure 14-2)

A. Arterial Supply

1. The abdominal aorta branches between vertebral level L1 and L2 into the **right renal artery** and **left renal artery.** The longer right renal artery passes posterior to the inferior vena cava (IVC) on its path to the right kidney. During its extrarenal course, each renal artery gives rise to the **inferior suprarenal arteries** and other branches that supply perinephric tissue, the renal capsule, and the proximal part of the ureter. Near the renal hilum, each renal artery divides into an **anterior division** and **posterior division**.

2. The anterior division branches into **four anterior segmental arteries**, which supply anterior segments of the kidney called the **apical segmental artery, anterosuperior segmental artery, anteroinferior segmental artery,** and **inferior segmental artery.** The posterior division continues as the **posterior segmental artery,** which supplies the posterior segment of the kidney. The segmental arteries are **end arteries** (i.e. they do not anastomose) and are distributed to various segments of the kidney. Segmental arteries have the following clinical importance:

   a. Because there is very little collateral circulation between segmental arteries (i.e. end arteries), an **avascular line (Brodel's white line)** is created between the anterior and posterior segments such that a longitudinal incision through the kidney will produce minimal bleeding. This approach is useful for surgical removal of renal (staghorn) calculi.

b. Ligation of a segmental artery results in necrosis of the entire segment of the kidney.

c. **Supernumerary (or aberrant) segmental arteries** are arteries that form during fetal development and persist in the adult. They may arise from either the renal artery (**hilar**) or directly from the aorta (**polar**). Ligation of a supernumerary segmental artery results in necrosis of the entire segment of the kidney.

3. The segmental arteries branch into **5 to 11 interlobar arteries.** The interlobar arteries branch into the **arcuate arteries,** which travel along the base of the renal pyramids at the corticomedullary junction. The arcuate arteries branch into the **interlobular arteries,** which travel through the cortex toward the capsule and branch into numerous **afferent arterioles.** Each afferent arteriole forms a capillary bed (or tuft) called the **renal glomerulus,** which is drained by an **efferent arteriole.**

4. The efferent arteriole of renal glomeruli from cortical and midcortical nephrons branches into a **cortical peritubular capillary bed.** The efferent arteriole of renal glomeruli from juxtamedullary nephrons branches into **12 to 25 descending vasa recta,** which are long, straight capillaries that run to varying depths of the medulla. The ends of the descending vasa recta give rise to a **medullary peritubular capillary bed.**

B. Venous Drainage

1. **From the Kidney Surface and Capsule.** The venous ends a capillary bed near the kidney surface and capillaries of the kidney capsule drain into **stellate veins.** Stellate veins drain into **interlobular veins.** The interlobular veins drain into **arcuate veins.**

2. **From the Kidney Cortex.** The venous ends of the cortical peritubular capillary bed converge to drain into **interlobular veins.** The interlobular veins drain into **arcuate veins.**

3. **From the Kidney Medulla.** The venous ends of the medullary capillary bed converge to form the **ascending vasa recta,** which completes the hairpin loop. The ascending vasa recta drains into both the **interlobular veins** and **arcuate veins.**

4. The arcuate veins drain into **interlobar veins,** which anastomose and converge to form several renal veins that unite in a variable fashion to form the **renal vein.** The veins draining the kidney have no segmental organization like the arterial supply described above. The renal veins lie anterior to the renal arteries at the renal hilum. The longer left renal vein passes anterior to the aorta on its path to the IVC. The renal veins ultimately drain into the IVC.

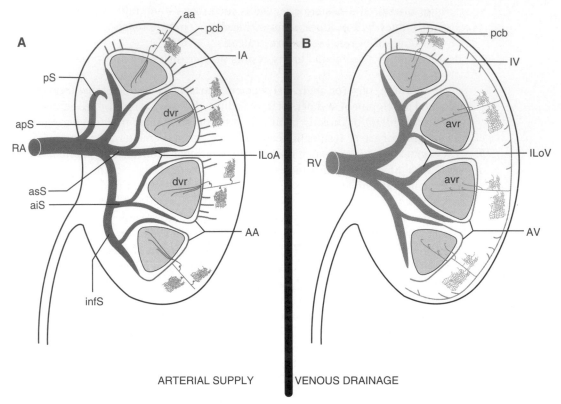

A

aa
pcb
IA
pS
apS
dvr
RA
ILoA
asS
dvr
aiS
AA
infS

B

pcb
IV
avr
RV
ILoV
avr
AV

ARTERIAL SUPPLY | VENOUS DRAINAGE

● **Figure 14-2 Vasculature of the Kidney. (A) Arterial Supply of the Kidney. (B) Venous Drainage of the Kidney.** RA = renal artery, pS = posterior segmental artery, apS = apical segmental artery, asS = anterosuperior segmental artery, aiS = anteroinferior segmental artery, infS = inferior segmental artery, ILoA = interlobar artery, aa = afferent arteriole, pcb = peritubular capillary bed, AA = arcuate artery, dvr = descending vasa recta, avr = ascending vasa recta, AV = arcuate vein, IV = interlobular vein, IA = interlobular artery, ILoV = interlobar vein, RV = renal vein.

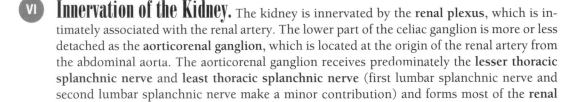

VI **Innervation of the Kidney.** The kidney is innervated by the **renal plexus**, which is intimately associated with the renal artery. The lower part of the celiac ganglion is more or less detached as the **aorticorenal ganglion**, which is located at the origin of the renal artery from the abdominal aorta. The aorticorenal ganglion receives predominately the **lesser thoracic splanchnic nerve** and **least thoracic splanchnic nerve** (first lumbar splanchnic nerve and second lumbar splanchnic nerve make a minor contribution) and forms most of the **renal plexus**. The renal plexus contains only **sympathetic components**. There is no (or at least very minimal) parasympathetic innervation of the kidney.

A. Parasympathetic. None (or at least very minimal).

B. Sympathetic. Preganglionic neuronal cell bodies are located in the **intermediolateral cell column** of the spinal cord. Preganglionic axons pass through the paravertebral ganglia (do not synapse) to become the **lesser thoracic splanchnic nerve, least thoracic splanchnic nerve, first lumbar splanchnic nerve**, and **second lumbar splanchnic nerve** and travel to the **aorticorenal ganglion**. Postganglionic neuronal cell bodies are located in the aorticorenal ganglion. Postganglionic axons enter the **renal plexus** and are distributed to the **renal vasculature**, including the **juxtaglomerular cells**, where they play an important role in the regulation of blood pressure by effecting renin release. Postganglionic sympathetic axons release **norepinephrine (NE)** as a neurotransmitter, which binds to adrenergic receptors (a G-protein–linked receptor).

C. **Sensory Innervation.** Afferent (sensory) neurons whose cell bodies are located in the **dorsal root ganglion** run with the **least thoracic splanchnic nerve, first lumbar splanchnic nerve,** and **second lumbar splanchnic nerve** and relay pain information from the kidney to T12 through L2 spinal cord segments within the central nervous system (CNS). The pain associated with kidney disease may be referred over the **T12 through L2 dermatomes** (i.e. lumbar region, inguinal region, and anterosuperior thigh). Note that the sensory innervation runs with the sympathetic component.

Ⅶ Clinical Considerations

A. **Rotation of the Kidney.** During the relative ascent of the kidneys, the kidneys rotate 90 degrees medially so that the renal hilus is normally orientated in a medial direction.

B. **Ascent of the Kidney.** The fetal metanephros is located in the sacral region, whereas the adult kidneys are normally located at vertebral levels T12 through L3. The change in location (i.e. ascent) results from a disproportionate growth of the embryo caudal to the metanephros.

C. **Horseshoe kidney** occurs when the inferior poles of both kidneys fuse during fetal development. The horseshoe kidney gets trapped behind the **inferior mesenteric artery** as the kidney attempts to ascend toward the normal adult location.

D. **Duplication of renal pelvis and ureter** occurs when the ureteric bud prematurely divides before penetrating the metanephric mesoderm.

E. **Adult Polycystic Kidney Disease (PCKD).** Adult PCKD is most commonly caused (85% of cases) by an **autosomal dominant** mutation of the *ADPKD-1* gene, which is located on the **short arm (p arm) of chromosome 16 (16p)** and encodes for the protein **polycystin** (an integral membrane protein involved in cell-to-cell and cell-to-matrix interactions). Pathologic findings include bilaterally enlarged palpable kidneys; numerous cysts filled with a straw-colored fluid that distort the external contours of the kidney; cysts lined by simple cuboidal or columnar epithelium; cysts arising from any point along the nephron; association with cystic disease in other organs (especially the liver); and association with berry aneurysms within the circle of Willis. Clinical findings include symptoms that become apparent around 40 years of age; heaviness in the loins; bilateral flank and abdominal masses; hematuria; hypertension; azotemia; and uremia. These findings eventually lead to end-stage renal disease.

F. **Childhood Polycystic Kidney Disease (PCKD).** Childhood PCKD is caused by an **autosomal recessive** mutation of a gene linked to the **short arm (p arm) of chromosome 6 (6p)** and encodes for an as yet unidentified protein. Pathologic findings include bilaterally enlarged spongy kidneys that may impede delivery of the infant; numerous cysts that are present but do not distort the external contours of the kidney; cysts that arise from collecting ducts and tubules; cysts that are arranged in a radial pattern perpendicular to the kidney surface; and an association with congenital hepatic fibrosis. Clinical findings include that the condition leads to end-stage renal disease in which 75% of these infants die in the perinatal period.

G. **Genitourinary Tuberculosis.** The spread of tuberculosis leads to small granulomas within the kidney cortex usually near glomeruli. The infection will eventually destroy the renal papillae, which results in an irregular appearance of the minor calyces. Tuberculosis generally proceeds from the kidney toward the urinary bladder (kidney →

bladder) as opposed to schistosomiasis, which proceeds from the urinary bladder toward the kidney (urinary bladder → kidney).

H. **Renal Cell Carcinoma (RCC).** RCC is a malignant neoplasm involving the epithelium lining the renal tubules and ducts and is the most common cancer of the kidney. In 95% of cases, RCC is sporadic and unilateral. In 5% of cases, RCC is hereditary and arises in association with von Hippel-Lindau (VHL) disease, hereditary (autosomal dominant) clear cell carcinoma, or hereditary (autosomal dominant) papillary carcinoma and is multifocal and bilateral. Clinical findings include being more frequent in men; risk factors such as tobacco use and obesity; incidence that peaks at about 60 years of age; hematuria as the most common presenting sign; the classic triad of hematuria, flank pain, and a palpable abdominal mass observed in only 10% of patients; fever; weakness; malaise; weight loss; production of ectopic hormones (e.g. parathyroid-like hormone) leading to a number of paraneoplastic syndromes (e.g. hypercalcemia, polycythemia, hypertension, feminization or masculinization, or Cushing syndrome, one of the great mimics in medicine); and a tendency to metastasize (to lungs and bones) before giving any clinical signs. The major types of RCC are clear cell carcinoma (most common), papillary carcinoma, and chromophobe carcinoma.

I. **Wilms Tumor (WT; nephroblastoma).** WT is the **most common renal malignancy of childhood and** usually presents between 1 and 3 years of age. WT presents as a large, solitary, well-circumscribed mass that on cut section is soft, homogeneous, and tan-gray in color. WT is interesting histologically in that this tumor tends to recapitulate different stages of embryologic formation of the kidney so that three classic histologic areas are described: a stromal area; a blastemal area of tightly packed embryonic cells; and a tubular area. In 95% of the cases, the tumor is sporadic and unilateral. In 5% of the cases, the tumor arises in association with the WAGR (WAGR = Wilms, anivedia, genitourinary abnormalities, and mental retardation) syndrome, Denys-Drash syndrome, or the Beckwith-Wiedemann syndrome. WT is a neoplasm involving the *WT1* **gene** and the *WT2* **gene**, both located on the short arm of chromosome 11 (11p13). The *WT1* gene and the *WT2* gene are anti-oncogenes (or tumor suppressor genes) that encode proteins that suppress the cell cycle.

J. **Kidney Trauma.** Kidney trauma should be suspected in the following situations: fracture of the lower ribs, fracture of the transverse processes of the lumbar vertebrae, gunshot or knife wound over the lower rib cage, and after a car accident when seat belt marks are present. Right kidney trauma is associated with liver trauma whereas left kidney trauma is associated with spleen trauma. Clinical findings include flank mass or tenderness, flank ecchymosis, hypotension, and hematuria. One of the absolute indications for renal exploration is the presence of a **pulsatile or expanding retroperitoneal hematoma** found at laparotomy. The first structures that should be isolated during renal exploration are the **renal artery** and **renal vein** located superior to the inferior mesenteric artery.

K. **Surgical Approach to the Kidney.** An incision is made below and parallel to the 12th rib to prevent inadvertent entry into the pleural space. The incision may be extended to the front of the abdomen by traveling parallel to the inguinal ligament.

Ⅷ Ureter

A. **General Features.** The ureters are 25- to 30-cm-long muscular tubes whose peristaltic contractions convey urine from the renal pelvis to the urinary bladder. The ureters begin at the **ureteropelvic junction**, where the renal pelvis joins the ureter. Within the abdomen, the ureters descend retroperitoneal and anterior to the psoas major muscle, where they cross the pelvic inlet to enter the minor (or true) pelvis. Within the minor (or true) pelvis, the ureters descend retroperitoneal and anterior to the common iliac artery and vein, where they may be compromised by an aneurysm of the common iliac artery. The ureters end at the **ureterovesical junction** surrounded by the **vesical venous plexus**. The ureters end by traveling obliquely through the wall of the urinary bladder (i.e. the **intramural portion of the ureter**) and define the upper limit of the **urinary bladder trigone**. The intramural portion of the ureter functions as a check valve (**ureterovesical valve of Sampson**) to prevent urine reflux.

B. Ureter Relationships to Neighboring Structures. In the male, the ureters pass posterior to the **ductus deferens**. In the female, the ureters pass posterior and inferior to the **uterine artery**, which lies in the **transverse cervical ligament** (or **cardinal ligament of Mackenrodt**), and lie 1 to 2 cm lateral to the **cervix of the uterus**. During gynecologic operations (e.g. hysterectomy), the ureters may be inadvertently injured. The most common sites of injury are at the pelvic brim where the ureter is close to the ovarian blood vessels and where the uterine artery crosses the ureter along the side of the cervix.

C. Normal Constrictions of the Ureter. The ureters are normally constricted at three sites where kidney stones most commonly cause obstruction.
   1. At the ureteropelvic junction
   2. Where the ureters cross the pelvic inlet
   3. At the ureterovesical junction (along the intramural portion of the ureter)

D. Vasculature of the Ureter
   1. Arterial Supply. The arteries supplying the ureter are derived from the **abdominal aorta, renal artery, testicular artery, ovarian artery, common iliac artery, internal iliac artery, inferior vesical artery,** and **uterine artery**. Branches from these arteries supply different parts of the ureter along its course and are subject to much variation. The most constant arterial supply of the lower part of the ureter is the **uterine artery** in the female and the **inferior vesical artery** in the male. The longitudinal anastomosis between these branches may be weak so that inadvertent damage to one of these branches may lead to necrosis of a ureteral segment about 1 week postoperatively.
   2. Venous Drainage. The veins draining the ureter follow the arterial supply, although there is a conspicuous **vesical venous plexus** surrounding the end of the ureter.

E. Innervation of the Ureter. The ureter is innervated by the **ureteric plexus**. In the upper part of the ureter, the ureteric plexus receives input from the **renal plexus** and **abdominal aortic plexus**. In the intermediate part of the ureter, the ureteric plexus receives input from the **superior hypogastric plexus**. In the lower part of the ureter, the ureteric plexus receives input from the **inferior hypogastric plexus**. The ureteric plexus contains both **parasympathetic** and **sympathetic** components, although they do not play a major role in ureteral peristalsis but only a modulatory role.
   1. Parasympathetic
      a. **Upper Part of the Ureter.** Preganglionic neuronal cell bodies are located in the **dorsal nucleus of the vagus** and **nucleus ambiguus** of the medulla. Preganglionic axons run in the **vagus (cranial nerve [CN] X) nerve**. Postganglionic neuronal cell bodies are located in the ureteric plexus. Postganglionic axons are distributed to the upper part of the ureter.
      b. **Lower Part of the Ureter.** Preganglionic neuronal cell bodies are also located in the intermediolateral cell columns of the **S2 through S4** spinal cord segments.

Preganglionic axons travel to the ureteric plexus as the **pelvic splanchnic nerves.** Postganglionic neuronal cell bodies are located in the ureteric plexus. Postganglionic axons are distributed to the lower part of the ureter.

2. **Sympathetic**
   a. **Upper Part of the Ureter.** Preganglionic neuronal cell bodies are located in the **intermediolateral cell column** of the spinal cord. Preganglionic axons pass through the paravertebral ganglia (do not synapse) to become the **least thoracic splanchnic nerve, first lumbar splanchnic nerve, and second lumber splanchnic nerve** and travel to the **aorticorenal ganglion.** Postganglionic neuronal cell bodies are located in the aorticorenal ganglion. Postganglionic axons enter the ureteric plexus and are distributed to the upper part of the ureter.
   b. **Middle Part of the Ureter.** Preganglionic neuronal cell bodies are located in the **intermediolateral cell column** of the spinal cord. Preganglionic axons pass through the paravertebral ganglia (do not synapse) to become the **third lumbar splanchnic nerve and fourth lumbar splanchnic nerve** and travel to the **superior hypogastric plexus.** Postganglionic neuronal cell bodies are located in the superior hypogastric plexus. Postganglionic axons enter the ureteric plexus and are distributed to the middle part of the ureter.
   c. **Lower Part of the Ureter.** Preganglionic neuronal cell bodies are located in the **intermediolateral cell column** of the spinal cord. Preganglionic axons pass through the paravertebral ganglia (do not synapse) to become the **third lumbar splanchnic nerve and fourth lumbar splanchnic nerve** and travel to the **inferior hypogastric plexus** by way of the superior hypogastric plexus. Postganglionic neuronal cell bodies are located in the inferior hypogastric plexus. Postganglionic axons enter the ureteric plexus and are distributed to the lower part of the ureter.
   d. **Sensory Innervation.** Afferent (sensory) neurons whose cell bodies are located in the **dorsal root ganglion** run with the least thoracic splanchnic nerve, first lumbar splanchnic nerve, and second lumbar splanchnic nerve and relay pain information from most of the ureter to the T12 through L2 spinal segments within the CNS. The pain associated with ureter disease is mainly referred over the **T12 through L2 dermatomes** (i.e. lumbar region, inguinal region, and anterosuperior thigh).

F. **Clinical Considerations (Figure 14-3). Renal calculi ("kidney stones") obstruction** occurs most often at the three sites where the ureter normally constricts (see above), causing a **unilateral hydronephrosis.** Clinical findings include intermittent, excruciating pain in the flank area, abdomen, and testicular or vulvar region radiating onto the inner thigh depending on the the obstruction site; fever, hematuria, and decreased urine output may be present; and the patient assumes a posture with a severe ipsilateral costovertebral angle. There are four types of kidney stones:
   1. **Calcium oxalate calculi** are radiopaque. By urinalysis, they are colorless, octahedral-shaped crystals that look like small squares crossed by diagonal lines; rarely, they are dumbbell-shaped. They are the most common (80%) type of calculi and form when urine pH is less than 6.0 (acid pH) or neutral pH. Calcium oxalate calculi are associated with absorptive hypercalcemia, vitamin D intoxication, hyperparathyroidism, milk-alkali syndrome, and renal tubular acidosis, all of which result in **hypercalcemia;** diabetes; liver disease; or ethylene glycol poisoning.
   2. **Magnesium ammonium sulfate (struvite; triple phosphate) calculi** are radiopaque. By urinalysis, they are colorless, rectangular prism-shaped crystals. They are the second most common (15%) type of calculi, generally form staghorn calculi, and form when urine pH is greater than 7.4 (alkaline pH). Magnesium ammonium

sulfate calculi are associated with urinary tract infections by urea-splitting bacteria (e.g. *Proteus mirabilis, Proteus vulgaris, Providencia, Pseudomonas, Klebsiella, and Staphylococcus*).

3. **Uric acid calculi** are radiolucent. By urinalysis, they are yellow or red-brown diamond-shaped crystals. They are the third most common (5%) type of calculi and form when urine pH is less than 6.0 (acid pH). Uric acid calculi are associated with gout, leukemia, Lesch-Nyhan syndrome, and myeloproliferative disorders.

4. **Cystine calculi** are faintly radiopaque. By urinalysis, they are colorless, refractile, hexagonal-shaped crystals that may have a layered appearance. They are the least common (1%) type of calculi and form when urine pH is less than 6.0 (acid pH). Cystine calculi are caused by **cystinuria**, which is an autosomal recessive disorder that results in defective renal tubular reabsorption of the amino acids cystine, ornithine, arginine, and lysine.

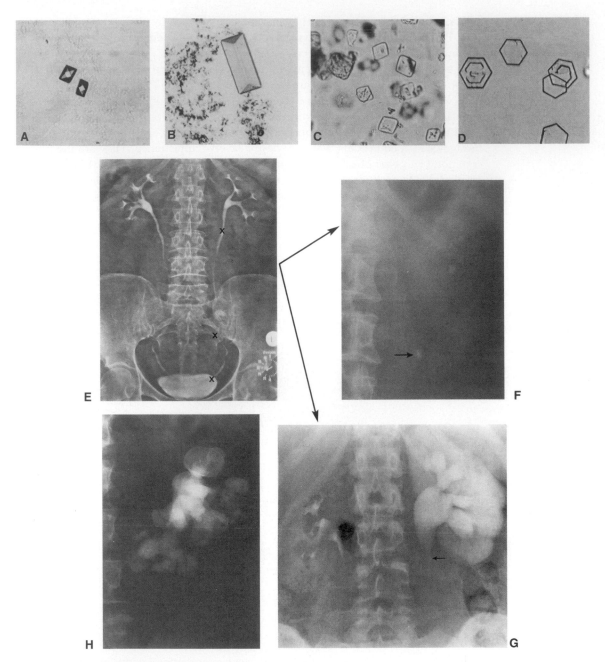

● **Figure 14-3 (A–D) Calculi (Kidney Stones). (A)** Photograph of calcium oxalate calculi shows that these kidney stones are colorless, octahedral-shaped crystals that look like small squares crossed by intersecting diagonal lines. **(B)** Photograph of magnesium ammonium sulfate (struvite or triple phosphate) calculi shows that these kidney stones are colorless, rectangular prism-shaped crystals. **(C)** Photograph of uric acid calculi shows that these kidney stones are yellow or red-brown in color and diamond prism-shaped crystals. **(D)** Photograph of cystine calculi shows that these kidney stones are colorless, refractile, hexagonal-shaped crystals that may have a layered appearance. **(E) IVU (intravenous urogram) of a Normal Kidney.** The normal collecting system of the kidney and the ureter are shown. The ureters are normally constricted at three sites (X) where kidney stones most commonly cause obstruction. **(F) AP Radiograph of Renal Calculi.** A kidney stone is shown (arrow) located at the ureteropelvic junction (junction of the renal pelvis and ureter). **(G) IVU of Renal Calculi.** Unilateral hydronephrosis (dilation of the collecting system) is shown caused by a kidney stone obstruction at the ureteropelvic junction (arrow). The classic findings of renal calculi on an IVP are very dense nephrogram in acute obstruction, a greatly delayed pyelogram, opacification of urine in an obstructed system takes hours, atrophy of kidney with reduced kidney parenchyma width in chronic obstruction. **(H) IVU of Staghorn Calculi.** Kidney stones may conform to the shape of part or all of the collecting system. Those kidney stones that fill at least two adjacent calyces are called staghorn calculi. Staghorn calculi are generally struvite calculi caused by bacterial infection.

Urinary Bladder (Figure 14-4)

A. General Features. The urinary bladder is a hollow structure with prominent smooth muscle walls that is a temporary reservoir for urine with a capacity of 120 to 320 mL. Micturition commonly occurs at about 280 mL. The bladder may store up to 500 mL of urine, but this is usually associated with pain. The size, shape, position, and relations vary according to its contents and the state of the neighboring viscera. The empty bladder is tetrahedral-shaped and consists of a **posterior surface (fundus or base), anterior surface, superior surface, apex,** and **neck.**

B. Urinary Bladder Relationships to Neighboring Structures

1. **Posterior Surface (fundus or base).** In the male, the posterior surface is related to the **rectovesical pouch, rectum, seminal vesicles,** and **ampulla of the ductus deferens.** In the female, the posterior surface is related to the **anterior wall of the vagina.**

2. **Anterior Surface.** In the male and female, the anterior surface is related to the **pubic symphysis** and **retropubic space (of Retzius).**

3. **Superior Surface.** In the male, the superior surface is related to the **peritoneal cavity** (completely covered by peritoneum), sigmoid colon, and terminal coils of the ileum. In the female, the superior surface is related to the **peritoneal cavity** (largely covered by peritoneum but is reflected posteriorly to the uterus forming the **vesicouterine pouch)** and **uterus.**

4. **Apex.** The apex is located posterior to the upper part of the pubic symphysis. In the male and female, the apex is related to the one **median umbilical ligament** or **urachus** (a remnant of the allantois in the fetus), the two **medial umbilical ligaments** (remnants of the right and left umbilical arteries in the fetus), and the two **lateral umbilical ligaments,** which are elevations formed by the right and left inferior epigastric arteries and veins.

5. **Neck.** The neck is the lowest region of the bladder and is located posterior to the lower part of the pubic symphysis. The neck is pierced by the **internal urethral orifice.** In the male, the neck is related to the **prostate gland** and **prostatic urethra.** In the female, the neck is related to the **urogenital diaphragm.**

C. Support of the Bladder

1. **Urogenital diaphragm**

2. **Pubovesical ligaments** are extensions of the **puboprostatic ligaments (in the male)** and **pubourethral ligaments (in the female).** The pubovesical ligaments extend from the lower portion of the pubic bone to the neck of the bladder.

3. **Median umbilical ligament** or **urachus** (a remnant of the allantois in the fetus) extends from the umbilicus to the apex of the bladder.

4. **False ligaments** are reflections or folds of peritoneum and include the **median umbilical fold, medial umbilical folds, superior false ligament, lateral false ligaments,** and **posterior false ligaments.**

D. Internal Anatomy of the Bladder. The majority of the internal surface of the empty bladder is **rough-surfaced** because the mucosa (transitional epithelium and lamina propria) is only loosely attached to the detrusor muscle. As the bladder fills with urine, these rough surfaces become smooth. However, the trigone of the bladder is always **smooth-surfaced** because the mucosa (transitional epithelium and lamina propria) is tightly attached to the detrusor muscle. The **trigone of the bladder** is located on the posterior surface of the bladder (fundus or base), and its limits are defined superiorly by the

openings of the ureters and inferiorly by the **internal urethral orifice**. Along the superior edge of the trigone is a ridge called the **interureteric crest** that connects the two openings of the ureter. The interureteric crest is produced by the continuation of the smooth muscle of the ureter into the detrusor muscle of the bladder.

E. Vasculature of the Urinary Bladder
  1. **Arterial Supply.** The arteries supplying the bladder include the **superior vesical artery** (a branch of the internal iliac artery), **inferior vesical artery** (a branch of the internal iliac artery), **obturator artery**, and **inferior gluteal artery**. In the female, branches of the **uterine artery** and **vaginal artery** also supply the bladder.
  2. **Venous Drainage.** The veins draining the bladder form a complicated venous plexus along the inferolateral portion of the bladder that ultimately drains into the **internal iliac vein** and the **prostatic venous plexus**.

F. Innervation of the Urinary Bladder. The bladder is innervated by the **vesical plexus**, which receives input from the **inferior hypogastric plexus**. The vesical plexus contains both **parasympathetic** and **sympathetic** components.
  1. **Parasympathetic.** Preganglionic neuronal cell bodies are located in the intermediolateral cell column of the **S2 through S4** spinal cord segments. Preganglionic axons travel to the vesical plexus as the **pelvic splanchnic nerves**. Postganglionic neuronal cell bodies are located in the vesical plexus and the bladder wall. Postganglionic axons are distributed to the detrusor muscle of the bladder where they cause **contraction of the detrusor muscle** and **relaxation of the internal urethral sphincter** (i.e. efferent limb of the micturition reflex).
  2. **Sympathetic.** Preganglionic neuronal cell bodies are located in the **intermediolateral cell column** of the spinal cord. Preganglionic axons pass through the paravertebral ganglia (do not synapse) to become the **lesser thoracic splanchnic nerve, least thoracic splanchnic nerve, first lumbar splanchnic nerve**, and **second lumbar splanchnic nerve** and travel to the **inferior hypogastric plexus** by way of the superior hypogastric plexus. Postganglionic neuronal cell bodies are located in the inferior hypogastric plexus. Postganglionic axons enter the vesical plexus and are distributed to the detrusor muscle of the bladder where they cause **relaxation of the detrusor muscle** and **contraction of the internal urethral sphincter** (although some investigators claim their action is strictly on the smooth muscle of blood vessels).
  3. **Sensory Innervation.** Sensory information from the bladder is carried by both parasympathetics (mainly) and sympathetics.
    a. **Parasympathetic.** Afferent (sensory) neurons whose cell bodies are located in the **dorsal root ganglion** run with the **pelvic splanchnic nerves** and relay **pain** and **stretch** information from the bladder to S2 through S4 spinal segments within the CNS. The **pain** associated with bladder disease may be referred over the **S2 through S4 dermatomes** (i.e. perineum and posterior thigh). The **stretch** information associated with bladder fullness from stretch receptors in the wall of the bladder is carried by afferent nerves that run with the pelvic splanchnic nerves and serve as the afferent limb in the micturition reflex.
    b. **Sympathetic.** Afferent (sensory) neurons whose cell bodies are located in the **dorsal root ganglion** run with the lesser thoracic splanchnic nerve, least thoracic splanchnic nerve, first lumbar splanchnic nerve, and second lumbar splanchnic nerve and relay pain information from the bladder to the T11 through L2 spinal cord segments with the CNS. The pain associated with bladder disease may be referred over the **T11 through L2 dermatomes** (i.e. lumbar region, inguinal region, and anterosuperior thigh).

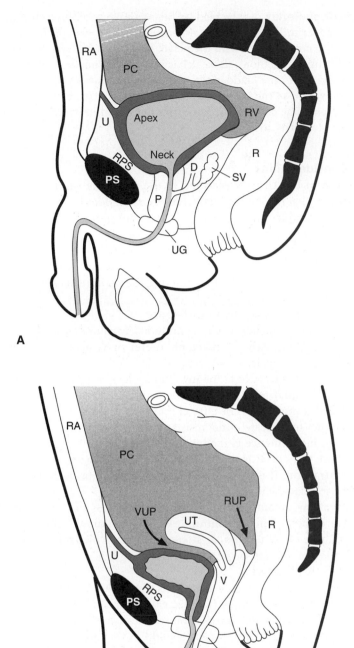

A

B

● **Figure 14-4 (A) Male Pelvis.** A sagittal section through the male pelvis demonstrating the various anatomic relationships of the urinary bladder. **(B) Female Pelvis.** A sagittal section through the female pelvis demonstrating the various anatomic relationships of the urinary bladder. RA = rectus abdominis muscle, U = urachus, RPS = retropubic space of Retzius, PS = pubic symphysis bone, P = prostate gland, PC = peritoneal cavity (shaded), RV = rectovesical pouch, R = rectum, D = ductus deferens, SV = seminal vesicle, UG = urogenital diaphragm, UB = urinary bladder, V = vagina, UT = uterus, VUP = vesicouterine pouch, RUP = rectouterine pouch of Douglas.

4. **Micturition Reflex.** As the bladder fills with urine, **stretch** information associated with bladder fullness from stretch receptors in the wall of the bladder is carried by afferent nerves that run with the pelvic splanchnic nerves and serve as the afferent limb in the micturition reflex. Pelvic splanchnic nerves are distributed to the detrusor muscle of the bladder where they cause **contraction of the detrusor muscle** and **relaxation of the internal urethral sphincter** (i.e. efferent limb of the micturition reflex). The **external urethral sphincter** is innervated by the **pudendal nerve** and is voluntarily relaxed.

G. Clinical Considerations

1. **Location of the Urinary Bladder.** In the adult, the empty bladder lies within the **minor (true) pelvis**. In the infant, the empty bladder lies within the **abdominal cavity**. As the bladder fills in the adult, it rises out of the minor pelvis above the pelvic inlet and may extend as high as the umbilicus. In acute retention of urine, a needle may be passed through the anterior abdominal wall (skin → superficial fascia [Camper's and Scarpa's] → linea alba → transversalis fascia → extraperitoneal fat → parietal peritoneum) without entering the peritoneal cavity to remove the urine (**suprapubic cystostomy**).

2. **Urine Leakage Caused by Incontinence**
    a. **Total incontinence** is the continuous involuntary loss of urine. It is most commonly caused by an **ectopic ureter** or **vesicovaginal fistula**. It is treated by surgical repair.
    b. **Stress incontinence** is the involuntary loss of urine associated with increases in abdominal pressure. It is most commonly caused by coughing, sneezing, Valsalva movement, or after childbirth. It is treated by ephedrine or phentolamine (to increase outlet resistance) or surgical repair.
    c. **Urge incontinence** is the involuntary loss of urine associated with an intense desire to void. It is most commonly caused by uncontrolled detrusor muscle contraction. It is treated by oxybutynin or imipramine (to stabilized detrusor muscle contraction).
    d. **Overflow incontinence** is the involuntary loss of urine as bladder overfilling overcomes sphincter control. It is most commonly caused by prostate cancer, stricture of the urethra, or atonic neurogenic bladder. It is treated by catheterization or surgery.

3. **Neurogenic Bladders**
    a. **Hypertonic neurogenic bladder** is a voiding dysfunction characterized by a **small urinary bladder** (i.e. decreased capacity) and **detrusor hyperreflexia** (overactivity of the detrusor muscle) causing thickened walls of the bladder ("pine tree bladder"). It causes voidings that are urgent and frequent. It is associated in general with upper motor neuron lesions (e.g. tumors of brain or spinal cord, upper spinal cord injury, cerebrovascular accidents, multiple sclerosis, or Parkinson's). It is treated with anticholinergics, catheterization, and surgical augmentation of the bladder.
    b. **Atonic neurogenic bladder** is a voiding dysfunction characterized by a **large urinary bladder** (i.e. increased capacity) and **detrusor areflexia** (underactivity of the detrusor muscle). It causes urine retention with subsequent overflow incontinence. It is associated in general with lower motor neuron lesions (e.g. spina bifida with meningomyelocele in the sacral region, sacral spinal cord injury, lumbar disk herniation impinging on sacral spinal nerves or the cauda equina, pelvic surgery or trauma damaging pelvic splanchnic nerves, diabetes

leading to peripheral neuropathy, tabes dorsalis, or syringomyelia). It is treated with catheterization or surgical diversion of urine.

4. **Urine Leakage Caused by Trauma (Figure 14-5)**

   a. **Rupture of the superior wall (dome)** results in an intraperitoneal extravasation of urine within the **peritoneal cavity**. It is caused by a compressive force on a full bladder.

   b. **Rupture of the anterior wall** results in an extraperitoneal extravasation of urine within the **retropubic space (of Retzius)**. It is caused by a fractured pelvis (e.g. car accident) that punctures the bladder.

   c. **Type I urethral injury** occurs when the posterior urethra is stretched but intact as a result of the rupture of the puboprostatic ligaments. Type I urethral injuries are rare.

   d. **Type II urethral injury** occurs when the posterior urethra is torn **above the urogenital diaphragm.** This results in an extraperitoneal extravasation of urine within the **retropubic space of Retzius**. It may be caused by a fractured pelvis (e.g. car accident) or improper insertion of a catheter.

   e. **Type III urethral injury** occurs when the anterior urethra (i.e. bulbous urethra) is torn **below the urogenital diaphragm** along with a disruption of the urogenital diaphragm so that the membranous urethra is torn also. Radiologists consider a type III urethral injury as a combined anterior–posterior urethral injury. This results in an extraperitoneal extravasation of urine within the **superficial perineal space** extending into the scrotal, penile, and anterior abdominal wall areas (urine will NOT extend into the thigh region or anal triangle). The superficial perineal space is located between Colles' fascia and dartos muscle and the external spermatic fascia. It is caused by a **straddle injury** (e.g. a boy slips off a bicycle seat and falls against the crossbar) and is the most common type of urine leakage injury. Clinical findings include blood at the urethral meatus, ecchymosis, painful swelling of the scrotal and perineal areas, and tender enlargement in the suprapubic region because of a full bladder.

   f. **Type IV urethral injury** occurs when the neck of the bladder and proximal prostatic urethra are injured. This may result in an extraperitoneal extravasation of urine within the **retropubic space of Retzius**. Type IV urethral injuries may be serious if the internal urethral sphincter is injured, which leads to incontinence.

   g. **Type V urethral injury** occurs when the penile urethra is torn. This is a pure anterior urethral injury. This results in an extraperitoneal extravasation of urine **beneath the deep fascia (of Buck)** and will be confined to the penis if the deep fascia of Buck is not torn. However, if the trauma also tears the deep fascia of Buck, then extravasation of urine will occur within the **superficial perineal space**. It is caused by a crushing injury to the penis.

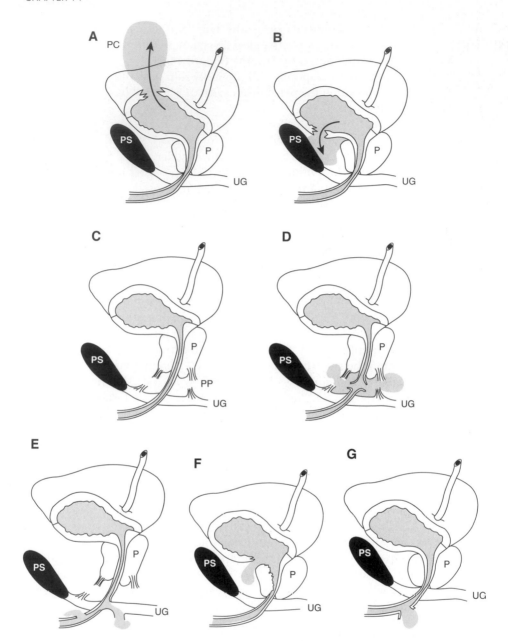

● **Figure 14-5 Urine Leakage as a Result of Trauma. (A) Rupture of Superior Wall of Urinary Bladder.** Diagram shows a rupture of the superior wall of the urinary bladder resulting in the extravasation of urine into the peritoneal cavity (PC). **(B) Rupture of Anterior Wall of Urinary Bladder. (C) Type I Urethral Injury.** Diagram shows a stretched but intact posterior urethra. Note the rupture of the puboprostatic ligaments (PP). **(D) Type II Urethral Injury.** Diagram shows a torn posterior urethra above the urogenital diaphragm resulting in the extravasation of urine into the retropubic space of Retzius. **(E) Type III Urethral Injury.** Diagram shows a torn bulbous urethra below the urogenital diaphragm along with a disruption of the urogenital diaphragm so that the membranous urethra is torn also. This results in extravasation of urine within the superficial perineal space. This is the most common type of urine leakage injury and is sometimes called a "straddle injury." **(F) Type IV Urethral Injury.** Diagram shows injury to the neck of the bladder and the proximal prostatic urethra that may result in extravasation of urine into the retropubic space of Retzius. **(G) Type V Urethral Injury.** Diagram shows a torn penile urethra that results in extravasation of urine beneath the deep fascia of Buck. PS = pubic symphysis, UG = urogenital diaphragm, P = prostate gland.

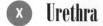

Urethra

A. Female Urethra. The female urethra is about 3 to 5 cm long and begins at the **internal urethral orifice** of the bladder where the detrusor muscle extends longitudinally into the urethra but does not form a significant internal urethral sphincter. The female urethra courses through the **urogenital diaphragm**, where it becomes related to the **deep transverse perineal muscle** and **sphincter urethrae muscle** (also called **external urethral sphincter**), both of which are skeletal muscles innervated by the **pudendal nerve.** The posterior surface of the female urethra fuses with the anterior wall of the vagina such that the **external urethral sphincter** does not completely surround the female urethra. This may explain the high incidence of stress incontinence in women, especially after childbirth. The female urethra terminates as the **navicular fossa** at the **external urethral orifice**, which opens into the **vestibule of the vagina** between the labia minora just below the clitoris. The female urethra develops endodermal outgrowths into the surrounding mesoderm to form the **urethral glands** and **paraurethral glands of Skene** (which are homologous to the prostate gland in the male). The paraurethral glands of Skene open on each side of the external urethral orifice. The vestibule of the vagina develops endodermal outgrowths into the surrounding mesoderm to form the **lesser vestibular glands** and the **greater vestibular glands of Bartholin** (which are homologous to the bulbourethral glands of Cowper in the male). The greater vestibular glands of Bartholin open on each side of the vaginal orifice.

B. Male Urethra. See Chapter 17 VI.

Radiology

A. Intravenous Urography (IVU) (Figure 14-6)

B. Retrograde Urography (RU) and Anterograde Urography (AU) (Figure 14-7)

C. Cystography (Figure 14-8)

D. Voiding Cystourethrography (Figure 14-9)

E. Ultrasonography, Angiography, Radioisotope Renography (Figure 14-10)

F. Magnetic Resonance (Figure 14-11)

G. Computed Tomography (Figure 14-12)

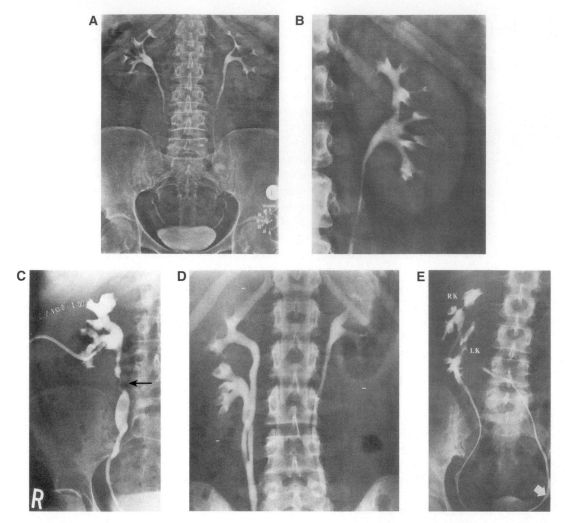

● **Figure 14-6 Intravenous Urograms. (A)** A normal intravenous urogram showing the collecting system, ureters, and urinary bladder. **(B)** A normal intravenous urogram shown the details of the collecting system and upper ureter of the left kidney. **(C)** An intravenous urogram shows a postsurgical stricture (arrow) of the ureter after calculi removal. **(D)** An intravenous urogram shows a congenital malformation called a ureteropelvic duplication of the right side. **(E)** An intravenous urogram shows a congenital malformation called crossed renal ectopia with kidney fusion. The left kidney (LK) is ectopic on the right side and is fused with the right kidney (RK). Note that the left ureter (arrow) inserts normally into the bladder.

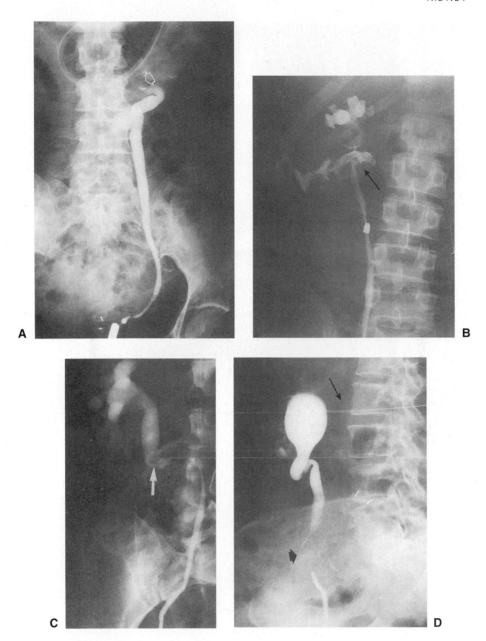

● **Figure 14-7 Urograms. (A)** A retrograde urogram shows an obstruction in the proximal ureter (arrow). **(B)** A retrograde urogram shows extravasation of contrast material at the ureteropelvic junction (arrow) because of a severed ureter. **(C)** A retrograde urogram shows a congenital malformation called a circumcaval ureter in which the ureter crosses posterior to and wraps around the inferior vena cava, causing a typical "reverse J" configuration of the ureter (arrow). **(D)** Anterograde urogram (nephrostogram) shows an obstruction in the middle portion of the ureter (thick arrow). Note the needle inserted directly into the kidney (thin arrow).

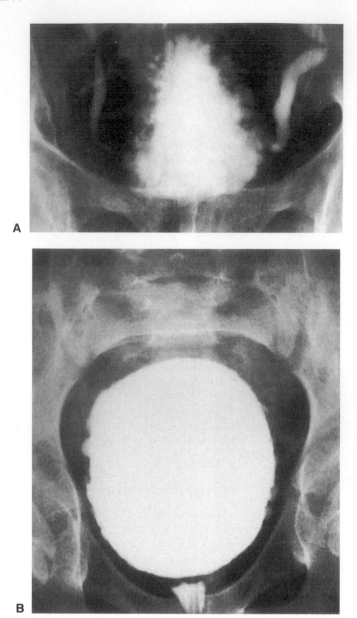

● **Figure 14-8 Cystograms. (A)** A cystogram shows a hypertonic neurogenic bladder, which is a voiding dysfunction characterized by a small urinary bladder and detrusor muscle hyperreflexia causing thickened walls of the bladder ("pine tree bladder"). **(B)** A cystogram shows an atonic neurogenic bladder, which is a voiding dysfunction characterized by a large urinary bladder and detrusor muscle areflexia.

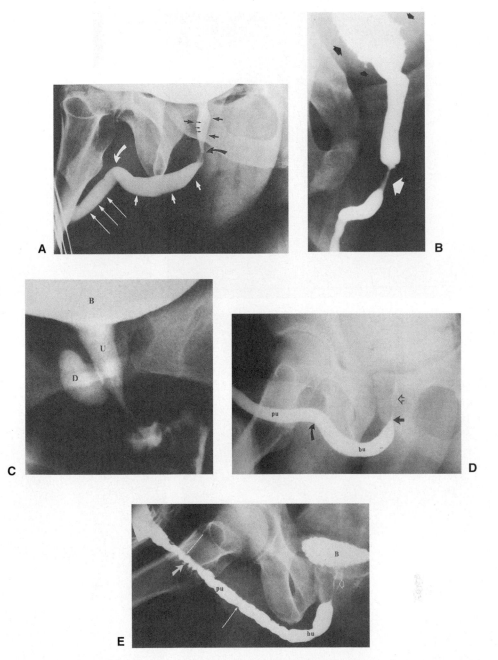

● **Figure 14-9 (A, B, C) Voiding Cystourethrograms. (A)** A normal voiding cystourethrogram in a male (right posterior projection) shows the prostatic urethra (large black arrows), the seminal colliculus (or verumontanum), which appears as a filling defect (small black arrows), and the short membranous urethra (curved black arrow). This makes up the posterior urethra. The bulbous urethra (short white arrows) and penile urethra (long white arrows) are also shown. The penoscrotal junction (curved white arrow) is shown. **(B)** A voiding cystourethrogram in a male shows a long stricture in the bulbous urethra (white arrow). Note the increased bladder trabeculations (black arrows) usually present with bladder-outlet obstruction. **(C)** A voiding cystourethrogram in a female shows a urethral diverticulum (D) along with the female urethra (U) and bladder (B). **(D, E) Retrograde Urethrograms. (D)** A normal retrograde urethrogram in a male shows the penile urethra (pu) and bulbous urethra (bu) demarcated by the suspensory ligament of the penis at the penoscrotal junction (curved arrow). Note that the urethra tapers to a point at the urogenital diaphragm marking the location of the membranous urethra (black arrow). The seminal colliculus (or verumontanum; open arrow) indicates the location of the prostatic urethra. **(E)** A retrograde urethrogram shows multiple strictures (long arrows) along the penile urethra (pu) and bulbous urethra (bu). Urethritis is evidenced by the filling of the urethral glands of Littre (short arrow). The seminal colliculus (verumontanum) is indicated by the open arrow). B = bladder.

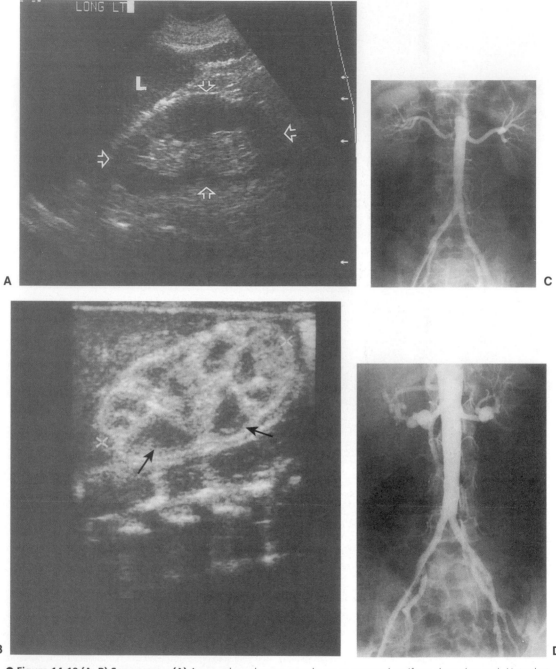

● **Figure 14-10 (A, B) Sonograms. (A)** A normal renal sonogram shows as a normal reniform shape (arrows). Note that the renal cortex and medulla are relatively sonolucent (i.e. appear black) whereas the collecting system (minor and major calyces) and renal pelvis produce echoes (i.e. appear white). L = liver. **(B)** A normal renal sonogram (longitudinal image) shows the outline of the kidney and the sonolucent renal pyramids (arrows). **(C, D) Aortograms. (C)** A normal aortogram shows the normal course and caliber of the abdominal aorta, which bifurcates at vertebral level L4. Note the normal branching of the right and left renal arteries. **(D)** An aortogram shows an abnormal caliber of the abdominal aorta along with bilateral renal artery aneurysms.

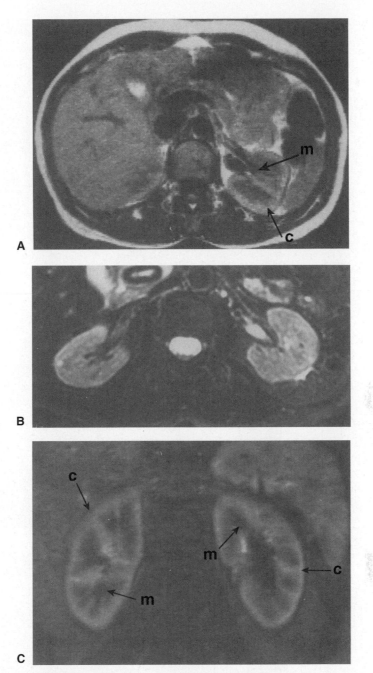

● **Figure 14-11 MRIs of the Kidneys. (A)** T_1-weighted spin-echo MRI shows a normal left kidney. Note that the renal cortex (c) can be easily distinguished from the renal medulla (m). **(B)** T_2-weighted spin-echo MRI shows a normal right and left kidney. Note that the entire renal parenchyma is bright so that the renal cortex cannot be distinguished from the renal medulla. **(C)** T_1-weighted gadolinium-enhanced MRI shows a normal right and left kidney. Note that the renal cortex (c) is quite enhanced and can be easily distinguished from the renal medulla (m).

A

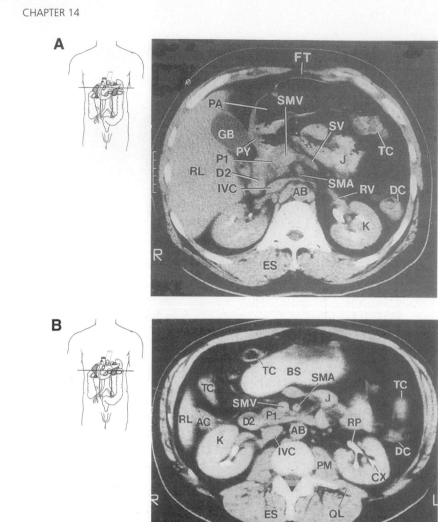

B

C

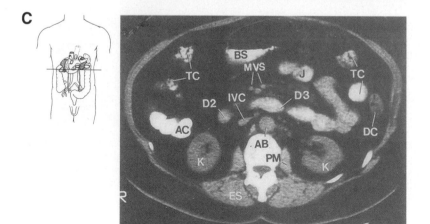

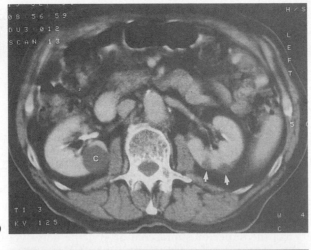

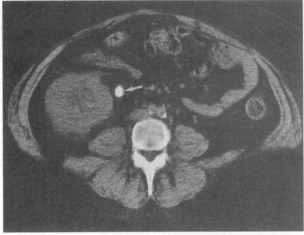

● **Figure 14-12 Computed Tomography (CT) Images. (A)** A normal CT image with contrast material at the upper border of vertebral level L2. **(B)** A normal CT image with contrast material at the lower border of vertebral level L2. **(C)** A normal CT image with contrast material at about vertebral level L3. **(D)** CT image shows a large cyst in the posterior portion of the right kidney (C) and two smaller cysts in the left kidney (arrows). **(E)** CT image shows a large, obstructing calculus ("kidney stone") in the ureter (arrow). AC = ascending colon, AB = abdominal aorta, BS = body of stomach, CX = renal calyx, DC = descending colon, D2 = second part of duodenum, D3 = third part of duodenum, D4 = fourth part of duodenum, ES = erector spinae muscle, FT = fat, GB = gallbladder, IVC = inferior vena cava, J = jejunum, K = kidney, MVS = superior mesenteric vessels, PA = antrum of stomach, PM = psoas major muscle, PV = portal vein, P1 = head of pancreas, QL = quadratus lumborum, RL = right lobe of liver, RP = renal pelvis, SMA = superior mesenteric artery, SMV = superior mesenteric vein, TC = transverse colon.

Chapter 15

Suprarenal (Adrenal) Glands

I **General Features (Figure 15-1).** The right suprarenal gland is shaped like a **pyramid** with its apex projecting superior and its base embracing the kidney. The left suprarenal gland is shaped like a **half-moon** covering the superior aspect of the kidney and extending inferiorly along the medial aspect of the kidney. The arterial supply is from the inferior phrenic artery via the **superior suprarenal artery**, the aorta via the **middle suprarenal artery**, and the renal artery via the **inferior suprarenal artery**. The venous drainage is to the **right suprarenal vein** (which empties into the inferior vena cava) and the **left suprarenal vein** (which empties into the left renal vein). The venous drainage is particularly important during an **adrenalectomy** because the suprarenal vein must be ligated as soon as possible to prevent catecholamine (epinephrine and norepinephrine) release into the circulation. In addition, the adrenal medulla receives venous blood draining the cortex that has a high concentration of cortisol. The synthesis of **phenylethanolamine-N-methyltransferase** (a key enzyme in the synthesis of epinephrine) is dependent on high levels of cortisol received via venous blood from the cortex.

II **Adrenal cortex** is derived embryologically from the mesoderm and is divided into three zones.

A. **Zona glomerulosa (ZG)** constitutes 15% of the cortical volume. The ZG secretes **aldosterone**, which is controlled by the **renin-angiotensin system**.

B. **Zona fasciculata (ZF)** constitutes 78% of the cortical volume. The ZF secretes **cortisol**, which is controlled by **corticotropin-releasing factor (CRF)** and **adrenocorticotropic hormone (ACTH)** from the hypothalamus and adenohypophysis, respectively.

C. **Zona reticularis (ZR)** constitutes 7% of the cortical volume. The ZR secretes **dehydroepiandrosterone (DHEA)** and **androstenedione**, which are controlled by **CRF** and ACTH from the hypothalamus and adenohypophysis, respectively.

D. **Clinical Considerations (Figure 15-2)**
1. **Primary Hyperaldosteronism**
   a. **Cause.** Elevated levels of aldosterone are commonly caused by an aldosterone-secreting adenoma (**Conn syndrome**) within the ZG or adrenal hyperplasia.
   b. **Symptoms.** Primary hyperaldosteronism is characterized clinically by hypertension, hypernatremia as a result of increased sodium ion reabsorption, weight gain as a result of water retention, hypokalemia as a result of increased K^+ secretion, and decreased plasma renin levels.
   c. **Treatment.** It is treated by surgery or **spironolactone**, which is an aldosterone receptor antagonist and therefore an effective antihypertensive and diuretic agent.

2. **Cushing Syndrome**
    a. **Cause.** Elevated levels of **cortisol** (i.e. hypercortisolism) are commonly caused by an ACTH-secreting adenoma within the adenohypophysis (70% of the cases; strictly termed **Cushing** *disease*), an adrenal adenoma (25% of the cases), or adrenal hyperplasia. An oat cell carcinoma of the lung may also ectopically produce ACTH. However, Cushing syndrome is most commonly caused by iatrogenic corticosteroid drug therapy.
    b. **Symptoms.** Cushing syndrome is characterized clinically by mild hypertension with cardiac hypertrophy, buffalo hump, osteoporosis with back pain, central obesity, moon facies, purple skin striae, skin ulcers (poor wound healing), thin wrinkled skin, amenorrhea, purpura, impaired glucose tolerance, and emotional disturbances.
    c. **Treatment. Ketoconazole** is an inhibitor of steroid biosynthesis that is used in the treatment of Cushing syndrome.
3. **Congenital Adrenal Hyperplasia**
    a. **Cause.** Congenital adrenal hyperplasia is caused most commonly by mutations in genes for enzymes involved in adrenocortical steroid biosynthesis (e.g. **21-hydroxylase deficiency, 11β-hydroxylase deficiency**). In 21-hydroxylase deficiency (90% of all cases), there is virtually no synthesis of the aldosterone or cortisol, so that intermediates are funneled into androgen biosynthesis, thereby elevating androgen levels.
    b. **Symptoms.** The elevated levels of androgens lead to **virilization of a female fetus,** ranging from mild clitoral enlargement to complete labioscrotal fusion with a phalloid organ. Increased urine 17-ketosteroids are found. Because cortisol cannot be synthesized, negative feedback to the adenohypophysis does not occur, so ACTH continues to stimulate the adrenal cortex resulting in **adrenal hyperplasia.**
    c. **Treatment.** Depending on the severity, treatment may include surgical reconstruction and steroid replacement.
4. **Primary Adrenal Insufficiency (Addison Disease)**
    a. **Cause.** Addison disease is commonly caused by autoimmune destruction of the adrenal cortex. Other causes include adrenal tuberculosis, fungal infections, and adrenal hemorrhage.
    b. **Symptoms.** It is characterized clinically by fatigue, anorexia, nausea, weight loss, hypoglycemia, hypotension, and hyperpigmentation of the skin because of increased secretion of melanocyte-stimulating hormone (MSH).
    c. **Treatment.** This condition is managed by steroid replacement therapy.
5. **Secondary Adrenal Insufficiency**
    a. **Cause.** Secondary adrenal insufficiency is caused by a disorder of the hypothalamus or adenohypophysis that reduces the secretion of ACTH. The most common cause is ACTH suppression because of iatrogenic corticosteroid drug therapy.
    b. **Symptoms.** It is clinically very similar to Addison disease except there is no hyperpigmentation of the skin.
    c. **Treatment.** This condition is managed by steroid replacement therapy.
6. **Adrenal Cortical Carcinoma.** About 80% of adrenal cortical carcinomas are functional, invade locally, and cannot be completely surgically resected as micrometastases to organs occur. Most patients survive for only 1 to 3 years. An adrenal cortical carcinoma that is not functional generally tends to be highly malignant.

Ⅲ Adrenal Medulla

A. General Features. The adrenal medulla contains chromaffin cells that are modified postganglionic sympathetic neurons derived embryologically from neural crest cells. Preganglionic sympathetic axons (via splanchnic nerves) synapse on chromaffin cells and cause chromaffin cells to secrete catecholamines. The secretion product is 90% epinephrine and 10% norepinephrine.

B. Clinical Considerations (Figure 15-3)

1. **Pheochromocytoma** is a relatively rare neoplasm (usually not malignant) of **neural crest origin** that contains both epinephrine and norepinephrine.

   a. **Characteristics.** Pheochromocytoma occurs within families (mainly in adults) as part of the **MEN type IIa syndrome** (pheochromocytoma, hyperparathyroidism, and medullary carcinoma of the thyroid) or associated with **von Recklinghausen neurofibromatosis**. It is generally found in the region of the adrenal gland but is also found in extra-adrenal sites (e.g. near the aortic bifurcation called the **organ of Zuckerkandl**).

   b. **Symptoms.** It is associated with persistent or paroxysmal hypertension, anxiety, tremor, profuse sweating, pallor, chest pain, and abdominal pain.

   c. **Diagnosis.** Increased urine vanillylmandelic acid (VMA) and metanephrine levels, inability to suppress catecholamines with clonidine, and hyperglycemia are common laboratory findings.

   d. **Treatment.** Pheochromocytoma is treated by surgery or **phenoxybenzamine** (an α-adrenergic antagonist).

2. **Neuroblastoma** is an extracranial neoplasm containing primitive neuroblasts of **neural crest origin** and is associated with the amplification of the **N-*myc*** oncogene.

   a. **Characteristics.** Neuroblastoma is the most common solid tumor in children and may metastasize to the bone marrow, liver, and orbit. These tumors are found in extra-adrenal sites usually along the sympathetic chain ganglia (60%) or within the adrenal medulla (40%).

   b. **Symptoms.** It is associated with **opsoclonus** (rapid, irregular movements of the eye in the horizontal and vertical directions ("dancing eyes").

   c. **Diagnosis.** A neuroblastoma contains small cells arranged in **Homer-Wright pseudorosettes**. Increased urine VMA and metanephrine levels are found.

   d. **Treatment** includes surgical excision, radiation, and chemotherapy.

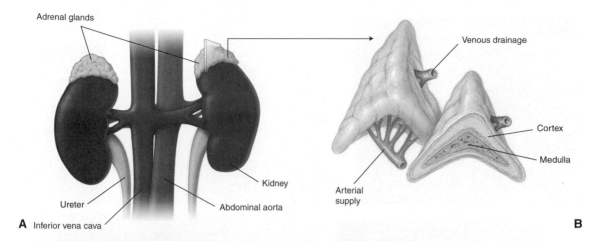

A

B

C

LABORATORY FINDINGS USED TO DIAGNOSE SUPRARENAL GLAND DISORDERS[a]

Clinical Condition	Suppression With Dexamethasone Test[b]	Plasma Levels			
		Aldosterone	Cortisol	Androgens	ACTH
Primary hyperaldosteronism (Conn syndrome)		High			
Cushing syndrome					
ACTH adenoma	Positive		High		High
Adrenal adenoma	Negative		High		Low
Normal patient	Positive		Normal		Normal
Congenital adrenal hyperplasia 21-Hydroxylase deficiency 11β-Hydroxylase deficiency		Low	Low	High	High
Addison disease (primary adrenal insufficiency)		Low	Low	Low	High
Secondary adrenal insufficiency		Normal	Low	Low	Low

[a]Many clinical vignette questions will include the plasma levels of various hormones or the results of a dexamethasone test. Knowing which hormones are increased, decreased, normal, or not applicable in certain clinical conditions will be of great assistance in your diagnosis and in answering the question.
[b]Dexamethasone suppression test is based on the ability of dexamethasone (a synthetic glucocorticoid) to inhibit ACTH and cortisol secretion. If the adenohypophysis–adrenal cortex axis is normal, dexamethasone will inhibit ACTH and cortisol secretion by negative feedback.
ACTH = adrenocorticotropic hormone.

● **Figure 15-1 Gross Anatomy (A) and Cut Section (B) of the Suprarenal Glands. (C) Laboratory findings used to diagnose suprarenal gland disorders.**

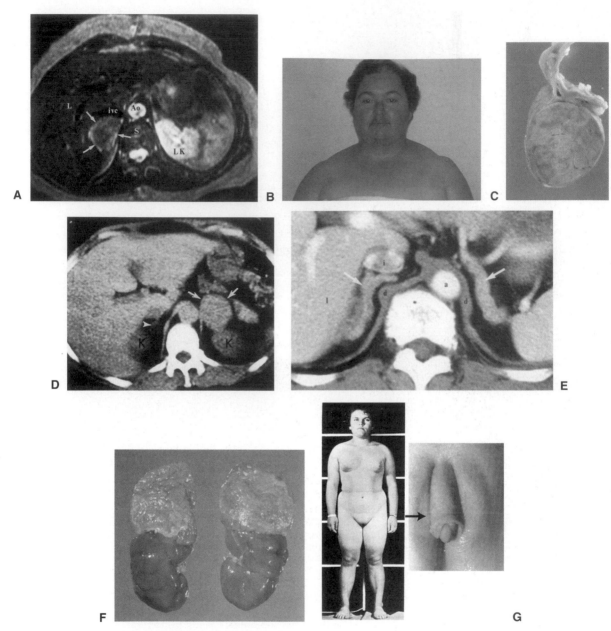

● **Figure 15-2 (A) Conn Syndrome.** MRI shows a right adrenal mass (arrows) that proved to be a benign hyperfunctioning adenoma causing Conn syndrome. Ao = aorta, ivc = inferior vena cava, L = liver, LK = left kidney, S = spine. **(B–E) Cushing Syndrome. (B)** Photograph shows a woman with an ACTH-secreting pituitary adenoma with a moon face, buffalo hump, and increased facial hair. **(C)** Photograph of an adrenal adenoma (cut surface) shows mottled yellow appearance with a rim of compressed normal adrenal tissue. **(D)** CT scan of Cushing syndrome caused by adrenal adenoma. A large mass (arrows) is shown in the left adrenal gland located posterior to the pancreas and anterior to the kidney (K). The normal right adrenal gland is shown (arrowhead). An adrenal adenoma usually occurs unilaterally, whereas adrenal hyperplasia occurs bilaterally. **(E)** CT scan of Cushing syndrome caused by adrenal hyperplasia. Both adrenal glands are enlarged (arrows) while maintaining their normal anatomic shape. Note that except for the increased size, the adrenal glands appear normal, which may confound the diagnosis. In some cases of adrenal hyperplasia, the adrenal glands may demonstrate bilateral nodularity. d = crura of diaphragm, l = right lobe of the liver, i = inferior vena cava, a = aorta. **(F, G) Congenital Adrenal Hyperplasia. (F)** Photograph shows the markedly enlarged adrenal glands from a 7-week-old infant who died of severe salt-wasting congenital adrenal hyperplasia. **(G)** Photograph shows a patient (XX genotype) with female pseudointersexuality as a result of congenital adrenal hyperplasia. Masculinization of female external genitalia is apparent with fusion of the labia majora and enlarged clitoris.

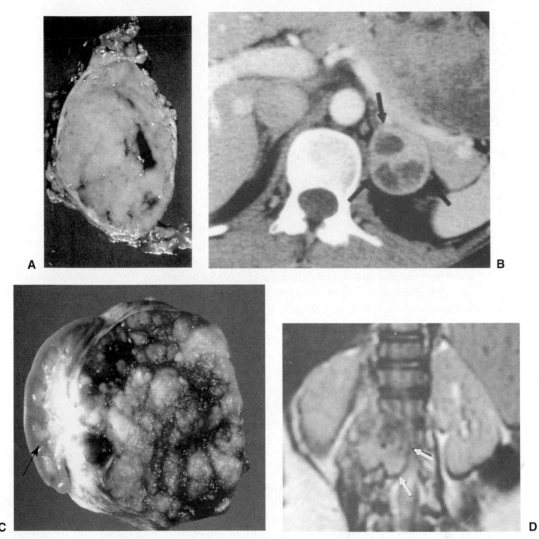

● **Figure 15-3 (A, B) Pheochromocytoma. (A)** Gross photograph of a pheochromocytoma. Pheochromocytomas vary in size from 3 to 5 cm in diameter. They are gray-white to pink-tan in color. Exposure of the cut surface often results in darkening of the surface because of formation of yellow-brown adrenochrome pigment. **(B)** CT scan shows a 3-cm pheochromocytoma in the left adrenal gland that contains focal areas of necrosis (arrows). **(C, D) Neuroblastoma**. **(C)** Gross photograph of a neuroblastoma. Neuroblastomas vary in size from 1 cm to filling the entire abdomen. They are generally soft and white to gray-pink in color. As the size increases, the tumors become hemorrhagic and undergo calcification and cyst formation. Note the nodular appearance of this tumor with the kidney apparent on the left border (arrow). **(D)** MRI shows a neuroblastoma on the right side just medial to the ipsilateral kidney extending into the vertebral column (arrows).

Chapter 16

Female Reproductive System

① Ovaries (Figure 16-1)

A. General Features. The ovaries are almond-shaped structures that are located **posterior** to the broad ligament. They are attached to the lateral pelvic wall by the **suspensory ligament of the ovary** (a region of the broad ligament), which contains the ovarian artery, vein, and nerve. The surface of the ovaries is not covered by peritoneum, but rather by a simple cuboidal epithelium called the **germinal epithelium**. The arterial supply is from the abdominal aorta via the **ovarian arteries** and the internal iliac artery via **ascending branches of the uterine arteries**, which anastomose with each other. The venous drainage via a **pampiniform plexus of veins** is to the **right ovarian vein** (which empties into the inferior vena cava [IVC]) and the **left ovarian vein** (which empties into the left renal vein).

B. Clinical Considerations

1. **Ovarian Cancer (Figure 16-2A).** Ovarian cancer may develop from oocytes (oocyte or germ cell tumors), follicular cells (follicular cell tumors or sex cord cell tumors), stromal cells (stromal cell tumors), or germinal epithelium (germinal epithelium tumors). The most common type is a **germinal epithelium tumor**, which is a malignant transformation of the germinal epithelium covering the ovary. The main lymphatic drainage of the ovary is to the deep **para-aortic lymph nodes** near the renal artery. An increased incidence of ovarian cancer occurs in women with **hereditary nonpolyposis colorectal cancer (HNPCC**; also called **Lynch syndrome II)**. Ovarian cancer is associated with mutations of the **p53 tumor suppressor gene**. **Carcinoembryonic antigen (CEA)** and **CA-125** (tumor markers) are useful in diagnosis. Some germ cell cancers produce **human chorionic gonadotropin (hCG)** and α-**fetoprotein (AFP)**, which may serve as markers. A palpable ovary or adnexal mass is generally suggestive of an ovarian neoplasm rather than an ovarian cyst.

2. **Ovarian Cysts.** Functional cysts in the ovary are so common as to be virtually physiologic and resolve spontaneously. A functional cyst is a physiologically and hormonally active cyst that has not yet involuted. They originate from either unruptured Graafian follicles or in Graafian follicles that have ruptured and immediately sealed. Ovarian cysts are nonneoplastic, fluid-filled cavities that may be solitary or multiple (up to 2 cm in diameter). There are three main types of cysts:

   a. **Follicular cysts** are generally large cysts (>2 cm) that may be diagnosed by palpation or ultrasound. Histologically, granulosa lutein cells can be identified if the pressure is not too great, and theca lutein cells may be conspicuous.

   b. **Corpus luteum cysts** are lined by a conspicuous rim of granulosa lutein cells.

     c. **Theca lutein cysts** are caused by elevated levels of **hCG** produced by the placenta during pregnancy. This causes a proliferation of theca lutein cells, which form small nodules in the ovary.

3. **Polycystic ovary syndrome (Figure 16-2B)** is characterized biochemically by increased levels of androgens and luteinizing hormone (LH) but decreased levels of follicle-stimulating hormone (FSH). This results in bilateral ovarian enlargement, cortical fibrosis, and multiple follicular cysts. Clinical findings include chronic anovulation with menstrual irregularities such as oligomenorrhea or amenorrhea; oily skin and acne; hirsutism; and obesity.

4. **Right side hydronephrosis** may indicate thrombosis of the right ovarian vein that constricts the ureter because the right ovarian vein crosses the ureter to enter the IVC.

5. **Ovarian pain** is often referred down the inner thigh via the obturator nerve.

Ⅱ   Uterine Tubes (Figure 16-1)

A. **General Features.** The uterine tube has four divisions: **infundibulum** (funnel-shaped and opens into the peritoneal cavity), **ampulla** (longest, widest part and is the site of fertilization), **isthmus**, and **intramural** (opens into the uterine cavity). The uterine tubes are supported by the **mesosalpinx**, which is a region of the broad ligament. The function of the uterine tubes is to convey fertilized and unfertilized oocytes to the uterine cavity by ciliary action and muscular contractions and to transport sperm in the opposite direction for fertilization to take place. The arterial supply is from the abdominal aorta via the **ovarian arteries** and the internal iliac artery via the **ascending branches of the uterine arteries**, which anastomose with each other. The venous drainage is to the **right ovarian vein** (which empties into the IVC), the **left ovarian vein** (which empties into the left renal vein), and the **uterine veins**.

B. **Clinical Considerations**

1. **Acute and chronic salpingitis (Figure 16-2C)** is a bacterial infection (most commonly *Neisseria gonorrhea* or *Chlamydia trachomatis*) of the uterine tube with acute inflammation (neutrophil infiltration) or chronic inflammation, which may lead to scarring of the uterine tube predisposing to **ectopic tubal pregnancy**. Salpingitis is probably the most common cause of female sterility.

2. **Ectopic tubal pregnancy (Figure 16-2D)** most often occurs in the **ampulla** of the uterine tube. Risk factors include salpingitis, pelvic inflammatory disease, pelvic surgery, or exposure to DES (diethylstilbestrol). Clinical signs include sudden onset of abdominal pain, which may be confused with appendicitis in a young woman, last menses 60 days ago, and positive hCG test; culdocentesis shows intraperitoneal blood.

Ⅲ   Uterus (Figure 16-1)

A. **General Features.** The uterus is divided into four regions called the **fundus, cornu, body**, and **cervix**. The **fundus** is located superior to the cornu and contributes largely to the upper segment of the uterus during pregnancy. At term, the fundus may extend as high as the xiphoid process (vertebral level T9). The **cornu** is located near the entry of the uterine tubes. The **body** is located between the cornu and cervix. The **isthmus** is part of the body and is the dividing line between the body of the uterus and the cervix. The isthmus is the preferred site for a surgical incision during a delivery by cesarean section.

The **cervix** is located inferior to the body of the uterus and protrudes into the vagina. The cervix contains the **internal os, cervical canal**, and **external os.** The external os in a nulliparous woman is round. The external os in a parous woman is transverse. The arterial supply is from the internal iliac artery via the uterine arteries with a potential collateral supply from the ovarian arteries. The venous drainage via a uterine venous plexus is to the internal iliac veins → IVC.

B. Support of the Uterus. The uterus is supported by the following structures:
1. **Pelvic Diaphragm (levator ani muscles)**
2. **Urogenital Diaphragm**
3. **Urinary Bladder**
4. **Round ligament of the uterus,** which is a remnant of the gubernaculum in the embryo.
5. **Transverse cervical ligament (cardinal ligament of Mackenrodt),** which extends laterally from the cervix to the side wall of the pelvis. It is located at the base of the broad ligament and contains the **uterine artery** (a branch of the internal iliac artery).
6. **Uterosacral ligament,** which extends posteriorly from the cervix to the sacrum and is responsible for bracing the uterus in its normal **anteverted** position.
7. **Pubocervical ligament,** which extends anteriorly from the cervix to the pubic symphysis and helps to prevent a **cystocele** (a herniation of the urinary bladder into the anterior wall of the vagina).
8. **Broad ligament,** which is a double fold of parietal peritoneum that extends laterally from the uterus to the side wall of the pelvis.
   a. The broad ligament is divided into four regions: **mesosalpinx** (which supports the uterine tubes), **mesovarium** (which supports the ovary), **mesometrium** (which support the uterus), and the **suspensory ligament of the ovary.**
   b. The broad ligament contains the following structures: **ovarian artery, vein, and nerves; uterine tubes; ovarian ligament of the uterus** (which is a remnant of the gubernaculum in the embryo); **round ligament of the uterus** (which is a remnant of the gubernaculum in the embryo); **epoöphoron** (which is a remnant of the mesonephric tubules in the embryo); **paroöphoron** (which is a remnant of the mesonephric tubules in the embryo); **Gartner duct** (which is a remnant of the mesonephric duct in the embryo); **ureter** (which lies at the base of the broad ligament posterior and inferior to the uterine artery; during a hysterectomy, the ureters may be inadvertently ligated along with the uterine artery because of their close anatomic relationship); and the **uterine artery, vein, and nerves** (which lie at the base of the broad ligament within the transverse cervical ligament).

C. Position of the Uterus. The uterus is normally is an anteflexed and anteverted position, which places it in a nearly horizontal position lying on the superior wall of the urinary bladder. **Anteflexed** refers to the anterior bend of the uterus at the angle between the cervix and the body of the uterus. **Anteverted** refers to the anterior bend of the uterus at the angle between the cervix and the vagina.

D. Clinical Considerations
1. **Endometrial adenocarcinoma (Figure 16-2E)** is the most common gynecologic cancer in women and is linked to prolonged estrogen stimulation of the endometrium. Risk factors include exogenous estrogen treatment for menopause, obesity, diabetes, nulliparity, early menarche, and late menopause. This cancer grows in a diffuse or polypoid pattern and often involves multiple sites. The most

common histologic variant is composed entirely of glandular cells (called pure endometrial adenocarcinoma). Clinical features include perimenopausal or postmenopausal women who complain of abnormal uterine bleeding.

2. **Endometriosis (Figure 16-2F)** is the presence of endometrial glandular tissue in abnormal locations outside of the uterus. The ectopic sites most frequently involved include the ovary (80% of cases), uterine ligaments, rectovaginal septum, pouch of Douglas, pelvic peritoneum covering the uterus, uterine tubes, rectosigmoid colon, or bladder. Early foci of endometriosis on the ovary or peritoneal surface appear as red or bluish nodules ("**mulberry nodules**") about 1 to 5 mm in size. Because this ectopic endometrial tissue shows cyclic changes synchronous with the endometrium of the uterus (i.e. participates in the menstrual cycle), repeated bleeding leads to a deposition of hemosiderin, forming "**gunpowder mark**" lesions. In the ovary, repeated bleedings may lead to the formation of large (15 cm) cysts containing inspissated chocolate-colored material ("**chocolate cysts**"). Endometriosis results in infertility, dysmenorrhea, and pelvic pain (most pronounced at the time of menstruation).

3. **Uterine fibroids (leiomyoma; Figure 16-2G, H)** are a common benign neoplasm resulting from a proliferation of smooth muscle cells of the uterus, which may become calcified. The fibroids may be located within the myometrium of the uterus (intramural), beneath the endometrium (submucosa) where they may grow into the uterine cavity, or beneath the serosa (subserosal) where they may grow into the peritoneal cavity. This may result in infertility if the fibroids block the uterine tube or prevent implantation of the conceptus. Fibroids may be palpated as irregular, nodular masses protruding against the anterior abdominal wall.

4. **Primary amenorrhea** is the complete absence of menstruation in a woman from puberty.

5. **Secondary amenorrhea** is the absence of menstruation for at least 3 months in a woman who previously had normal menstruation. The most common cause of secondary amenorrhea is pregnancy, which can be determined by assaying urine **hCG**. Other pathologic causes of secondary amenorrhea include hypothalamic or pituitary malfunction (e.g. **anorexia nervosa**), ovarian disorders (e.g. **ovariectomy**), and end-organ disease (e.g. **Asherman syndrome**, in which the basal layer of the endometrium has been removed by repeated curettages). Secondary amenorrhea is evaluated clinically by assaying serum FSH and LH levels along with a progesterone challenge. Bleeding after a **progesterone withdrawal test** indicates that the endometrium was primed by estrogen, thereby indicating that the hypothalamic–pituitary axis and the ovaries are functioning normally.

6. **Menorrhagia** is excessive bleeding at menstruation in either the amount of blood or number of days. It is usually associated with a leiomyoma (fibroids).

7. **Dysmenorrhea** is excessive pain during menstruation. It is commonly associated with endometriosis and an increased level of prostaglandin F in the menstrual fluid.

8. **Metrorrhagia** is bleeding that occurs at irregular intervals. It is commonly associated with cervical carcinoma or cervical polyps.

9. **Prepubertal bleeding** is bleeding that occurs before menarche. It is commonly associated with vaginitis, infection, sexual abuse, or embryonal rhabdomyosarcoma.

10. **Postmenopausal bleeding** occurs approximately 1 year after the cessation of the menstrual cycle. It is commonly associated with malignant tumors of the uterus.

IV **Cervix.** The cervix is the lower part of the uterus that measures about 2.5 to 3.0 cm in length. The cervix is divided into a **supravaginal portion** (lying above the vaginal vault) and a **vaginal portion (portio vaginalis)**, which protrudes into the vagina. The junction between the cervix and uterus is at the **internal os**. Histologically, the cervical wall consists of:

A. A **simple columnar epithelium**, which invaginates into the cervical stroma to form **mucus-secreting cervical glands**. This epithelium and cervical glands do not slough off during the menstrual cycle and are relatively unaffected by the menstrual cycle except that the cervical mucus produced during the proliferative phase is **watery** and the cervical mucus produced during the secretory phase is **viscous**.

B. The wall of the cervix is predominately **connective tissue** with very little smooth muscle (very different compared with the uterine wall, which is predominately smooth muscle). During pregnancy, the cervix undergoes little or no expansion. However, during childbirth, the connective tissue becomes pliable (called "**cervical softening**") because of the action of **relaxin**.

V Ectocervix. The outer epithelial surface of the vaginal portion of the cervix (portio vaginalis) is called the **ectocervix**. The epithelial surface lining the lumen of the **endocervical canal** is called the **endocervix**.

A. During prepuberty, the **ectocervix** is covered by a **nonkeratinized, stratified squamous epithelium** that is continuous with the vaginal epithelium.

B. The **endocervical canal** connects the uterine cavity with the vaginal cavity and extends from the internal os to the **external os**. The endocervical canal is lined by **simple columnar epithelium**, which invaginates into the cervical stroma to form **mucus-secreting cervical glands**.

C. At puberty, the simple columnar epithelium of the endocervical canal extends onto the ectocervix. However, exposure of the simple columnar epithelium to the acidic (pH = 3) environment of the vagina induces a transformation from columnar to squamous epithelium (i.e. **squamous metaplasia**) and the formation of a **transformation zone**.

D. The transformation zone is the site of **Nabothian cysts**, which develop as stratified squamous epithelium grows over the mucus-secreting simple columnar epithelium and entraps large amounts of mucus.

E. The transformation zone is the most common site of **squamous cell carcinoma of the cervix** (**Figure 16-2I**), which is usually preceded by epithelial changes called **cervical intraepithelial neoplasia (CIN)** diagnosed by a Pap smear. **Human papillomavirus (HPV)** has also been linked as an important factor in cervical oncogenesis and is often tested for. Cervical carcinoma may spread to the side wall of the pelvis, where the ureters may become obstructed, leading to hydronephrosis. The most common site of lymph node spread (i.e. sentinel nodes) is to the obturator lymph nodes.

VI Vagina (Figure 16-1)

A. General Features. The vagina is a fibromuscular tube that is kept moist by mucus produced by **cervical glands** that drain down through the cervical canal and additional mucus produced by the **greater vestibular glands (of Bartholin)** and **lesser vestibular glands**. The vagina extends from the cervix to the vestibule of the vagina. The vagina is the longest part of the birth canal, and its distension during childbirth is limited by the ischial spines and sacrospinous ligaments. The arterial supply is from the internal iliac artery via **vaginal branches of uterine arteries** to the superior portion of the vagina and the **internal pudendal artery** to the middle and lower portions of the vagina. The venous drainage via the vaginal venous plexus along the sides of the vagina, which is continuous with the uterine venous plexus, is to the internal iliac veins → IVC. The vagina forms a recess around the cervix called the **fornix**. The fornix is divided into three regions:

1. **Anterior fornix** is located anterior to the cervix and is related to the **vesicouterine pouch**. The urinary bladder is palpable through the anterior fornix during a digital examination.

2. **Lateral fornices** are located lateral to the cervix.

3. **Posterior fornix** is located posterior to the cervix and is related to the rectouterine pouch (of Douglas). The rectum, sacral promontory (S1 vertebral body), and coccyx are palpable through the posterior fornix during digital examination. The posterior fornix is a site for culdocentesis.

B. Clinical Considerations

1. **Culdocentesis** is a procedure in which a needle is passed through the posterior fornix into the rectouterine pouch of the peritoneal cavity to obtain a fluid sample for analysis or collect oocytes for in vitro fertilization. It provides diagnostic information for many gynecologic conditions (e.g. pelvic inflammatory disease, ectopic tubal pregnancy).

2. **Cystocele** is the herniation of the urinary bladder into the anterior wall of the vagina.

3. **Rectocele** is the herniation of the rectum into the posterior wall of the vagina.

4. **Bartholin cyst (Figure 16-2J)** is caused by an obstruction of the duct from the greater vestibular glands of Bartholin.

5. **Vaginitis** is a chronic infection most often caused by *Trichomonas vaginalis* (15% of cases), *Candida albicans* (25%), or *Gardnerella vaginalis* (30%). The vaginal epithelium is resistant to bacterial, fungal, and protozoan invasion so that the pathogens remain within the lumen of vagina.

    a. *Trichomonas vaginalis* is a **flagellated protozoan** that is sexually transmitted. It produces a vaginitis characterized by an inflammatory vaginal smear with numerous neutrophils, a fiery-red appearance of the vaginal and cervical mucosa ("strawberry mucosa"), and a **thin, gray-white, frothy, purulent, malodorous discharge (pH > 4.5)**. Postcoital bleeding is a common complaint. The organism is best seen in fresh preparations diluted with warm saline in which the tumbling motility of the organism can be observed.

    b. *Candida albicans* is a **yeast** that produces pseudohyphae and true hyphae in tissues. It produces superficial white patches or large fluffy membranes that easily detach, leaving a red, irritated underlying surface and a **thick, white, "cottage cheese" discharge (pH < 4.5)**. The organism can be observed on KOH preparations of the discharge.

    c. *Gardnerella vaginalis* (a **gram-negative bacillus**) is a bacterial infection generally called **bacterial vaginosis** in which higher than normal levels of the bacteria are present. It is not sexually transmitted. It produces a vaginitis characterized by no inflammatory vaginal smear, no changes in the mucosa, and a **thin, homogeneous, somewhat adherent, fishy-odor discharge (pH > 4.5)**. The discharge gives a positive amine test ("whiff test"; fishy amine smell) when mixed with KOH. A vaginal smear will show increased number of bacteria and "clue cells," which are squamous cells with a clumped nucleus and a folded cytoplasm covered with bacteria.

VII **External Genitalia (Figure 16-1)**

A. **Labia majora** are two folds of hairy skin with underlying fat pads.

B. **Labia minora** are two folds of hairless skin located medial to the labia majora that enclose the vestibule of the vagina. Each labium minus is continuous anteriorly with the **prepuce of the clitoris** and the **frenulum of the clitoris**. Each labium minus is continuous posteriorly with the **fourchette**, which connects the labia minora with the **vaginal introitus (entry)**.

C. **Vestibule of the vagina** is the space between the labia minora. It contains the **urethral orifice**; **paraurethral glands (of Skene)**; **vaginal introitus (entry)**, which is incompletely covered by the **hymen**; **greater vestibular glands (of Bartholin)**; and **lesser vestibular glands**.

D. **Clitoris.** Although the clitoris is homologous with the penis, the clitoris has NO corpus spongiosum and does NOT transmit the urethra.
   1. **Body of the clitoris** is formed by two **corpora cavernosa**, which are continuous with the crura of the clitoris.
   2. **Glans of the clitoris** is formed by the fusion of the **vestibular bulbs**.

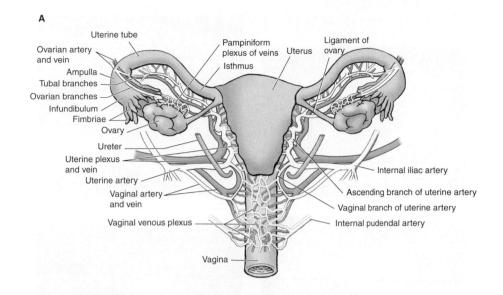

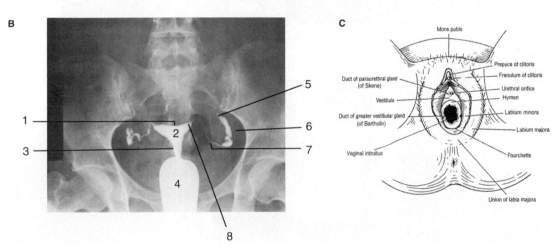

● **Figure 16-1 Female Pelvis. (A) Diagram of the Arterial Supply and Venous Drainage of the Ovaries, Uterine Tubes, Uterus, and Vagina. (B)** AP radiograph of the female pelvis after injection of a radiopaque compound into the uterine cavity (hysterosalpingography). 1 = fundus of uterus, 2 = uterine cavity, 3 = isthmus of uterus, 4 = cervical canal (dilated and stretched), 5 = infundibulum of uterine tube, 6 = ampulla of uterine tube, 7 = isthmus of uterine tube, 8 = opening of uterine tube. **(C) Diagram of the Female Genitalia.**

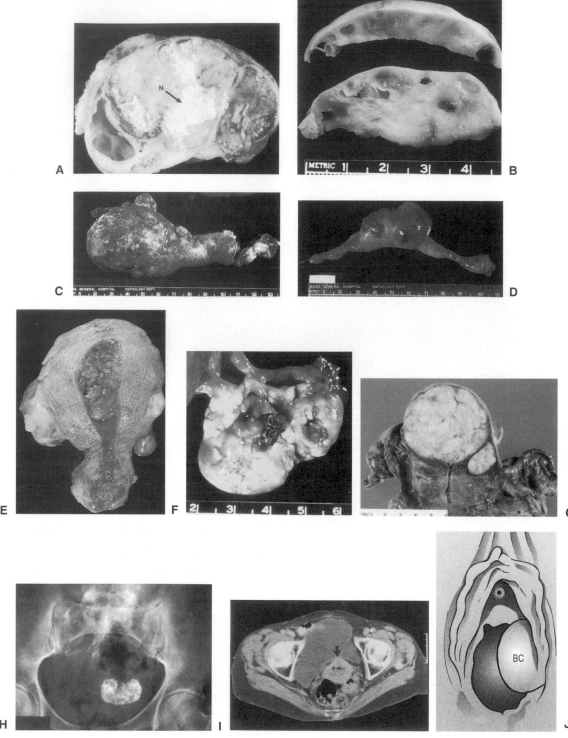

● **Figure 16-2 (A) Malignant Serous Cystadenocarcinoma of the Ovary.** Malignant serous cystadenocarcinoma of the ovary derived from germinal epithelium. Photograph shows an enlarged ovary containing a solid tumor that exhibits extensive necrosis (N). **(B) Polycystic Disease of the Ovary.** Photograph shows the cut sections of an ovary with numerous cysts embedded in a sclerotic stroma. **(C) Salpingitis.** Photograph shows the uterine tube is markedly distended, the fimbriated end is closed, and there is hemorrhage on the serosal surface. **(D) Ectopic Tubal Pregnancy.** Photograph shows an enlarged uterine tube as a result of the growing embryo. **(E) Endometrial Adenocarcinoma.** Photograph shows an opened uterine cavity to reveal a partially necrotic, polypoid endometrial cancer. **(F) Endometriosis.** Photograph shows an ovary with red and bluish nodules ("mulberry nodules"). **(G, H) Uterine Fibroids (Leiomyoma).** **(G)** Photograph shows a bisected uterus to reveal prominent, sharply circumscribed, fleshy tumor. **(H)** Radiograph shows a calcified mass just to the left of the midline. Calcifications in fibroids are often popcornlike in appearance. A very large fibrinoid may occupy the entire pelvic cavity or may even extend into the abdomen. **(I) Squamous Cell Carcinoma of the Cervix.** CT scan shows a mass (large arrow) immediately posterior to the urinary bladder. A small amount of gas is present within the mass (small arrow) secondary to necrosis. Note the posterior margin of the urinary bladder. **(J) Bartholin Cyst.** Diagram shows a Bartholin cyst (BC) on the left side of the vestibule of the vagina. This cyst is caused by an obstruction of the duct from the greater vestibular glands of Bartholin.

Chapter 17

Male Reproductive System

❶ Testes (Figures 17-1, 17-2)

A. **General Features.** The testes (plural) **produce spermatozoa** and **secrete male androgens** (i.e. testosterone, which is converted to dihydrotestosterone [DHT] and 5α-androstanediol) via **Leydig cells.** The testes are paired, ovoid organs located in the scrotum. Each mature adult testis (singular) is 4 to 5 cm in length, 2.5 cm in width, and 3 cm in thickness, and weighs about 11 to 17 g. The right testis is commonly slightly larger and heavier than the left. The testes are surrounded incompletely (medially, laterally, and anteriorly, but not posteriorly) by a sac of peritoneum called the **tunica vaginalis.** Beneath the tunica vaginalis, the testes are surrounded by a thick connective tissue capsule called the **tunica albuginea** because of its whitish color. Beneath the tunica albuginea, the testes are surrounded by a highly vascular layer of connective tissue called the **tunica vasculosa.** The tunica albuginea projects connective tissue septae inward toward the mediastinum that divides the testis into about 250 lobules, each of which contains one to four highly coiled **seminiferous tubules.** These septae converge toward the midline on the posterior surface, where they meet to form a ridgelike thickening called the **mediastinum.** The septae are continuous with the interstitial connective tissue that contains the Leydig (interstitial) cells. The testes contain the **seminiferous tubules, straight tubules, rete testes, efferent ductules,** and **Leydig (interstitial) cells.** The arterial blood supply is from the abdominal aorta via the **testicular arteries.** There is a rich collateral arterial blood supply from the internal iliac artery via the **artery of the ductus deferens,** the inferior epigastric artery via the **cremasteric artery,** and the femoral artery via the **external pudendal artery.** The collateral circulation is sufficient to allow ligation of the testicular artery during surgery. Venous drainage is to the **right testicular vein** (which empties into the inferior vena cava [IVC]) and the **left testicular vein** (which empties into the left renal vein). This is important in males in whom the appearance of a **left-side testicular varicocele** may indicate occlusion of the left testicular vein or left renal vein as a result of a malignant tumor of the kidney. The testicular veins are formed by the union of the veins of the **pampiniform plexus.** Lymphatic drainage of the testes is to **deep lumbar nodes** near the renal hilus, which is important clinically in evaluating the spread of testicular cancer. Note that the lymphatic drainage of the scrotum is to **superficial inguinal nodes.**

B. **Clinical Considerations**
   1. **Cryptorchidism (Figure 17-4A)** occurs when the testes begin to descend along the normal pathway but fail to reach the scrotum (versus an **ectopic testis,** which descends along an abnormal pathway). The undescended testes are generally found within the **inguinal canal** or **abdominal cavity near the deep inguinal ring.** Bilateral cryptorchidism results in **sterility** because the cooler temperature of the scrotal sac

is necessary for spermatogenesis. Cryptorchidism is associated with increased incidence of cancer and torsion.

2. **Hydrocele of testes (Figure 17-4B)** occurs when a small patency of the processus vaginalis remains, so that peritoneal fluid can flow into the tunica vaginalis surrounding the testes.

3. **Varicocele (Figure 17-4C)** is an abnormal dilatation of the pampiniform plexus and testicular vein and usually presents as a palpable "bag of worms" scrotal swelling. It most often occurs on the left side (90%) because of compression of the left testicular vein by the sigmoid colon, which contains stored feces, and is often associated with infertility.

4. **Torsion (Figure 17-4D)** is the rotation of the testes about the spermatic cord usually toward the penis (i.e. medial rotation). An increased incidence occurs in men with testes in a horizontal position and a high attachment of the tunica vaginalis to the spermatic cord ("bell clapper deformity"). Torsion is a medical emergency because compression of the testicular vessels results in ischemic necrosis with 6 hours.

5. **Testicular lymphoma** is a malignant lymphoma that has metastasized to the testes and presents as a testicular mass. It is the most common form of testicular cancer in men older than 60 years of age.

6. **Yolk sac tumor** is the most common form of testicular cancer in infants and children up to 3 years of age. It is associated with **elevated α-fetoprotein levels**.

7. **Seminoma (Figure 17-4E)** is the most common type of germ cell neoplasm in men between 20 and 40 years of age and presents as a painless testicular mass (usually on the right side) or a nodularity. About 90% of testicular cancers arise from germ cells. Seminoma is associated with **elevated human chorionic gonadotropin (hCG) levels**.

8. **Testicular teratocarcinoma** is a germ cell neoplasm. In its early histologic stages, it may resemble a blastocyst with three primary germ layers (i.e. may be loosely referred to as "male pregnancy"). A testicular teratocarcinoma is composed of a collection of well-differentiated cells and structures from each of the primary germ layers (e.g. colon glandular tissue, cartilage, and squamous epithelium).

9. **5α-Reductase 2 deficiency** is caused by a mutation in the **5α-reductase 2 gene** that renders 5α-reductase 2 enzyme inactive. Normally, 5α-reductase 2 catalyzes the conversion of **testosterone (T)** → **DHT**. 5α-Reductase 2 deficiency produces the following clinical findings: underdevelopment of the penis and scrotum (microphallus, hypospadias, and bifid scrotum) and of the prostate gland. The epididymis, ductus deferens, seminal vesicle, and ejaculatory duct are normal. These clinical findings have led to inference that DHT is essential in the development of the penis and scrotum (external genitalia) and prostate gland in genotypic XY fetus. At puberty, these individuals demonstrate a striking virilization. An increased T:DHT ratio is diagnostic (normal = 5; 5α-reductase 2 deficiency = 20–60).

10. **17β-Hydroxysteroid dehydrogenase 3 (HSD) deficiency** is caused by a mutation in the **17β-HSD3 gene** that renders 17β-HSD3 enzyme inactive. Normally, 17β-HSD3 catalyzes the conversion of **androstenedione** → **testosterone**. This is the most common defect in androgen biosynthesis. 17β-HSD3 deficiency produces the following clinical findings: underdevelopment of the penis and scrotum (microphallus, hypospadias, and bifid scrotum) and of the prostate gland. The epididymis, ductus deferens, seminal vesicle, and ejaculatory duct are normal. The clinical findings in 17β-HSD3 deficiency and 5α-reductase 2 deficiency are very similar.

11. **Complete androgen insensitivity (CAIS; testicular feminization syndrome)** is caused by a mutation in the **androgen receptor (AR) gene** that renders AR inactive. Normally, AR is a **nuclear transcription factor** that is activated by androgens to

bind DNA promoter regions that regulate transcription of other genes. CAIS produces the following clinical findings: 46,XY genotype, testes, and normal-appearing female external genitalia; the uterus and uterine tubes are absent. These individuals present as normal-appearing females, and their psychosocial orientation is female despite their genotype.

Ⅱ **Epididymis (Figures 17-1, 17-2).** The epididymis is a very long (6 m) and highly coiled duct that is described as having a **head region, body region,** and **tail region. Sperm maturation (i.e. motility) and storage** occurs in the head and body of the epididymis. The tail of the epididymis is continuous with the ductus deferens. Histologically, the epididymis has an epithelial lining and muscular coat. The epididymis is lined by a pseudostratified columnar epithelium consisting of tall columnar **principal cells** and **basal cells.** The epididymis has a smooth luminal surface (in contrast to the saw-toothed pattern of the efferent ductules). The principal cells are characterized by stereocilia, apical invaginations, numerous pinocytotic vesicles, coated vesicles, lysosomes, well-developed rough endoplasmic reticulum, and Golgi. The principal cells have the following functions: resorption of testicular fluid begun in the efferent ductules; phagocytosis of degenerating sperm or spermatid residual bodies not phagocytosed by the Sertoli cells; and secretion of glycoproteins that bind to the surface of the cell membrane of the sperm, sialic acid, and glycerophosphocholine (which inhibits capacitation thus preventing sperm from fertilizing a secondary oocyte until the sperm enter the female reproductive tract). The basal cells act as a stem cell population to resupply the principal cells. In the head and body region of the epididymis, the muscular coat consists of a **circular layer of smooth muscle** that aids in the movement of sperm. In the tail region of the epididymis, the muscular coat consists of an **inner longitudinal layer, middle circular layer,** and **outer longitudinal layer of smooth muscle.** These three layers contract because of neural stimulation during sexual excitation and force sperm from the tail of the epididymis to the ductus deferens. This is the initial muscular component that contributes to the force of emission.

Ⅲ **Ductus Deferens (Figures 17-1, 17-2)**

A. General Features. The ductus deferens begins at the inferior pole of the testes, ascends to enter the spermatic cord, transits the inguinal canal, enters the abdominal cavity by passing through the deep inguinal ring, crosses the external iliac artery and vein, and enters the pelvis. The distal end of the ductus deferens enlarges to form the **ampulla,** where it is joined by a short duct from the seminal vesicle to form the **ejaculatory duct.** The epithelium of the ductus deferens is similar to the epididymis (i.e. **pseudostratified columnar epithelium with principal cells and basal cells**). The smooth muscular coat of the ductus deferens is similar to the tail region of the epididymis (i.e. **inner longitudinal layer, middle circular layer,** and **outer longitudinal layer of smooth muscle**), and contributes to the force of emission. The arterial supply is from the internal iliac artery via the **artery of the ductus deferens,** which anastomoses with the testicular artery. The venous drainage is to the **testicular vein** and the **distal pampiniform plexus.**

B. Clinical Consideration. Vasectomy: The scalpel will cut through the following layers in succession to gain access to the ductus deferens: skin → Colles' fascia and dartos muscle → external spermatic fascia → cremasteric fascia and muscle → internal spermatic fascia → extraperitoneal fat. The tunica vaginalis is not cut.

Ⅳ **Contents of the Spermatic Cord.** The contents of the spermatic cord include the following: ductus deferens, testicular artery, artery of the ductus deferens, cremasteric artery, pampiniform venous plexus, sympathetic and parasympathetic nerves, genitofemoral nerve, and lymphatics.

Ⅴ **Ejaculatory Duct (Figures 17-1, 17-2).** The distal end of the ductus deferens enlarges to form the ampulla, where it is joined by a short duct from the seminal vesicle to form the ejaculatory duct. The ejaculatory duct passes through the prostate gland and opens into the prostatic urethra at the seminal colliculus of the urethral crest. The epithelium is similar to the epididymis and ductus deferens. However, the ejaculatory duct has no smooth muscular coat. The force for emission is derived primarily by the smooth muscular coat of the tail region of the epididymis and ductus deferens.

Ⅵ **Urethra (Figures 17-2, 17-3).** In the male, the urethra is the terminal duct for both the urinary system (urine) and the reproductive system (sperm). The male urethra is about 18 to 20 cm long and begins at the internal urethral orifice of the bladder where the detrusor muscle extends longitudinally into the prostatic urethra and forms a complete collar around the neck of the bladder called the internal urethral sphincter. The male urethra is divided into five parts:

A. **Prostatic Urethra.** The prostatic urethra courses through and is surrounded by the **prostate gland**. The posterior wall has an elevation called the **urethral crest**. The **prostatic sinus** is a groove on either side of the urethral crest that receives most of the prostatic ducts from the prostate gland. At a specific site along the urethral crest there is an ovoid enlargement called the **seminal colliculus** (also called the **verumontanum**), where the ejaculatory ducts open and the **prostatic utricle** (a vestigial remnant of the paramesonephric duct in males that is involved in the embryologic development of the vagina and uterus) is found.

B. **Membranous Urethra.** The membranous urethra courses through the **urogenital diaphragm**, where it becomes related to the **deep transverse perineal muscle** and **sphincter urethrae muscle** (also called **external urethral sphincter**), both of which are skeletal muscle innervated by the **pudendal nerve**. The external urethral sphincter completely surrounds the male urethra. The prostatic urethra plus the membranous urethra is called the **posterior urethra** by radiologists.

C. **Bulbous Urethra.** The bulbous urethra courses through the **bulb of the penis** and develops endodermal outgrowths into the surrounding mesoderm to form the **bulbourethral glands of Cowper**. The bulbous urethra contains the openings of the bulbourethral glands of Cowper.

D. **Proximal Part of the Penile (spongy or cavernous) Urethra.** The proximal part of the penile urethra courses through and is surrounded by the **corpus spongiosum**. The proximal part of the penile urethra develops endodermal outgrowths into the surrounding mesoderm to form the **urethral glands of Littre**.

E. **Distal Part of the Penile Urethra.** The distal part of the penile urethra courses through the **glans penis** and terminates as the **navicular fossa** at the **external urethral orifice**, which opens onto the surface of the glans penis. The bulbous urethra plus the proximal and distal parts of the penile urethra is called the **anterior urethra** by radiologists.

Seminal Vesicles (Figures 17-1, 17-2). The seminal vesicles are highly coiled tubular diverticula that originate as evaginations of the ductus deferens distal to the ampulla. The mucosa (epithelium and lamina propria) is thrown into highly convoluted folds, forming labyrinth-like cul-de-sacs, all of which open into a central lumen. The **lamina propria** consists of connective tissue. The **muscular coat** consists of an inner circular layer and outer longitudinal layer. Contraction of the smooth muscle during emission discharges the secretory product (seminal fluid) into the ejaculatory duct. The **adventitia** consists of connective tissue. The seminal vesicles are lined by a **pseudostratified columnar epithelium** consisting of **columnar cells** and **basal cells**. The columnar cells have numerous microvilli, rough endoplasmic reticulum, Golgi, lipid droplets, secretory granules, and lipochrome pigment. These are characteristics of cells active in secretion. The secretion product is a whitish-yellow viscous material that contains **fructose** (the principal metabolic substrate for sperm) and **other sugars**, **choline**, **proteins**, **amino acids**, **ascorbic acid**, **citric acid**, and prostaglandins. Seminal vesicle secretion (i.e. seminal fluid) accounts for 70% of the volume of the ejaculated semen. The characteristic pale yellow color of semen is caused by the **lipochrome pigment** secreted by the columnar cells. In **forensic medicine**, the presence of fructose (which is not produced elsewhere in the body) and choline crystals is used to determine the presence of semen. The basal cells are stem cells.

 Bulbourethral (BU) Glands of Cowper (Figures 17-1, 17-2). The BU glands are located in the deep perineal space embedded in the skeletal muscles of the urogenital diaphragm (i.e. deep transverse perineal muscle and sphincter urethrae muscle) and adjacent to the membranous urethrae. The ducts of the BU glands open into the penile urethra. The BU glands are compound tubuloalveolar glands (resemble mucus-secreting glands) surrounded by a connective tissue capsule that extends septae that divide the BU glands into many lobules. The compound tubuloalveolar glands are lined by a simple cuboidal epithelium. The epithelium produces a clear, mucouslike, slippery fluid that contains **galactose**, **galactosamine**, **galacturonic acid**, **sialic acid**, and **methylpentose**. This fluid makes up a major portion of the preseminal fluid (or preejaculate fluid) and probably serves to lubricate the penile urethra.

 Prostate Gland (Figures 17-1, 17-2, 17-5A, B)

A. General Features. The prostate gland is located between the base of the urinary bladder and the urogenital diaphragm. The anterior surface of the prostate is related to the retropubic space. The posterior surface of the prostate is related to the seminal vesicles and rectum. The prostate gland can be easily palpated by a digital examination via the rectum. The prostate gland consists of five lobes: **right and left lateral lobes**, **right and left posterior lobes**, and a **middle lobe**. The prostate gland is a collection of 30 to 50 compound tubuloalveolar glands that are arranged in three zones: the **peripheral zone** (contains the largest glands and highest number of glands), **central zone**, and **transitional (periurethral) zone**. The compound tubuloalveolar glands are lined by a simple columnar epithelium (however, it may vary from pseudostratified to cuboidal epithelium). The prostatic epithelium contains basal cells, secretory cells, and endocrine cells. The basal cells are the stem cell or proliferative compartment of the prostatic epithelium normally dividing and maturing into secretory cells. The secretory cells contain rough endoplasmic reticulum, Golgi, small clear secretory vacuoles, and lysosomes. The epithelium produces the prostatic fluid, which contains **citric acid**, **prostatic acid phosphatase (PAP)**, **prostaglandins**, **fibrinogen**, and **prostatic-specific antigen (PSA)**. Serum levels of PSA and PAP are used as a diagnostic tool for prostatic carcinoma. PSA is a serine protease that liquefies semen after ejaculation. The endocrine cells are randomly scattered and contain serotonin, somatostatin, calcitonin, and bombesin. The lumen of the glands contains corpora amylacea (or prostatic concretions), which are calcified or precipitated prostatic fluid, the significance of which is not understood. The number of prostatic concretions increases with age. The prostate gland is surrounded by a capsule consisting of connective tissue and smooth muscle. The capsule is highly vascularized (important in carcinoma metastasis). The capsule (both connective tissue and smooth muscle) extends into the prostate gland, forming the stroma. The arterial supply is from the internal iliac artery via the **inferior vesical artery**.

The venous drainage follows two pathways. The first is to the **prostatic venous plexus** → **internal iliac veins** → **inferior vena cava (IVC)**. This may explain the metastasis of prostatic cancer to the heart and lungs. The second is to the **prostatic venous plexus** → **vertebral venous plexus** → **cranial dural sinuses**. This may explain the metastasis of prostatic cancer to the vertebral column and brain.

B. Clinical Considerations

1. **Benign Prostatic Hyperplasia (BPH; Figure 17-5C). BPH** is characterized by hyperplasia of the **transitional (periurethral) zone**, which generally involves the lateral and middle lobes and develops in all men. Hyperplasia of epithelial and fibromuscular stromal cells leads to the formation of soft, yellow-pink nodules. BPH compresses the prostatic urethra and obstructs urine flow. The hyperplasia may be caused by increased sensitivity of the prostate gland to **DHT**. BPH is NOT premalignant. Clinical signs include increased frequency of urination, nocturia, dysuria, difficulty starting and stopping urination, dribbling, and a sense of incomplete emptying of bladder. Treatment may include 5α-reductase inhibitors (e.g. **finasteride [Proscar]**) to block conversion of T → DHT, or α-adrenergic antagonists (e.g. **terazosin, prazosin, doxazosin**) to inhibit prostate gland secretion.

2. **Prostatic Carcinoma (PC; Figure 17-5D–F).** PC is most commonly found in the **peripheral zone**, which generally involves the posterior lobes (which can be palpated on a digital rectal examination). Neoplastic epithelial cells lead to the formation of yellow, firm, gritty tumors that invade nearby structures. Because PC begins in the peripheral zone, by the time urethral blockage occurs (i.e. patient complains of difficulty in urination), the carcinoma is in an advanced stage. Clinical signs include usually asymptomatic until the advanced stages, indurated mass on digital rectal examination, obstructive uropathy, and low back or pelvic pain. **Prostatic intraepithelial neoplasia (PIN)** is frequently associated with PC. Serum **PSA levels** are diagnostic. Metastasis to bone (e.g. lumbar vertebrae, pelvis) is frequent. Treatment may include **leuprolide (Lupron)**, which is a gonadotropin-releasing hormone agonist that inhibits the release of follicle-stimulating hormone and luteinizing hormone when administered in a continuous fashion, thereby inhibiting secretion of testosterone, **cyproterone (Androcur)** or **flutamide (Eulexin)**, which are androgen receptor antagonists, radiation, or prostatectomy.

X External Genitalia

A. Scrotum (See Chapter 8)

B. Penis (Figure 17-3).
The penis consists of three columns of erectile tissue bounded together by the **tunica albuginea**: one **corpus spongiosum** and two **corpora cavernosa**. The penis is supported by the **suspensory ligament**, which arises from the linea alba and inserts into the deep fascia (of Buck). The arterial supply is from the internal pudendal

artery via the **deep artery of the penis** (involved in the erection of the penis) and **dorsal artery of the penis**. The venous drainage follows two pathways. The first is to the **deep dorsal vein of the penis** → prostatic venous plexus → internal iliac vein → IVC. The second is to the **superficial dorsal vein of the penis** → external pudendal vein → great saphenous vein → femoral vein → external iliac vein → IVC. The penis is innervated by the pudendal nerve via the **dorsal nerve of the penis**.

1. **Corpus Spongiosum.** The corpus spongiosum begins as the **bulb of the penis** and ends as the **glans penis**. It is ventrally situated in the penis and transmits the urethra. During erection, the corpus spongiosum does not get as turgid as the corpora cavernosa.

2. **Corpora Cavernosa.** The corpora cavernosa begin as the **crura of the penis** and end proximal to the **glans penis**. They are dorsally situated in the penis.

3. **Erectile Tissue of the Penis.** The erectile tissue of the penis found within the corpus spongiosum and corpora cavernosa consists of vascular channels that are lined by endothelium. The walls of these channels consist of connective tissue and smooth muscle. Within the walls, blood vessels and small nerves can be found.

C. **Clinical Considerations**

1. **Hypospadias (Figure 17-4F)** occurs when the urethral folds fail to fuse completely, resulting in the external urethral orifice opening onto the ventral surface of the penis. It is generally associated with a poorly developed penis that curves ventrally, known as **chordee**.

2. **Epispadias (Figure 17-4H)** occurs when the external urethral orifice opens onto the dorsal surface of the penis. It is generally associated with exstrophy of the bladder.

XI ● Erection, Secretion, Emission, and Ejaculation

A. **Erection.** Erection of the penis is controlled by the parasympathetic nervous system via the **pelvic splanchnic nerves (S2 through S4)**, which dilate blood vessels supplying the erectile tissue. This engorges the corpora cavernosa and corpus spongiosum with blood, compresses the veins, which impedes venous return, and causes a full erection. The erection of the penis is also maintained by the somatic nervous system via the **perineal branch of the pudendal nerve**, which contracts the **bulbospongiosus muscles** and **ischiocavernosus muscles**. This compresses the erectile tissue of the bulb of the penis and the crura of the penis and helps to maintain the erection.

B. **Secretion.** Secretion from the seminal vesicles, bulbourethral glands of Cowper, and the prostate gland is controlled by the parasympathetic nervous system via the **pelvic splanchnic nerves (S2 through S4)**, which stimulate the secretory activity of these glands.

C. **Emission.** Emission from the penis is controlled by the sympathetic nervous system via the **L3 and L4 lumbar splanchnic nerves** and the **sacral splanchnic nerves (L5 and S1 through S3)**, which contract the smooth muscle of the tail region of the epididymis, ductus deferens, seminal vesicle, and prostate gland, thus promoting movement of sperm and fluid, and contracts the internal urethral sphincter (i.e. smooth muscle), thus preventing reflux of sperm and fluid into the urinary bladder.

D. **Ejaculation.** Ejaculation from the penis is controlled by the somatic nervous system via the **pudendal nerve**, which contracts the **bulbospongiosus muscle** (i.e. skeletal muscle) to propel sperm and fluid and relaxes the **sphincter urethrae muscle** located within the deep perineal space (i.e. skeletal muscle; also called the external urethral sphincter).

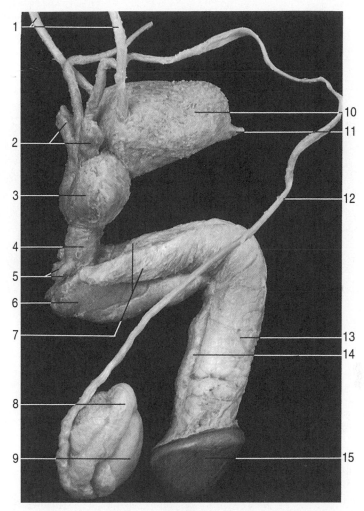

● **Figure 17-1 The Male Reproductive System.** 1 = ureter, 2 = seminal vesicle, 3 = prostate gland, 4 = membranous urethra, 5 = bulbourethral (Cowper) glands, 6 = bulb of the penis, 7 = left and right crura of the penis, 8 = epididymis, 9 = testes, 10 = urinary bladder, 11 = apex of the urinary bladder, 12 = ductus deferens, 13 = corpus cavernosum, 14 = corpus spongiosum, 15 = glans penis.

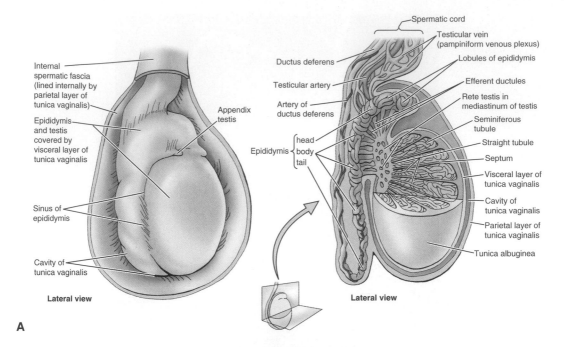

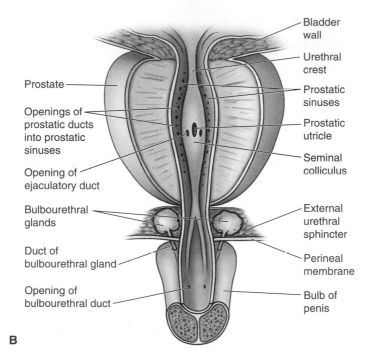

● **Figure 17-2 (A) Anatomy of the Testes and Epididymis. (B) Anatomy of the Interior of the Male Bladder and Urethra.**

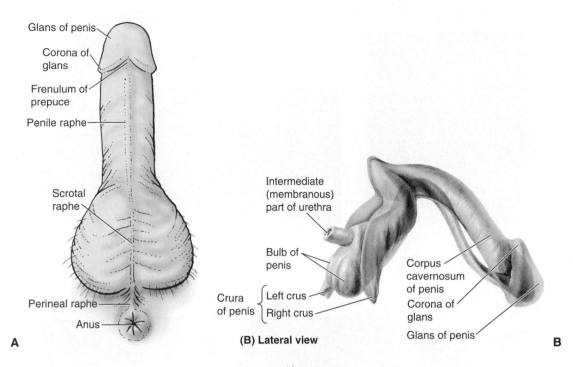

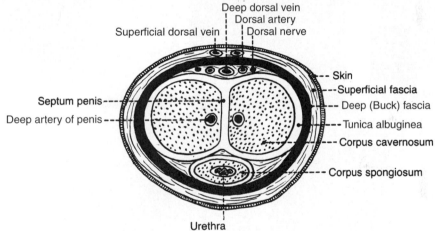

● Figure 17-3 (A) Urethral Surface of a Circumcised Penis (inferior view). (B) Internal Structure of the Penis. (C) Cross-Section of the Penis.

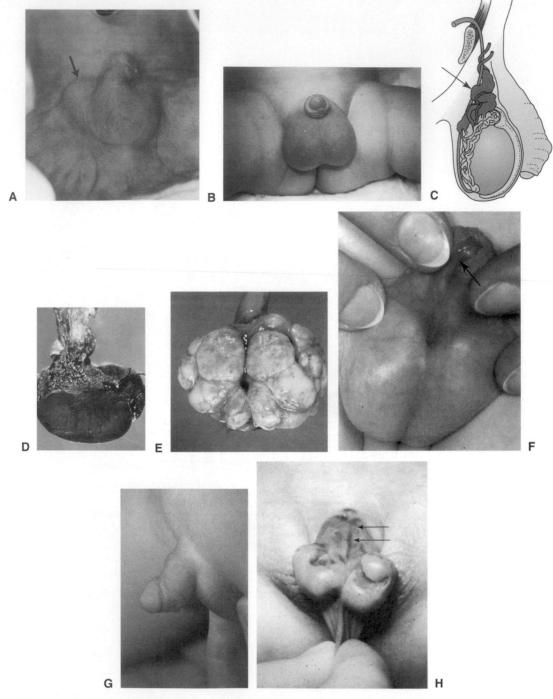

● **Figure 17-4 (A) Cryptorchidism.** Photograph shows that both testes have not descended into the scrotal sac. The undescended right testis is apparent (arrow). **(B) Hydrocele.** Photograph shows a bilateral hydrocele. **(C) Varicocele.** Diagram shows the abnormal dilatation of the pampiniform plexus of veins (arrow). **(D) Torsion.** Photograph shows the cut section of the testis from a man who experienced sudden excruciating scrotal pain. Note the diffuse hemorrhage and necrosis of the testis and adnexal structures. **(E) Seminoma.** Photograph shows the cut surface of a nodular tumor that is tan with punctate hemorrhages in an otherwise solid mass. **(F) Hypospadias.** Photograph shows the urethral opening on the ventral surface of the penis (arrow). **(G) Chordee.** Photograph shows that the penis is poorly developed and bowed ventrally. **(H) Epispadias.** Photograph shows the urethral opening on the dorsal surface of the penis (arrows), whereby the penis is almost split in half.

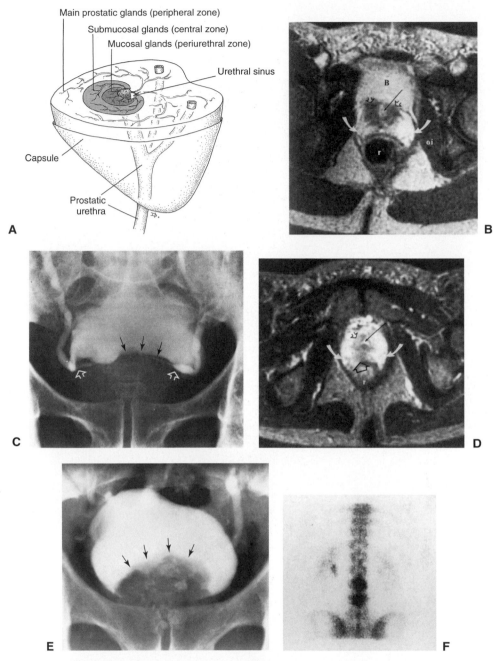

● **Figure 17-5 (A) Prostate Gland.** Diagram of the prostate gland indicating the relationship of the peripheral zone, central zone, and the periurethral zone to the prostatic urethra. **(B) Normal Prostate Gland.** MRI shows a high-intensity peripheral zone (curved arrows), the urethra (long arrow), and the lower-intensity central zone (open arrows). B = bladder, r = rectum, oi = obturator internus muscle. **(C) Benign Prostatic Hyperplasia.** IVP radiograph shows elevation of the base of the bladder by a smooth half-moon filling defect (arrowheads). This causes a deformity in the pathway of the ureter such that the ureters end in a hook ("fish-hooking" phenomena; open arrows). **(D–F) Prostatic Carcinoma. (D)** MRI shows a low-intensity prostate carcinoma (large open arrow) in the peripheral zone (curved arrows). The urethra (long arrow) and the dark central zone are apparent. r = rectum. **(E)** IVP radiograph shows elevation of the base of the bladder by an irregular filling defect (arrows). **(F)** A radionuclide bone scan shows increased tracer uptake in L3 and L4 vertebrae indicating metastatic spread of prostatic carcinoma.

Chapter 18

Pelvis

I **Bones of the Pelvis (Figures 18-1, 18-2).** The bony pelvis is a basin-shaped ring of bone that consists of the following:

A. Coxal (hip) Bone. There are two coxal bones, and each coxal bone is formed by the fusion of the **ischium**, **ilium**, and **pubis**, which join at the acetabulum (an incomplete cup-shaped cavity) of the hip joint.

   1. Ilium. The ilium forms the lateral part of the hip bone and joins the ischium and pubis to form the acetabulum and ala. It comprises the anterior-superior iliac spine, anterior-inferior iliac spine, posterior iliac spine, greater sciatic notch, iliac fossa, and gluteal lines.

   2. Ischium. The ischium joins the ilium and superior ramus of the pubis to form the acetabulum. The ramus of the ischium joins the inferior pubic ramus to form the ischiopubic ramus. It comprises the ischial spine, ischial tuberosity, and lesser sciatic notch.

   3. Pubis. The pubis forms the anterior part of the acetabulum and the anteromedial part of the hip bone. It comprises the body, superior ramus, and inferior ramus.

B. Sacrum. The sacrum is formed by the fusion of the S1 through S5 vertebrae and is the posterior portion of the bony pelvis. The sacrum contains the **dorsal sacral foramina**, which transmit the dorsal primary rami of the sacral spinal nerves; the **ventral sacral foramina**, which transmit the ventral primary rami of the sacral spinal nerves; and the **sacral hiatus**, which is formed as a result of the failure of the laminae of the S5 vertebrae to fuse. The pedicles form the **sacral cornua**, which are important landmarks in locating the sacral hiatus for administration of caudal anesthesia.

C. Coccyx (tail bone). The coccyx is formed by the fusion of the Co1 through Co4 vertebrae.

II **Greater and Lesser Sciatic Foramina.** The **sacrotuberous ligament** (which runs from the sacrum to the ischial tuberosity) and **sacrospinous ligament** (which runs from the sacrum to the ischial spine) help define the borders of the foramina.

A. Greater sciatic foramen is divided into the **suprapiriformis recess** and **infrapiriformis recess** by the piriformis muscle. This foramen transmits the following important structures as they exit the pelvic cavity to enter the gluteal and thigh regions: **superior gluteal vein, artery, and nerve; piriformis muscle; inferior gluteal vein, artery, and nerve; sciatic nerve; internal pudendal vein and artery; and pudendal nerve.**

B. Lesser sciatic foramen transmits the following important structures as they reenter the pelvic cavity and proceed to the perineum: **internal pudendal vein and artery** and

pudendal nerve. Note that the internal pudendal vein, internal pudendal artery, and pudendal nerve exit the pelvic cavity via the greater sciatic foramen and then reenter the pelvic cavity through the lesser sciatic foramen and proceed to the perineum.

III **Pelvic inlet (pelvic brim)** is defined by the **sacral promontory (S1 vertebra)** and the **linea terminalis.** The linea terminalis includes the **pubic crest,** the **iliopectineal line,** and the **arcuate line.** The pelvic inlet divides the pelvic cavity into two parts: the **major (false) pelvic cavity,** which lies above the pelvic inlet between the iliac crests and is actually part of the abdominal cavity, and the **minor (true) pelvic cavity,** which lies below the pelvic inlet and extends to the pelvic outlet. The pelvic inlet is oval-shaped in females and heart-shaped in males. The measurements of the pelvic inlet include the following:

A. True conjugate diameter is the distance from the sacral promontory to the superior margin of the pubic symphysis. This diameter is measured radiographically on a lateral projection.

B. Diagonal conjugate diameter is the distance from the sacral promontory to the inferior margin of the pubic symphysis. This diameter is measured during an obstetric examination.

IV **Pelvic outlet** is defined by the **coccyx, ischial tuberosities, inferior pubic ramus,** and **pubic symphysis.** This outlet is closed by the **pelvic diaphragm** and **urogenital diaphragm.** The pelvic outlet is diamond-shaped in both females and males. The pelvic outlet is divided into the **anal triangle** and **urogenital triangle** by a line passing through the ischial tuberosities. The measurements of the pelvic outlet include the following:

A. Transverse diameter is the distance between the ischial tuberosities.

B. Interspinous diameter is the distance between the ischial spines. The ischial spines may present a barrier to the fetus during childbirth if the interspinous diameter is less than 9.5 cm.

V **Comparison of the Female and Male Pelvis (Table 18-1)**

TABLE 18-1	COMPARISON OF THE FEMALE AND MALE PELVIS
Female Pelvis	**Male Pelvis**
Thin and light	Thick and heavy
Pelvic inlet is oval-shaped	Pelvic inlet is heart-shaped
Pelvic outlet is diamond-shaped	Pelvic outlet is diamond-shaped
Pelvic outlet is comparatively larger because of everted ischial tuberosities	Pelvic outlet is comparatively small
Major (false) pelvic cavity is shallow	Major (false) pelvic cavity is deep
Minor (true) pelvic cavity is wide and shallow; cylindrical	Minor (true) pelvic cavity is narrow and deep; tapering
Subpubic angle (pubic arch) is wide (>80°)	Subpubic angle (pubic arch) is narrow (<70°)
Greater sciatic notch is wide (~90°)	Greater sciatic notch is narrow (~70°); inverted V
Sacrum is short and wide	Sacrum is long and narrow
Obturator foramen is triangular-shaped	Obturator foramen is round-shaped

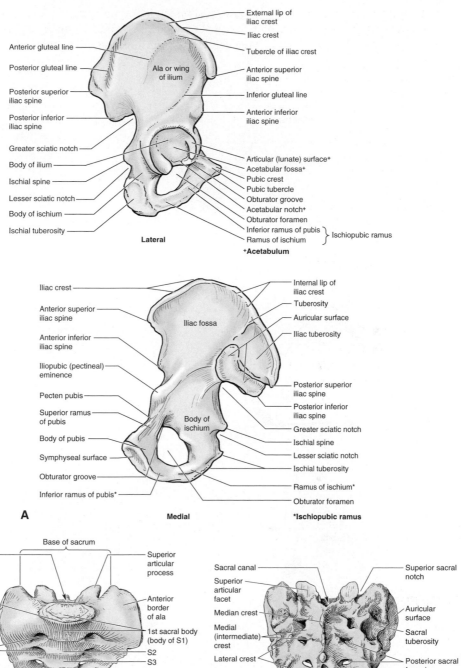

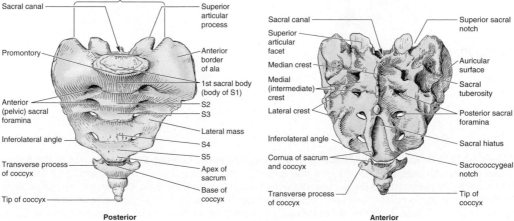

● **Figure 18-1 Bones of the Pelvis (A)** The right coxal bone (lateral and medial views). **(B)** The sacrum and coccyx.

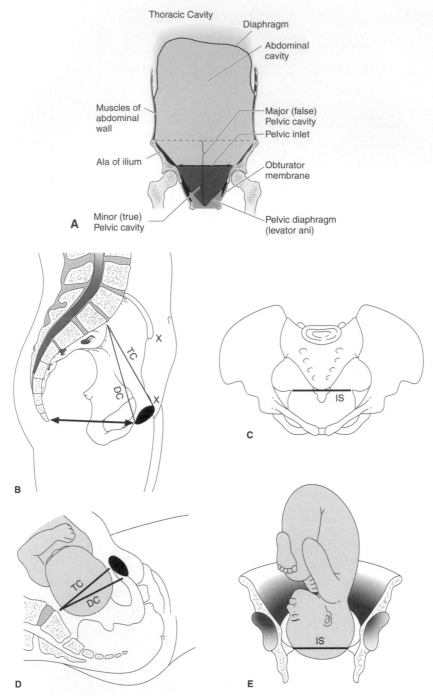

● **Figure 18-2 (A) Relationships of Thoracic, Abdominal, and Pelvic Cavities. (B) Lateral View of the Pelvis.** The diameter of the pelvic inlet is measured by the true conjugate (TC) diameter and the diagonal conjugate (DC) diameter. The opening of the pelvic outlet is shown (line with arrows) extending from the pubic symphysis to the coccyx. Note also that in the natural position of the bony pelvis, the anterior superior iliac spine and the pubic tubercle lie in the same vertical plane (see Xs). **(C) Superior View of the Pelvis.** The diameter of the pelvic outlet is measured by the transverse diameter (not shown) and the interspinous (IS) diameter. **(D) Lateral View of the Pelvis.** Note that during childbirth the fetal head must pass through the pelvic inlet. The TC and DC diameters mea-sure the diameter of the pelvic inlet. **(E) Frontal View of the Pelvis.** Note that during childbirth the fetal head must pass through the pelvic outlet. The IS diameter measures the diameter of the pelvic outlet. The TC, DC, and IS diameters are important during childbirth when the fetus must travel through the birth canal, which consists of the pelvic inlet → minor pelvis → cervix → vagina → pelvic outlet.

VI ## Muscles of the Pelvis (Figure 18-3). The muscles of the pelvis include the **obturator internus muscle**, the **piriformis muscle**, the **coccygeus muscle**, and the **levator ani muscles** (**iliococcygeus, pubococcygeus**, and **puborectalis muscles**).

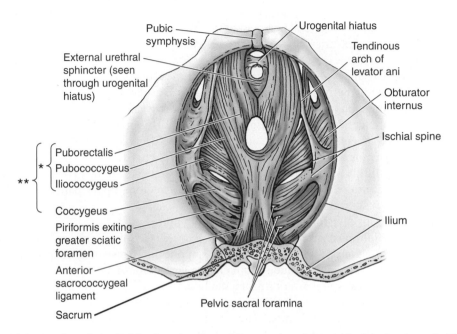

● **Figure 18-3 Muscles of the Pelvis.** Superior view of the muscles of the pelvis. * = levator ani, ** = pelvic diaphragm (floor).

VII # Arterial Supply

A. Internal Iliac Artery. The internal iliac artery arises from the bifurcation of the common iliac artery. The internal iliac artery is commonly divided into an **anterior division** and a **posterior division**.

1. Anterior division gives off the following branches:

    a. **Inferior gluteal artery** exits the pelvis via the infrapiriformis recess of the greater sciatic foramen (i.e. inferior to the piriformis muscle). This artery supplies the pelvic diaphragm, piriformis, quadratus femoris, uppermost hamstrings, gluteus maximus, and the sciatic nerve.

    b. **Internal pudendal artery** exits the pelvis via the infrapiriformis recess of the greater sciatic foramen (i.e. inferior to the piriformis muscle), enters the perineum via the lesser sciatic foramen, and courses to the urogenital triangle via the pudendal canal. This artery supplies the perineum (main artery of the perineum) including the skin and muscles of the anal triangle and the urogenital triangle and the erectile bodies.

    c. **Umbilical artery** runs along the lateral pelvic wall and alongside the bladder for a short distance then obliterates to form the **medical umbilical ligament**. The umbilical artery gives rise to the **superior vesical artery**, which supplies the superior part of the urinary bladder.

d. **Obturator artery** runs along the lateral pelvic wall and exits the pelvis via the obturator canal. This artery supplies the pelvic muscles, muscles of the medial compartment of the thigh, head of the femur, and ilium.

e. **Vaginal Artery (female) or Inferior Vesical Artery (male).** The **vaginal artery** in the female supplies the anterior and posterior walls of the vagina, vestibular bulb, and adjacent rectum. The **inferior vesical artery** in the male runs in the lateral ligament of the bladder and supplies the fundus of the bladder, prostate gland, seminal vesicle, ductus deferens, and lower part of the ureter.

f. **Uterine Artery (female) or Artery of the Ductus Deferens (male).** The **uterine artery** in the female runs medially in the base of the broad ligament to reach the junction of the cervix and body of the uterus and runs in front of and above the ureter near the lateral fornix of the vagina. This uterine artery supplies the uterus, ligaments of the uterus, uterine tube, ovary, cervix, and vagina. The artery of the ductus deferens in the male supplies the ductus deferens.

g. **Middle rectal artery** runs medially and descends in the pelvis. The middle rectal artery supplies the lower part of the rectum, upper part of the anal canal, prostate gland, and seminal vesicles.

2. **Posterior division** gives off the following branches:

a. **Iliolumbar artery** ascends anterior to the sacroiliac joint and posterior to the psoas major muscle. This artery supplies the psoas major, iliacus, quadratus lumborum, and cauda equina in the vertebral canal.

b. **Lateral sacral artery** runs medially in front of the sacral plexus and give rise to branches that enter the anterior sacral foramina and then emerge from the posterior sacral foramina. This artery supplies the meninges, roots of the sacral nerves, and muscles and skin overlying the sacrum.

c. **Superior gluteal artery** exits the pelvis via the suprapiriformis recess of the greater sciatic foramen (i.e. superior to the piriformis muscle). This artery supplies the piriformis, gluteal muscles, and tensor fascia lata.

B. Median sacral artery arises from the posterior aspect of the abdominal aorta and runs close to the midline over the L4 and L5 vertebrae, sacrum, and coccyx. The median sacral artery gives rise to **medial sacral arteries.** This median sacral artery supplies the posterior part of the rectum, lower lumbar vertebrae, sacrum, and coccyx.

C. Superior rectal artery is a continuation of the inferior mesenteric artery and descends into the pelvis between the layers of the sigmoid mesocolon. This artery supplies the superior part of the rectum.

D. Ovarian Artery (female) or Testicular Artery (male). The ovarian artery in the female arises from the abdominal aorta and reaches the ovary through the suspensory ligament of the ovary. This artery supplies the ureter, ovary, and ampulla of the uterine tube. The testicular artery in the male arises from the abdominal aorta and then runs in the inguinal canal to enter the scrotum. This artery supplies the ureter, testis, and epididymis.

Ⅷ Venous Drainage

A. Pelvic Venous Plexuses. The pelvic venous plexuses within the minor (true) pelvic cavity are formed by intercommunicating veins surrounding the pelvic viscera and include the **rectal venous plexus, vesical venous plexus, prostatic venous plexus, uterine venous**

plexus, and **vaginal venous plexus**. These pelvic venous plexuses drain venous blood via a number of different pathways as follows:

1. Pelvic venous plexuses → internal iliac veins, which join the external iliac veins to form the common iliac veins → common iliac veins join to form the inferior vena cava (IVC). This is the main venous drainage pathway.
2. Pelvic venous plexuses → median sacral vein → common iliac vein → inferior vena cava.
3. Pelvic venous plexuses → ovarian veins → inferior vena cava.
4. Pelvic venous plexuses → superior rectal vein → inferior mesenteric vein → portal vein.
5. Pelvic venous plexuses → lateral sacral veins → internal vertebral venous plexus → cranial dural sinuses.

B. Other Venous Drainage
   1. **Iliolumbar veins** lying with the iliac fossae within the major (false) pelvic cavity usually drain directly into the common iliac veins.
   2. **Superior gluteal veins** drain into the internal iliac veins and are its largest tributary except during pregnancy when the uterine veins become larger.

IX Nerves (Figure 18-4)

A. Sacral Plexus. The components of the sacral plexus include:
   1. **Rami** are the **L4 through L5 (lumbosacral trunk) and S1 through S4 ventral primary rami** of spinal nerves.
   2. **Divisions (anterior and posterior)** are formed by rami dividing into anterior and posterior divisions.
   3. **Branches.** The major terminal branches are:
      a. **Superior gluteal nerve (L4 through S1)** innervates the gluteus medius, gluteus minimus, and tensor fascia lata muscles.
      b. **Inferior gluteal nerve (L5 through S2)** innervates the gluteus maximus muscle.
      c. **Nerve to piriformis (S1 and S2)** innervates the piriformis muscle.
      d. **Common fibular nerve (L4 through S2).**
      e. **Tibial nerve (L4 through S3).** The tibial nerve and common fibular nerve comprise the **sciatic nerve** (see Chapter 21).
      f. **Nerve to the quadratus femoris and inferior gemellus (L5 through S1)** innervates the quadratus femoris and inferior gemellus muscles.
      g. **Nerve to the obturator internus and superior gemellus (L5 through S2)** innervates the obturator internus and superior gemellus muscles.
      h. **Posterior femoral cutaneous nerve (S1 through S3)** innervates the skin of the buttocks, thigh, and calf (sensory). This nerve gives rise to the **inferior cluneal nerves** and **perineal branches**.
      i. **Perforating cutaneous nerve (S2 and S3)** innervates the skin in the perineal area.
      j. **Pudendal nerve (S2 through S4)** passes through the greater sciatic foramen, crosses the ischial spine, and enters the perineum with the internal pudendal artery through the pudendal canal. This nerve gives rise to the **inferior rectal nerve, perineal nerve,** and the **dorsal nerve of the penis (or clitoris)**.
      k. **Nerve to the levator ani and coccygeus (S3 and S4)** innervates the levator ani muscles and the coccygeus muscle.
      l. **Perineal branch of spinal nerve S4** innervates the skin of the perineum (sensory).

B. Coccygeal Plexus. The components of the coccygeal plexus include:
1. **Rami** are the S4 and S5 **ventral primary rami** of the spinal nerves.
2. **Coccygeal nerve** innervates the coccygeus muscle, part of the levator ani muscles, and the sacrococcygeal joint.
3. **Branches.** There is one branch from the coccygeal plexus called the **anococcygeal nerve**, which innervates the skin between the tip of the coccyx and the anus.

C. Autonomic Components
1. **Superior hypogastric plexus** is a continuation of the intermesenteric plexus from the inferior mesenteric ganglion below the aortic bifurcation and receives the L3 and L4 lumbar splanchnic nerves. This plexus contains ganglionic neuronal cell bodies on which preganglionic sympathetic axons of the L3 and L4 lumbar splanchnic nerves synapse. The superior hypogastric plexus descends anterior to the L5 vertebra and ends by dividing into the **right hypogastric nerve** and **left hypogastric nerve**.
2. **Right and left hypogastric nerves** descend on either side lateral to the rectum and join the right or left inferior hypogastric plexus, respectively.
3. **Right and left inferior hypogastric plexuses** are located against the posterolateral pelvic wall lateral to the rectum, vagina, and base of the bladder. The right and left inferior hypogastric plexuses are formed by the union of the **right or left hypogastric nerves**, the **sacral splanchnic nerves (L5 and S1 through S3)**, and the **pelvic splanchnic nerves (S2 through S4)**. This plexus contains ganglionic neuronal cell bodies on which preganglionic sympathetic axons of the sacral splanchnic nerves (L5 and S1 through S3) synapse.
4. **Sacral sympathetic trunk** is a continuation of the paravertebral sympathetic chain ganglia in the pelvis. The sacral trunks descend on the inner surface of the sacrum medial to the sacral foramina and converge to form the small median **ganglion impar** anterior to the coccyx.

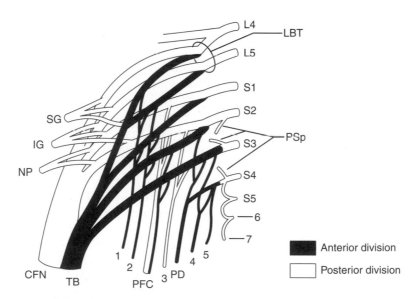

● **Figure 18-4 Nerves of the Pelvis.** Sacral plexus and coccygeal plexus. CFN = common fibular nerve, IG = inferior gluteal nerve, LBT = lumbosacral trunk, NP = nerve to piriformis, PD = pudendal nerve, PFC = posterior femoral cutaneous nerve, PSp = pelvic splanchnic nerves, SG = superior gluteal nerve, TB = tibial nerve, 1 = nerve to quadratus femoris and inferior gemellus muscles, 2 = nerve to obturator internus and superior gemellus muscles, 3 = perforating cutaneous nerve, 4 = nerve to levator ani and coccygeus muscles, 5 = perineal branch of S4 nerve, 6 = coccygeal nerve, 7 = anococcygeal nerve.

Support of the Pelvic Organs. The pelvic organs are supported by the following muscles and ligaments:

A. **Pelvic Diaphragm (floor).** The pelvic diaphragm is composed of the following muscles:
   1. **Coccygeus muscle**
   2. **Levator ani muscles,** which consists of:
      a. Iliococcygeus
      b. Pubococcygeus
      c. Puborectalis. This muscle forms a U-shaped sling around the anorectal junction causing a 90-degree perineal flexure. This muscle is important in maintaining fecal continence.
      d. Pubovaginalis. In the female, the pubovaginalis forms a U-shaped sling around the vagina. This muscle can be exercised to increase vaginal tension during intercourse.

B. **Urogenital Diaphragm.** The urogenital diaphragm is composed of the following muscles:
   1. **Deep transverse perineal muscle**
   2. **Sphincter urethra muscle**

C. **Transverse cervical ligament (cardinal ligament of Mackenrodt)** is a condensation of endopelvic fascia, which extends laterally from the cervix to the side wall of the pelvis.

D. **Uterosacral ligament** is a condensation of endopelvic fascia, which extends posteriorly from the cervix to the sacrum.

E. **Pubocervical ligament** is a condensation of endopelvic fascia, which extends anteriorly from the cervix to the pubic symphysis.

Clinical Considerations

A. **Pelvic relaxation** is the weakening or loss of support of pelvic organs as a result of damage of the pelvic diaphragm, urogenital diaphragm, transverse cervical ligament (cardinal ligament of Mackenrodt), uterosacral ligament, or pubocervical ligament. This may result in **cystocele** (prolapse of urinary bladder into the anterior vaginal wall), **rectocele** (prolapse of rectum into posterior wall of vagina), or **uterine prolapse** (prolapse of uterus into vaginal vault). It is caused by multiple childbirths; birth trauma; increased intraabdominal pressure as a result of obesity, heavy lifting, or chronic cough; or menopausal loss of muscle tone. Clinical signs include a heavy sensation in the lower abdomen that exacerbates on heavy lifting or prolonged standing, increased frequency of urination with burning sensation because of urine stagnation and bacterial proliferation, and urine leakage with coughing or sneezing (i.e. stress incontinence).

B. **The Pelvic Ring.** The pelvic ring consists of the sacrum and the two coxal bones that have resilient articulations in which small degrees of movement are possible between the sacroiliac (SI) joint and the pubic symphysis. The **sacrum is the keystone of the femoral-sacral arch** that supports the vertebral column over the legs. The **anterior and posterior SI ligaments** attach the upper sacrum to the ilium. The **sacrotuberous ligament** and the **sacrospinous ligament** attach the lower sacrum to the ischium. The functional stability of the pelvic ring depends on these ligaments.

C. **Pudendal nerve block (Figure 18-5)** provides perineal anesthesia during forceps childbirth delivery by anesthetizing the pudendal nerve. A 1% lidocaine solution is injected transvaginally or just lateral to the labia majora **around the tip of the ischial spine** and **through the sacrospinous ligament.** The pain of childbirth is transmitted by the pudendal nerve through sensory fibers of **S2 through S5** spinal nerves. The pudendal nerve passes out of the pelvic cavity through the greater sciatic foramen, travels around the posterior surface of the ischial spine, and reenters the pelvic cavity through the lesser sciatic foramen. The pudendal nerve travels within the fascia of the obturator internus muscle (called the **pudendal canal of Alcock)** and divides into the **inferior rectal nerve, perineal nerve,** and **dorsal nerve of the penis (or clitoris).** To obtain complete anesthesia of the perineal region, the **ilioinguinal nerve** (which branches into the **anterior labial nerves),** the **genitofemoral nerve,** and the **perineal branch of the posterior femoral cutaneous nerve** are anesthetized.

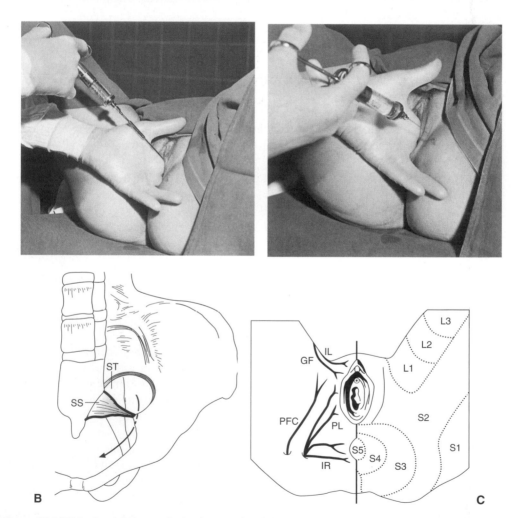

● **Figure 18-5 (A) Pudendal Nerve Block.** Photographs of the clinical administration of a pudendal nerve block both transvaginally and lateral to the labia majora. The ischial spine is a good anatomic landmark. **(B) Pudendal Nerve Pathway.** Diagram indicating the path of the pudendal nerve (curved arrow) as it passes out of the pelvic cavity through the greater sciatic foramen (posterior to the ischial spine) and returns to the pelvic cavity through the lesser sciatic foramen as it proceeds to the perineum. ST = sacrotuberous ligament, SS = sacrospinous ligament. **(C) Diagram of the Perineum in the Lithotomy Position.** The posterior labial nerves (PL) and inferior rectal nerves (IR), which are terminal branches of the pudendal nerve, are shown. In addition, the ilioinguinal nerve (IL), genitofemoral nerve (GF), and perineal branch of the posterior femoral cutaneous nerve (PFC) are indicated.

XII Radiology. AP radiograph of Male Pelvis (Figure 18-6)

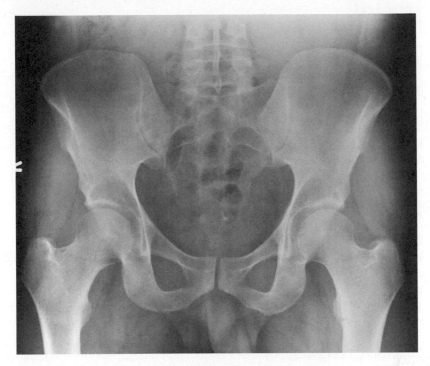

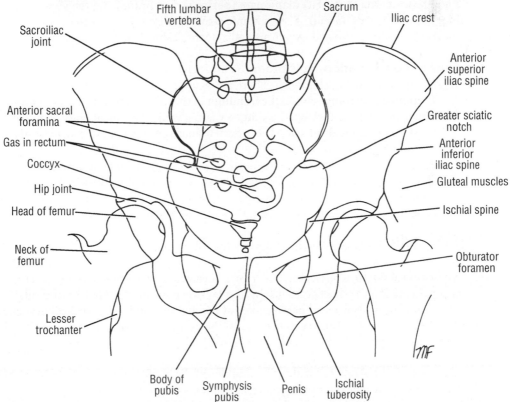

● **Figure 18-6 Male Pelvis. (A)** AP radiograph of the male pelvis. **(B)** Diagrammatic representation of the radiograph in A.

Chapter 19

Perineum

I **Perineum (Figure 19-1).** The perineum is a part of the pelvic outlet located inferior to the pelvic diaphragm. The perineum is diamond-shaped and can be divided by a line passing through the ischial tuberosities into two triangles: the **urogenital (UG) triangle** and the **anal triangle**.

II **Urogenital (UG) Triangle.** The UG triangle comprises the following:

A. Deep Perineal Space. The deep perineal space is a space that lies between the **superior fascia of the UG diaphragm** and the **inferior fascia of the UG diaphragm (perineal membrane)**. This space contains a number of structures that completely occupy it. The anatomic structures found within the deep perineal space of the male and female are indicated in **Table 19-1**. One of those structures is the **UG diaphragm**, which consists of the **deep transverse perineal muscle** and the **sphincter urethrae muscle**.

B. Superficial Perineal Space. The superficial perineal space is a space that lies between the **inferior fascia of the UG diaphragm (perineal membrane)** and the **superficial perineal fascia (Colles' fascia)**. The anatomic structures found within the superficial perineal space of the male and female are indicated in **Table 19-1**.

C. Clinical Consideration. Episiotomy is an incision of the perineum to enlarge the vaginal opening during childbirth. There are two types of episiotomies.
  1. **Median episiotomy** starts at the **frenulum of the labia minora** and proceeds directly downward cutting through the **skin → vaginal wall → perineal body → superficial transverse perineal muscle**. The external anal sphincter muscle may be inadvertently cut.
  2. **Mediolateral episiotomy** starts at the frenulum of the labia minora and proceeds at a 45-degree angle cutting through the **skin → vaginal wall → bulbospongiosus muscle**. This procedure has a higher risk of bleeding in comparison with a median episiotomy but creates more room than a median episiotomy.

III **Anal Triangle.** The anal triangle comprises the following:

A. Ischiorectal Fossa. The ischiorectal fossa is located on either side of the anorectum and is separated from the pelvic cavity by the levator ani muscle. This fossa contains ischiorectal fat, inferior rectal nerves, inferior rectal artery and vein, perineal branches of the posterior femoral cutaneous nerve, and the pudendal canal (Alcock's canal), which transmits the pudendal nerve and the internal pudendal artery and vein.

B. Muscles of the Anal Triangle. The muscles of the anal triangle include obturator internus, external anal sphincter, levator ani, and coccygeus muscles.

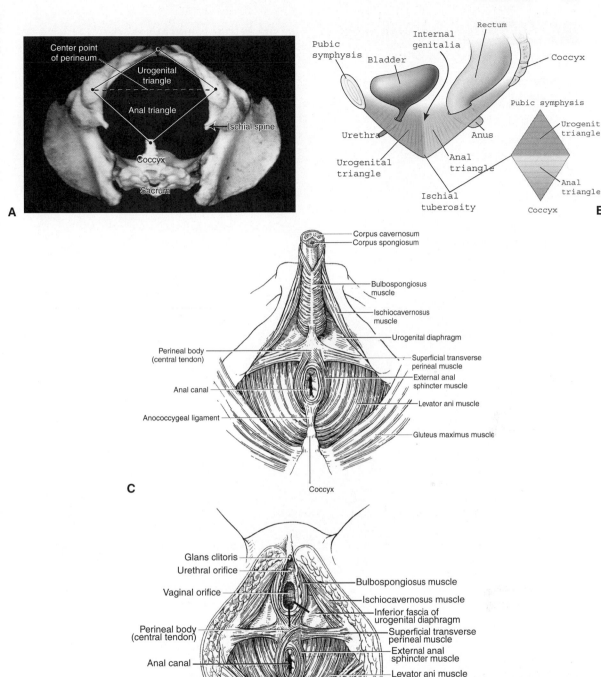

● **Figure 19-1 (A) Osseous Boundaries of the Perineum.** The diamond-shaped perineum extends from the pubic symphysis to the coccyx. Note that a transverse line joining the anterior ends of the ischial tuberosities divides the perineum into two unequal triangular areas, the urogenital triangle anteriorly and the anal triangle posteriorly. The midpoint of the transverse line indicates the site of the perineal body (central perineal tendon). **(B) Lateral Diagram of the Perineum.** Lateral diagram of the perineum shows that the urogenital triangle and the anal triangle do not occupy the same plane. **(C) Muscles of the Male Perineum. (D) Muscles of the Female Perineum.** Note the two incision lines for a median and mediolateral episiotomy (thick black lines).

TABLE 19-1	STRUCTURES WITHIN THE DEEP AND SUPERFICIAL PERINEAL SPACES
Male	**Female**

Structures Within the Deep Perineal Space

Male	Female
Membranous urethra	Membranous urethra
	Vagina
Urogenital diaphragm	Urogenital diaphragm
Deep transverse perineal muscle	Deep transverse perineal muscle
Sphincter urethrae muscle	Sphincter urethrae muscle
Branches of internal pudendal artery	Branches of internal pudendal artery
Artery of the bulb	Artery of the bulb
Dorsal artery of the penis	Dorsal artery of the clitoris
Deep artery of the penis	Deep artery of the clitoris
Branches of pudendal nerve	Branches of pudendal nerve
Dorsal nerve of the penis	Dorsal nerve of the clitoris
Bulbourethral glands (of Cowper)	No glands

Structures within the Superficial Perineal Space

Male	Female
Penile (spongy) urethra	External urethra
	Vestibule of the vagina
Bulbospongiosus muscle	Bulbospongiosus muscle
Ischiocavernosus muscle	Ischiocavernosus muscle
Superficial transverse perineal muscle	Superficial transverse perineal muscle
Branches of internal pudendal artery	Branches of the internal pudendal artery
Perineal artery → posterior scrotal arteries	Perineal artery → posterior labial arteries
Dorsal artery of the penis	Dorsal artery of the clitoris
Deep artery of the penis	Deep artery of the clitoris
Branches of pudendal nerve	Branches of pudendal nerve
Perineal nerve → posterior scrotal nerves	Perineal nerve → posterior labial nerves
Dorsal nerve of the penis	Dorsal nerve of the clitoris
Bulb of the penis	Vestibular bulb
Crura of the penis	Crura of the clitoris
Perineal body	Perineal body
	Round ligament of the uterus
Duct of the bulbourethral gland	Greater vestibular glands (of Bartholin)

Chapter 20

Upper Limb

I **Bones.** The bones of the upper limb include the clavicle, scapula, humerus, radius, ulna, carpal bones (scaphoid, lunate, triquetrum, pisiform, trapezium, trapezoid, capitate, and hamate), metacarpals, and phalanges (proximal, middle, and distal).

II **Muscles**

A. **Anterior axioappendicular muscles** include the pectoralis major, pectoralis minor, subclavius, and serratus anterior.

B. **Posterior axioappendicular and scapulohumeral muscles** include the trapezius, latissimus dorsi, levator scapulae, rhomboid major and minor, deltoid, supraspinatus, infraspinatus, teres minor, teres major, and subscapularis.

C. **Muscles of the anterior (flexor) compartment of the arm** include the biceps brachii, brachialis, and coracobrachialis.

D. **Muscles of the posterior (extensor) compartment of the arm** include the triceps and anconeus.

E. **Muscles of the anterior (flexor) compartment of the forearm** include the pronator teres, flexor carpi radialis, palmaris longus, flexor carpi ulnaris, flexor digitorum superficialis, flexor digitorum profundus, flexor pollicis longus, and pronator quadratus.

F. **Muscles of the posterior (extensor) compartment of the forearm** include the brachioradialis, extensor carpi radialis longus, extensor carpi radialis brevis, extensor digitorum, extensor digiti minimi, extensor carpi ulnaris, supinator, extensor indicis, abductor pollicis longus, extensor pollicis longus, extensor pollicis brevis.

G. **Intrinsic muscles of the hand** include the opponens pollicis, abductor pollicis brevis, flexor pollicis brevis, adductor pollicis, abductor digiti minimi, flexor digiti minimi brevis, opponens digiti minimi, lumbricals (first through fourth), dorsal interossei (first through fourth), and palmar interossei (first through third).

ⓘ Arterial Supply (Figures 20-1 and 20-2)

A. Subclavian artery extends from the **arch of the aorta** to the **lateral border of the first rib**. The subclavian artery gives off the following branches:

  1. **Internal thoracic artery** is continuous with the **superior epigastric artery**, which anastomoses with the **inferior epigastric artery** (a branch of the external iliac artery). This may provide a route of collateral circulation if the abdominal aorta is blocked (e.g. postductal coarctation of the aorta).
  2. **Vertebral artery**
  3. **Thyrocervical trunk** has three branches:
      a. **Suprascapular artery**, which participates in collateral circulation around the shoulder.
      b. **Transverse cervical artery**, which participates in collateral circulation around the shoulder.
      c. **Inferior thyroid artery**

B. Axillary artery is a continuation of the subclavian artery and extends from the **lateral border of the first rib** to the **inferior border of the teres major muscle**. The tendon of the pectoralis minor muscle crosses the axillary artery anteriorly and divides the axillary artery into three distinct parts (i.e. the first part is medial, the second part is posterior, and the third part is lateral to the muscle). The axillary artery gives off the following branches:

  1. **First Part**
      a. Superior thoracic artery
  2. **Second Part**
      a. **Thoracoacromial artery** is a short, wide trunk that divides into four branches: acromial, deltoid, pectoral, and clavicular.
      b. Lateral thoracic artery
  3. **Third Part**
      a. Anterior humeral circumflex artery
      b. Posterior humeral circumflex artery
      c. Subscapular artery, which gives off the **circumflex scapular artery** and the thoracodorsal artery.

C. Brachial artery is a continuation of the axillary artery and extends from the **inferior border of the teres major muscle** to the **cubital fossa** where it ends in the cubital fossa opposite the neck of the radius. The brachial artery gives off the following branches:

  1. **Deep brachial artery.** A fracture of the humerus at midshaft may damage the **deep brachial artery and radial nerve** as they travel together on the posterior aspect of the humerus in the radial groove. The deep brachial artery ends by dividing into the **middle collateral artery** and **radial collateral artery**.
  2. **Superior ulnar collateral artery** runs with the ulnar nerve posterior to the medial epicondyle and anastomoses with the posterior ulnar recurrent artery to participate in collateral circulation around the elbow.
  3. **Inferior ulnar collateral artery** anastomoses with the anterior ulnar recurrent artery to participate in collateral circulation around the elbow.
  4. **Radial artery** gives off the following branches:
      a. **Recurrent radial artery** anastomoses with the radial collateral artery.
      b. **Palmar carpal branch**
      c. **Dorsal carpal branch**
      d. **Superficial palmar branch** completes the superficial palmar arch.

    e.   **Princeps pollicis artery** divides into two **proper digital arteries** for each side of the thumb.

    f.   **Radialis indicis artery**

    g.   **Deep palmar arch** is the main termination of the radial artery and anastomoses with the deep palmar branch of the ulnar artery. It gives rise to three **palmar metacarpal arteries**, which join the common palmar digital arteries from the superficial arch.

  5. **Ulnar artery** gives off the following branches:

    a.   **Anterior ulnar recurrent artery**

    b.   **Posterior ulnar recurrent artery**

    c.   **Common interosseous artery**, which divides into the **anterior interosseous artery** and **posterior interosseous artery**. The posterior interosseous artery gives rise to the **recurrent interosseous artery**.

    d.   **Palmar carpal branch**

    e.   **Dorsal carpal branch**

    f.   **Deep palmar branch** completes the deep palmar arch.

    g.   **Superficial palmar arch** is the main termination of the ulnar artery and anastomoses with the superficial palmar branch of the radial artery. It gives rises to three **common palmar digital arteries**, each of which divides into **proper palmar digital arteries**, which run distally to supply the adjacent sides of the fingers.

D. **Collateral circulation** exists in the upper limb in the following regions:

  1. **Collateral circulation around the shoulder** involves the following pathways:

    a.   Thyrocervical trunk → transverse cervical artery → circumflex scapular artery → subscapular artery → axillary artery.

    b.   Thyrocervical trunk → supracapular artery → circumflex scapular artery → subscapular artery → axillary artery.

  2. **Collateral circulation around the elbow** involves the following pathways:

    a.   Superior ulnar collateral artery → posterior ulnar recurrent artery.

    b.   Inferior ulnar collateral artery → anterior ulnar recurrent artery.

    c.   Middle collateral artery → recurrent interosseus artery.

    d.   Radial collateral artery → recurrent radial artery.

  3. **Collateral circulation in the hand** involves the following pathway: superficial palmar arch → deep palmar arch.

E. **Clinical Considerations**

  1. **Subclavian steal syndrome** refers to retrograde flow in the vertebral artery as a result of an ipsilateral subclavian artery stenosis. The subclavian artery stenosis results in lower pressure in the distal subclavian artery. As a result, blood flows from the contralateral vertebral artery to the basilar artery and then in a retrograde direction down the ipsilateral vertebral artery away from the brainstem. Although this may have deleterious neurologic effects, the reversed vertebral artery blood flow serves as an important collateral circulation for the arm in the setting of a significant stenosis or occlusion of the subclavian artery. The most common cause for a subclavian steal syndrome is atherosclerosis. Subclavian steal is more common on the left side probably because of a more acute origin of the subclavian artery that results in increased turbulence and accelerated atherosclerosis.

  2. **Placement of Ligatures.** A surgical ligature may be placed on the subclavian artery or axillary artery **between the thyrocervical trunk** and **subscapular artery**. A surgical ligature may also be placed in the on the brachial artery **distal to the inferior ulnar collateral artery**. A surgical ligature may NOT be placed on the axillary artery between the **subscapular artery** and the **deep brachial artery**.

3. **Bleeding Control.** To control profuse bleeding caused by trauma of the axilla (e.g. a stab or bullet wound), the third part of the axillary artery may be compressed against the humerus in the inferior part of the lateral wall of the axilla. If compression is required more proximally, the first part of the axillary artery may be compressed at its origin by downward pressure in the angle between the clavicle and the inferior attachment of the sternocleidomastoid muscle.

4. **Percutaneous arterial catheterization** uses the brachial artery (if the femoral artery approach is unavailable). The **left brachial artery** is preferred because approaching from the left side allows access to the descending aorta without crossing the right brachiocephalic trunk and left common carotid arteries, thereby reducing the risk of stroke.

5. **Blood Pressure.** The brachial artery is used to measure blood pressure by inflating a cuff around the arm, which compresses and occludes the brachial artery against the humerus. A stethoscope is placed over the cubital fossa, and the air in the cuff is gradually released. The first audible sound indicates systolic pressure. The point at which the pulse can no longer be heard indicates the diastolic pressure. To control profuse bleeding as a result of trauma, the brachial artery may be compressed near the middle of the arm medial to the humerus.

6. **Access for chronic hemodialysis** most commonly uses the **radial artery** and the **cephalic vein.**

7. The **Allen test** is a test for occlusion of either the ulnar or radial artery. Blood is forced out of the hand by making a tight fist and then the physician compresses the ulnar artery. If blood fails to return to the palm and fingers after the fist is opened, then the uncompressed radial artery is occluded.

8. **Deep Laceration.** The deep palmar arch lies posterior to the tendons of the flexor digitorum superficialis and flexor digitorum profundus muscles. Therefore, a deep laceration at the metacarpal-carpal (MC) joint that cuts the deep palmar arch will also compromise flexion of the fingers.

9. **Laceration of the palmar arches** results in profuse bleeding. Because of the collateral circulation between the superficial and palmar arches, it is usually not sufficient to ligate either the ulnar or radial artery. It may be necessary to compress the brachial artery proximal to the elbow to prevent blood from reaching both the ulnar and radial arteries.

10. **Raynaud syndrome** is an idiopathic condition characterized by intermittent bilateral attacks of ischemia of the fingers with cyanosis, paresthesia, and pain. This may also be brought about by cold temperature or emotional stimuli. Because arteries are innervated by postganglionic sympathetic neurons, a cervicodorsal **presynaptic sympathectomy** may be performed to dilate the digital arteries to the fingers.

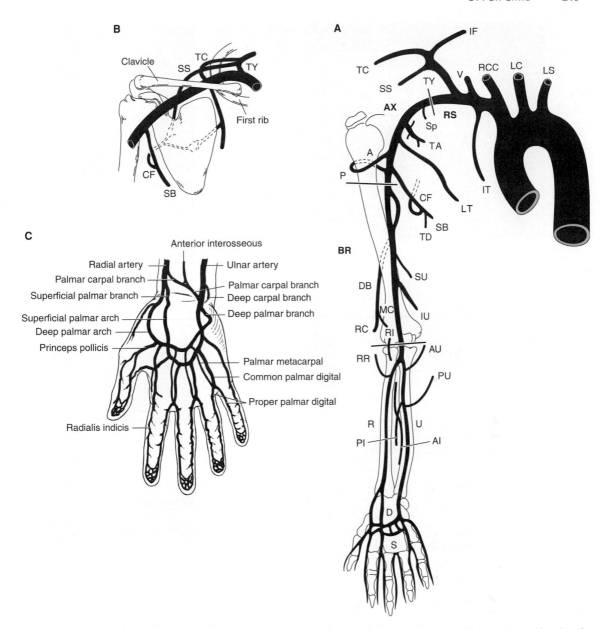

● **Figure 20-1 (A) Arterial Supply of the Upper Limb.** The lines from proximal to distal indicate the lateral border of the first rib, inferior border of the teres major muscle, and the cubital fossa, respectively. You should be able to identify an artery and then know what nerve runs with the artery. **(B) Diagram of the Collateral Circulation Around the Shoulder. (C) Arterial Supply of the Hand.** A = anterior circumflex humeral artery, AI = anterior interosseous artery, AU = anterior ulnar recurrent artery, AX = axillary artery, BR = brachial artery, CF = circumflex scapular artery, D = deep palmar arch, DB = deep brachial artery (runs with the radial nerve), IF = inferior thyroid artery, IT = internal thoracic artery, IU = inferior ulnar collateral artery, LC = left common carotid artery, LS = left subclavian artery, LT = lateral thoracic artery (runs with the long thoracic nerve), MC = middle collateral branch, P = posterior circumflex humeral artery (runs with the axillary nerve), PI = posterior interosseous artery, PU = posterior ulnar recurrent artery, R = radial artery, RC = radial collateral branch, RCC = right common carotid artery, RI = recurrent interosseous artery, RR = radial recurrent artery, RS = right subclavian artery, S = superficial palmar arch, SB = subscapular artery, Sp = superior thoracic artery, SS = suprascapular artery, SU = superior ulnar collateral artery, TA = thoracoacromial artery, TC = transverse cervical artery, TD = thoracodorsal artery, TY = thyrocervical trunk, U = ulnar artery (runs with the ulnar nerve), V = vertebral artery.

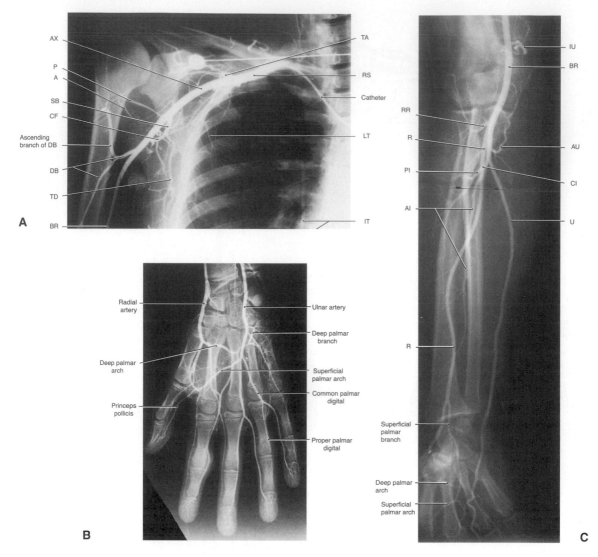

● **Figure 20-2 (A) Axillary Arteriogram.** AX = axillary artery, A = anterior circumflex humeral artery, AI = anterior interosseous artery, AU = anterior ulnar recurrent artery, BR = brachial artery, CF = circumflex scapular artery, CI = common interosseous artery, DB = deep brachial artery (runs with the radial nerve), IT = internal thoracic artery, IU = inferior ulnar collateral artery, LT = lateral thoracic artery (runs with the long thoracic nerve), P = posterior circumflex humeral artery (runs with the axillary nerve), PI = posterior interosseous artery, R = radial artery, RR = radial recurrent artery, RS = right subclavian artery, SB = subscapular artery, TA = thoracoacromial artery, TD = thoracodorsal artery, U = ulnar artery (runs with the ulnar nerve). **(B) Brachial Arteriogram. (C) Arteriogram of the Hand.**

IV Venous Drainage

A. **Superficial Veins of the Upper Limb.** The **dorsal venous network** located on the dorsum of the hand gives rise to the cephalic vein and basilic vein. The **palmar venous network** located on the palm of the hand gives rise to the median antebrachial vein.

   1. **Cephalic vein** courses along the anterolateral surface of the forearm and arm and then between the deltoid and pectoralis major muscles along the deltopectoral groove and enters the clavipectoral triangle. The cephalic vein pierces the costocoracoid membrane and empties into the axillary vein.

   2. **Basilic vein** courses along the medial side of the forearm and arm. The basilic vein pierces the brachial fascia and merges with the venae comitantes of the axillary artery to form the axillary vein.

   3. **Median cubital vein** connects the cephalic vein to the basilic vein over the cubital fossa. The median cubital vein lies superficial to the bicipital aponeurosis and is used for intravenous injections, blood transfusions, and withdrawal.

   4. **Median antebrachial vein** courses on the anterior aspect of the forearm and empties into the basilic vein of the median cubital vein.

B. **Deep veins of the upper limb** follow the arterial pattern of the arm leading finally to the **axillary vein.**

C. **Communicating venous system** is a network of **perforating veins** that connect the superficial veins with the deep veins.

V Cutaneous Nerves of the Upper Limb

A. **Supraclavicular nerve** arises from the cervical plexus (C3, C4) and innervates the skin over the upper pectoral, deltoid, and outer trapezius areas.

B. **Medial brachial cutaneous nerve** arises from the medial cord of the brachial plexus and innervates the medial side of the forearm.

C. **Medial antebrachial cutaneous nerve** arises from the medial cord of the brachial plexus and innervates the medial side of the forearm.

D. **Lateral brachial cutaneous nerve** arises from the axillary nerve and innervates the lateral side of the arm.

E. **Lateral antebrachial cutaneous nerve** arises from the musculocutaneous nerve and innervates the lateral side of the forearm.

F. **Posterior brachial and antebrachial cutaneous nerves** arise from the radial nerve and innervate the posterior side of the arm and forearm, respectively.

G. **Intercostobrachial nerve** arises from intercostal nerve 2 and innervates the medial side of the arm.

H. **Median nerve** arises from the medial and lateral cord of the brachial plexus and innervates the skin of the lateral palm of the hand along with the palmar and distal dorsal aspects of the lateral three and one half digits (thumb, index finger, middle finger, and half of the ring finger).

I.   **Ulnar nerve** arises from the medial cord of the brachial plexus and innervates the skin of the medial palm and medial dorsum of the hand along with the palmar and distal dorsal aspects of the medial one and one half digits (half of the ring finger and little finger).

J.   **Superficial branch of the radial nerve** arises from radial nerve and innervates the skin of lateral dorsum of the hand along with the proximal dorsal aspects of the lateral three and one half digits (thumb, index finger, middle finger, and half of the ring finger).

VI   Brachial Plexus (Figures 20-3, 20-4). The components of the brachial plexus include:

A.   **Rami** are the C5 through T1 ventral primary rami of spinal nerves and are located between the **anterior scalene** and **middle scalene muscles**.

B.   **Trunks (upper, middle, lower)** are formed by the joining of rami and are located in the **posterior triangle of the neck**.

C.   **Divisions (three anterior and three posterior)** are formed by trunks dividing into anterior and posterior divisions, are located **deep to the clavicle**, and are named according to their relationship to the **axillary artery**.

D.   **Cords (lateral, medial, posterior)** are formed by joining of the anterior and posterior divisions and are located in the **axilla deep to the pectoralis minor muscle**.

E.   **Branches.** The five major terminal branches are:
1.   **Musculocutaneous nerve (C5 through C7)**
2.   **Axillary nerve (C5 and C6)**
3.   **Radial nerve (C5 through T1)**
4.   **Median nerve (C5 through T1)**
5.   **Ulnar nerve (C8 and T1)**

F.   **Clinical Consideration. Injuries to the Brachial Plexus**
1.   **Erb-Duchenne or upper trunk injury** involves the C5 and C6 ventral primary rami. It is caused by a violent stretch between the head and shoulder (i.e. adduction traction of the arm with hyperextension of the neck). This damages the **musculocutaneous nerve** (innervates the biceps brachii and brachialis muscles), **suprascapular nerve** (innervates the infraspinatus muscle), **axillary nerve** (innervates the teres minor muscle), and **phrenic nerve** (which innervates the diaphragm). Clinical signs include the arm is pronated and medially rotated (**"waiter's tip hand"**). This occurs because the biceps brachii muscle (which is a supinator of the forearm) is weakened so that the pronator muscles dominate and the infraspinatus muscle (which is a lateral rotator of the arm) is weakened so that the medial rotator muscles dominate; and **ipsilateral paralysis of the diaphragm** because of involvement of the C5 component of the phrenic nerve.
2.   **Klumpke or lower trunk injury** involves the C8 and T1 ventral primary rami. It is caused by a sudden pull upward of the arm (i.e. abduction injury). This damages the **median nerve, ulnar nerve** (both of which innervate muscles of the forearm and hand), and **sympathetics of the T1 spinal nerve**. Clinical signs include **loss of function of the wrist and hand** and **Horner's syndrome**, in which **miosis** (constriction of the pupil as a result of paralysis of dilator pupillae muscle), **ptosis** (drooping of the eyelid as a result of paralysis of superior tarsal muscle), and **hemianhydrosis** (loss of sweating on one side) occur.

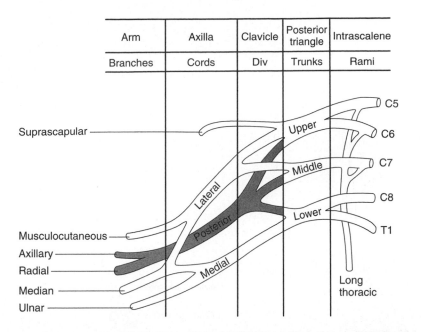

	Arm	Axilla	Clavicle	Posterior triangle	Intrascalene
	Branches	Cords	Div	Trunks	Rami

Suprascapular

Upper
Middle
Lower

C5
C6
C7
C8
T1

Lateral
Posterior
Medial

Musculocutaneous
Axillary
Radial
Median
Ulnar

Long thoracic

A

Injury	Injury Description	Nerves Damaged	Clinical Sign
Erb-Duchenne (C5 and C6 Upper Trunk)	Violent stretch between the head and shoulder (i.e. adduction traction of the arm and hyperextension of the neck)	Musculocutaneous Suprascapular Axillary Phrenic	Arm is pronated and medially rotated (Waiter's tip) Ipsilateral paralysis of diaphragm
Klumpke (C8 and T1 Lower Trunk)	Sudden pull upward of the arm (i.e. abduction injury)	Median Ulnar Sympathetics of T1 spinal nerve	Loss of function of the hand and wrist Horner's syndrome[a]

[a]Clinical signs of Horner's syndrome include miosis (constriction of the pupil caused by paralysis of dilator pupillae muscle), ptosis (drooping of eyelid caused by paralysis of superior tarsal muscle), and hemianhydrosis (loss of sweating on one side).

B

● **Figure 20-3 (A) Diagram of the Brachial Plexus.** Diagram of the brachial plexus showing the rami, trunks, divisions, cords, and five major terminal branches along with their respective anatomic positions. For example, during surgery in the posterior triangle of the neck, the trunks of the brachial plexus may be damaged. The posterior divisions, cords, and branches are shaded. The suprascapular nerve and long thoracic nerve are also shown. **(B) Diagram Indicating the Erb-Duchenne Injury and Klumpke Injury to the Brachial Plexus.**

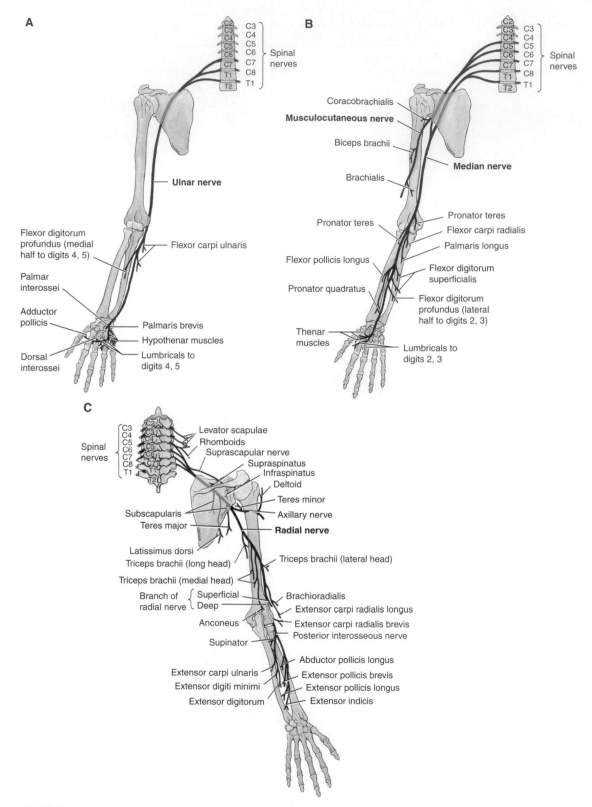

A

C2
C3
C4
C5
C6
C7
T1
T2

C3
C4
C5
C6
C7
C8
T1

Spinal nerves

Ulnar nerve

Flexor digitorum profundus (medial half to digits 4, 5)

Flexor carpi ulnaris

Palmar interossei

Adductor pollicis

Palmaris brevis

Hypothenar muscles

Dorsal interossei

Lumbricals to digits 4, 5

B

C2
C3
C4
C5
C6
C7
T1
T2

C3
C4
C5
C6
C7
C8
T1

Spinal nerves

Coracobrachialis

Musculocutaneous nerve

Biceps brachii

Median nerve

Brachialis

Pronator teres

Pronator teres

Flexor carpi radialis

Palmaris longus

Flexor pollicis longus

Flexor digitorum superficialis

Pronator quadratus

Flexor digitorum profundus (lateral half to digits 2, 3)

Thenar muscles

Lumbricals to digits 2, 3

C

C3
C4
C5
C6
C7
C8
T1

Spinal nerves

C2
C3
C4
C5
C6
C7
T1
T2

Levator scapulae

Rhomboids

Suprascapular nerve

Supraspinatus

Infraspinatus

Deltoid

Teres minor

Axillary nerve

Radial nerve

Subscapularis

Teres major

Latissimus dorsi

Triceps brachii (long head)

Triceps brachii (lateral head)

Triceps brachii (medial head)

Branch of radial nerve { Superficial / Deep }

Brachioradialis

Extensor carpi radialis longus

Anconeus

Extensor carpi radialis brevis

Supinator

Posterior interosseous nerve

Abductor pollicis longus

Extensor carpi ulnaris

Extensor pollicis brevis

Extensor digiti minimi

Extensor pollicis longus

Extensor digitorum

Extensor indicis

● **Figure 20-4 Innervation of the Upper Limb Muscles. (A) Anterior View.** Ulnar nerve. **(B) Anterior View.** Median and musculocutaneous nerves. **(C) Posterior View.** Radial nerve.

VII Nerve Lesions (Table 20-1)

A. Long thoracic nerve injury may be caused by a stab wound or removal of lymph nodes during a mastectomy. Paralysis of the serratus anterior muscle occurs so that abduction of the arm past the horizontal position is compromised. In addition, the arm cannot be used to push with. To test the serratus anterior muscle clinically, the patient is asked to face a wall and push against it with both arms. The medial border and inferior angle of the scapula on the injured side will become prominent, called "**winging of the scapula.**"

B. Axillary nerve injury may be caused by a fracture of the surgical neck of the humerus or anterior dislocation of the shoulder joint. Paralysis of the deltoid muscle occurs so that abduction of the arm to the horizontal position is compromised. Paralysis of the teres minor muscle occurs so that lateral rotation of the arm is weakened. Sensory loss occurs on the lateral side of the upper arm. To test the deltoid muscle clinically, the patient's arm is abducted to the horizontal, and then the patient is asked to hold that position against a downward pull.

C. Radial nerve injury may be caused by a fracture of the humerus at midshaft, a badly fitted crutch, or falling asleep with the arm draped over a chair. Paralysis of the muscles in the extensor compartment of the forearm occurs so that extension of the wrist and digits is lost and supination is compromised. Extension of the forearm is preserved because innervation to the triceps muscle is generally intact. Sensory loss occurs on the posterior arm, posterior forearm, and lateral aspect of the dorsum of the hand. Clinically, the hand will be flexed at the wrist and lie flaccid in a condition known as "**wrist drop.**"

D. Median nerve injury at the elbow or axilla may be caused by a supracondylar fracture of the humerus. Paralysis of the muscles in the flexor compartment of the arm occurs so that flexion of the wrist is weakened, the hand will deviate to the ulnar side on flexion, flexion of the index and middle fingers at the distal (DIP) and proximal (PIP) interphalangeal joints is lost, and pronation is lost. Paralysis of lumbricals 1 and 2 occurs so that flexion of the index and middle fingers at the metacarpophalangeal (MP) joint is lost. Paralysis of abductor pollicis brevis, opponens pollicis, and flexor pollicis brevis muscles occurs so that abduction, opposition, and flexion of the thumb are lost. Sensory loss occurs on the palmar and dorsal aspects of the index, middle, and half of the ring fingers and palmar aspect of the thumb. Clinically, a flattening of the thenar eminence will occur in a condition known as "**ape hand,**" and when the patient is asked to make a fist the index and middle fingers tend to remain straight while the ring and little finger flex in a condition known as "**benediction hand.**" To test the integrity of the median nerve (motor) the patient maintains an O with the thumb and index finger while the physician tries to pass a probe between them. This procedure tests the function of the opponens pollicis muscle.

E. Median nerve injury at the wrist may be caused by a slashing of the wrist in a suicide attempt or carpal tunnel syndrome. No paralysis of the muscles in the flexor compartment of the arm occurs. Paralysis of lumbricals 1 and 2 occurs so that flexion of the index and middle fingers at the MP joint is weakened. Paralysis of abductor pollicis brevis, opponens pollicis, and flexor pollicis brevis muscles occurs so that abduction and opposition of the thumb are lost (flexion of thumb remains because the flexor pollicis longus muscle is spared). Sensory loss occurs on the palmar and dorsal aspects of the index, middle, and half of the ring fingers and the palmar aspect of the thumb.

Clinically, a flattening of the thenar eminence will occur in a condition known as **"ape hand."**

F. **Ulnar nerve injury at the elbow or axilla** may be caused by a fracture of the medial epicondyle of the humerus. Paralysis of the flexor carpi ulnaris muscle occurs so that the hand will deviate to the radial side on flexion. Paralysis of the medial part of the flexor digitorum profundus muscle occurs so that flexion of the ring and little finger at the DIP joint is lost. Paralysis of lumbricals 3 and 4 occurs so that flexion of the ring and little fingers at the MP joint is lost and extension of the ring and little fingers at the DIP and PIP joints is lost. Paralysis of the palmar and dorsal interosseous muscles occurs so that abduction and adduction of the fingers are lost; flexion of fingers at the MP joint is lost; and extension of fingers at the DIP and PIP joints is lost. Paralysis of the adductor pollicis muscle occurs so that adduction of the thumb is lost. Paralysis of the abductor digiti minimi, flexor digiti minimi, and opponens digiti minimi muscles occurs so that little finger movements are lost. Sensory loss occurs on the palmar and dorsal aspects of half of the ring finger and the little finger. Clinically, a mild **"clawhand"** is observed. To test the integrity of the ulnar nerve (motor), the patient holds a piece of paper between the middle finger and ring finger as the physician tries to remove it. This tests the function of the interosseus muscles.

G. **Ulnar nerve injury at the wrist** may be caused by a slashing of the wrist in a suicide attempt. There is no paralysis of the flexor carpi ulnaris muscle. There is no paralysis of the medial part of the flexor digitorum profundus muscle. Paralysis of lumbricals 3 and 4 occurs so that flexion of the ring and little fingers at the MP joint is lost and extension of the ring and little fingers at the DIP and PIP joints is lost. Paralysis of the palmar and dorsal interosseous muscles occurs so that abduction and adduction of the fingers are lost; flexion of fingers at the MP joint is lost; and extension of fingers at the DIP and PIP joints is lost. Paralysis of the adductor pollicis muscle occurs so that adduction of the thumb is lost. Paralysis of the abductor digiti minimi, flexor digiti minimi, and opponens digiti minimi muscles occurs so that little finger movements are lost. Sensory loss occurs on the palmar and dorsal aspects of half the ring finger and the little finger. Clinically, a severe **"clawhand"** is observed because of the unopposed action of the flexor digitorum profundus.

TABLE 20-1	NERVE LESIONS		
Nerve Injury	**Injury Description**	**Impairments**	**Clinical Aspects**
Long thoracic nerve	Stab wound Mastectomy	Abduction of arm past horizontal is compromised	Test: Push against a wall causes winging of scapula
Axillary nerve	Surgical neck fracture of humerus Anterior dislocation of shoulder joint	Abduction of arm to horizontal is compromised Sensory loss on lateral side of upper arm	Test: Abduct arm to horizontal and ask patient to hold position against a downward pull
Radial nerve	Midshaft fracture of humerus Badly fitted crutch Arm draped over a chair	Extension of wrist and digits is lost Supination is compromised Sensory loss on posterior arm, posterior forearm, and lateral aspect of dorsum of hand	Wrist drop
Median nerve at elbow	Supracondylar fracture of humerus	Flexion of wrist is weakened Hand will deviate to ulnar side on flexion Flexion of index and middle fingers at DIP, PIP, and MP joints is lost Abduction, opposition, and flexion of thumb are lost Sensory loss on palmar and dorsal aspects of the index, middle, and half of the ring fingers and palmar aspect of thumb	Ape hand Benediction hand
Median nerve at wrist	Slashing of wrist Carpal tunnel syndrome	Flexion of index and middle fingers at MP joint is weakened Abduction and opposition of thumb are lost Sensory loss same as at elbow	Test: Make an O with thumb and index finger
Ulnar nerve at elbow	Fracture of medial epicondyle of humerus	Hand will deviate to radial side upon flexion Flexion of ring and little finger at DIP is lost Flexion at MP joint and extension at DIP and PIP joints of ring and little finger are lost Adduction and abduction of fingers are lost Adduction of thumb is lost Little finger movements are lost Sensory loss on palmar and dorsal aspects of half of ring finger and little finger	Claw hand
Ulnar nerve at wrist	Slashing of wrist	Flexion at MP joint and extension at DIP and PIP joints of ring and little finger are lost Adduction and abduction of fingers are lost Adduction of thumb is lost Little finger movements are lost Sensory loss same as at elbow	Test: Hold paper between middle and ring fingers

DIP = distal interphalangeal, MIP = middle interphalangeal, MP = metacarpophalangeal, PIP = proximal interphalangeal.

Shoulder Region (Figure 20-5)

A. The Axilla. The axilla is a pyramid-shaped region located between the upper thoracic wall and the arm. The medial wall of the axilla is the upper ribs and the serratus anterior muscle. The lateral wall of the axilla is the humerus. The posterior wall of the axilla is the subscapularis, teres major, and latissimus dorsi muscles. The anterior wall of the axilla is the pectoralis major and pectoralis minor muscles. The base of the axilla is the axillary fascia. The apex of the axilla is the space between the clavicle, scapula, and rib 1.

B. Spaces
1. The **quadrangular space** (transmits the **axillary nerve** and **posterior humeral circumflex artery**) is bounded superiorly by the teres minor and subscapularis muscles, inferiorly by the teres major muscle, medially by the long head of the triceps, and laterally by the surgical neck of the humerus.
2. The **upper triangular space** (transmits the **circumflex scapular artery**) is bounded superiorly by the teres minor muscle, inferiorly by the teres major muscle, and laterally by the long head of the triceps.
3. The **lower triangular space** (transmits the **radial nerve** and **deep brachial artery**) is bounded superiorly by the teres major muscle, medially by the long head of the triceps, and laterally by the medial head of the triceps.

C. Glenohumeral Joint
1. **General Features.** The glenohumeral joint is the articulation of the head of the humerus with the glenoid fossa of the scapula. This joint has two prominent bursae: the **subacromial bursa** (separates the tendon of the supraspinatus muscle from the deltoid muscle) and the **subscapular bursa** (separates the scapular fossa and the tendon of the subscapularis muscle). The "**rotator cuff**" (along with the **tendon of the long head of the biceps brachii muscle**) contributes to the stability of the glenohumeral joint by holding the head of the humerus against the glenoid surface of the scapula. The rotator cuff is formed by the tendons of the following muscles (SITS acronym):
   a. **Subscapularis muscle** innervated by the subscapular nerve.
   b. **Infraspinatus muscle** innervated by the suprascapular nerve.
   c. **Teres minor muscle** innervated by the axillary nerve.
   d. **Supraspinatus muscle** innervated by the suprascapular nerve.
2. **Clinical Considerations**
   a. **Anterior/inferior dislocation of the humerus** ("shoulder dislocation") is the most common direction of a shoulder dislocation. The head of the humerus lies anterior and inferior to the **coracoid process** of the scapula and may damage the **axillary nerve** or **axillary artery.** The dislocation occurs because of the shallowness of the glenoid fossa. Impaction of the anterior-inferior surface of the glenoid labrum on the posterolateral aspect of the humeral head after it dislocates may cause a depressed humeral head fracture called the **Hill-Sachs lesion.** Clinical signs include loss of normal round contour of the shoulder, a palpable depression under the acromion, and a palpable head of the humerus in the axilla.
   b. **Rotator Cuff Injury (also called subacromial bursitis or painful arc syndrome). Rotator cuff tendinitis** most commonly involves the **tendon of the supraspinatus muscle** and the **subacromial bursa.** It presents in middle-aged men with pain on lifting the arm above the head. **Acute rotator cuff tear** pres-

ents as acute onset of pain with inability to lift arm above the head after a traumatic event. The most common rotator cuff tear is an isolated tear of the **supraspinatus tendon** at its insertion at the greater tuberosity. Partial thickness tears are more common than full thickness tears.

D. Acromioclavicular Joint

  1. General Features. The acromioclavicular joint is the articulation of the lateral end of the clavicle with the acromion of the scapula. This joint is stabilized by **the coracoacromial ligament, coracoclavicular ligament** (subdivided into the **conoid** and **trapezoid ligaments**), and the **acromioclavicular ligament**.

  2. Clinical Considerations

   a. **Acromioclavicular subluxation ("shoulder separation")** is a common injury caused by a downward blow at the tip of the shoulder. There are three grades of shoulder separation: **grade I**, in which there is no ligament tearing and no abnormal joint spaces (i.e. minor sprain); **grade II**, in which the acromioclavicular ligament is torn and the acromioclavicular space is 50% wider than the normal, contralateral shoulder; and **grade III**, in which the coracoclavicular ligament and acromioclavicular ligament are torn, and the coracoclavicular space and acromioclavicular space are 50% wider than the normal contralateral shoulder. Clinical signs include injured arm hangs noticeably lower than normal arm, noticeable bulge at tip of shoulder because of upward displacement of clavicle, pushing down on the lateral end of the clavicle and releasing causes a rebound ("piano key sign"), and radiograph with a 10-pound weight shows a marked separation of the acromion from the clavicle in a grade II and III.

   b. **Fracture of the clavicle** most commonly occurs at the middle one third of the clavicle. This fracture results in the upward displacement of the proximal fragment because of the pull of the sternocleidomastoid muscle and downward displacement of the distal fragment because of the pull of the deltoid muscle and gravity. The subclavian artery, subclavian vein, and divisions of the brachial plexus that are located deep to the clavicle may be put in jeopardy.

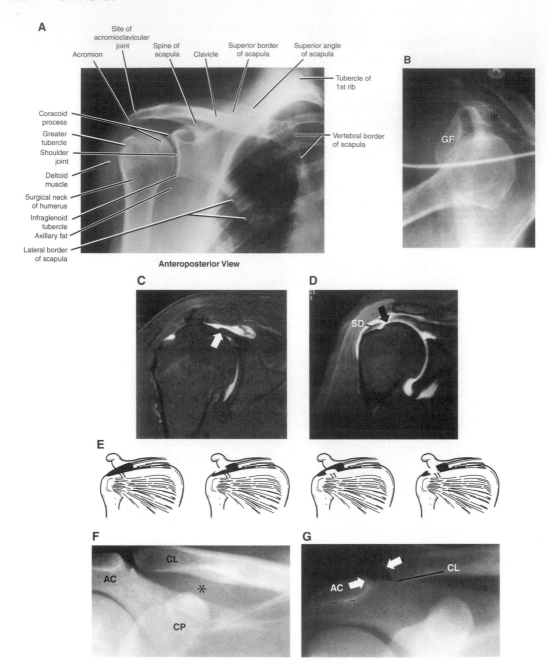

● **Figure 20-5 (A) AP Radiograph of Shoulder Region. (B) AP Radiograph of Anterior Dislocation of Shoulder.**
The humeral head is displaced out of the glenoid fossa (GF) inferior to the coracoid process (*) of the scapula. **(C–E)**
Rotator Cuff Injury. (C) Full-thickness tear of the supraspinatus and infraspinatus tendons. An oblique coronal T_2-
weighted fat-suppressed MRI shows retraction of the supraspinatus tendon (arrow) and superior subluxation of the
humeral head. **(D)** MR arthrogram shows a complete tear of the rotator cuff (arrow). The bright contrast medium flows
from the glenohumeral joint space into the subdeltoid bursa (SD), which does not occur in a normal intact rotator cuff.
(E) Diagram of various tears of the supraspinatus tendon. **(F, G) Acromioclavicular Subluxation ("Shoulder**
Separation"). (F) AP radiographs shows a normal adult shoulder. The acromioclavicular ligament (arrowhead) and the
coracoclavicular ligament (*) are shown. CL = clavicle, AC = acromion, CP = coracoid process. **(G)** Type II acromioclavicular separation. AP radiograph (weight-bearing) shows the acromion (AC; dashed line) more inferior to the clavicle (CL;
solid line). The acromioclavicular space (arrows) is abnormally widened but the coracoclavicular space in normal.

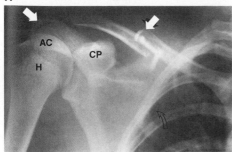

● **Figure 20-5 (Continued). (H) Fracture of the Clavicle.** AP radiograph shows a fracture of the middle one third of the clavicle (arrows). Note the upward displacement of the proximal fragment and the downward displacement of the distal fragment. AC = acromion, CP = coracoid process, H = head of the humerus.

IX Elbow Region (Figure 20-6)

A. Elbow joint consists of three articulations among the humerus, ulna, and radius.
   1. **Humeroulnar joint** is reinforced by the **ulnar collateral ligament.** The actions of flexion and extension of the forearm occur at this joint. A tear of this ligament will permit abnormal **abduction** of the forearm.
   2. **Humeroradial joint** is reinforced by the **radial collateral ligament.** The actions of flexion and extension of the forearm occur at this joint. A tear of this ligament will permit abnormal **adduction** of the forearm.
   3. **Radioulnar joint** is reinforced by the **annular ligament.** The actions of pronation and supination of the forearm occur at this joint.

B. Clinical Considerations
   1. **Nursemaid's Elbow.** A severe distal traction of the radius (e.g. a parent yanking the arm of a child) can cause **subluxation of the head of the radius** from its encirclement by the **annular ligament.** The reduction of nursemaid's elbow involves applying direct pressure posteriorly on the head of the radius while simultaneously supinating and extending the forearm. This manipulation effectively "screws" the head of the radius into the annular ligament. Clinical signs: child presents with a flexed and pronated forearm held close to the body.
   2. **Lateral epicondylitis (tennis elbow)** is inflammation of the **common extensor tendon** of the wrist where it originates on the lateral epicondyle of the humerus.
   3. **Medial epicondylitis (golfer's elbow)** is inflammation of the **common flexor tendon** of the wrist where it originates on the medial epicondyle of the humerus.
   4. **Tommy John surgery** (named after the famous Chicago White Sox baseball pitcher) replaces or augments a torn ulnar collateral ligament. When this ligament is torn, it is impossible to throw a ball with force and speed. A replacement tendon is taken from the hamstring muscle and wrapped in a figure-eight pattern through holes drilled in the humerus and ulna.
   5. **Supracondylar fracture of the humerus** places the contents of the cubital fossa in jeopardy, specifically the median nerve (see Table 20-1) and brachial artery. The contents of the cubital fossa include the **median nerve, brachial artery, biceps brachii tendon, median cubital vein** (superficial to the bicipital aponeurosis), and **radial nerve** (lying deep to the brachioradialis muscle).
   6. **Little Leaguer's elbow** is the avulsion of the medial epicondyle by violent or multiple contractions of the flexor forearm muscles (e.g. strenuous or repeated throwing of a ball).
   7. **Dislocation of the elbow** is most commonly a posterior dislocation of the radius and ulna with respect to the distal end of the humerus. Depending on the magni-

tude and direction of the dislocating force, fractures of the distal humerus, coronoid process of the ulna, or radial head may occur.

8. **Fracture of the olecranon** may result from a fall on the forearm with the elbow flexed, in which case the fracture is transverse; or it may result from a fall directly on the olecranon process itself, in which case the fracture is comminuted.

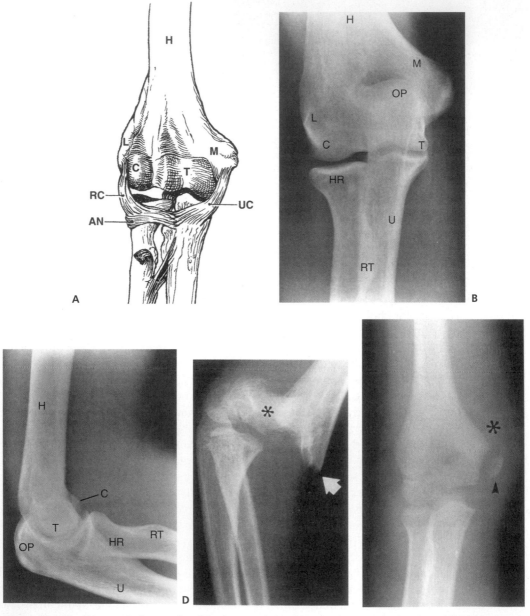

● **Figure 20-6 (A–C) Normal Elbow Joint. (A)** Diagram of the elbow region. Note the location of the ligaments that support the elbow joint. **(B)** AP radiograph of the right elbow joint. **(C)** Lateral radiograph of the right elbow joint. **(D) Supracondylar Fracture.** Lateral radiograph of a supracondylar fracture of the humerus shows a fracture site (arrow) with posterior displacement of the distal fragment (*) as well as the radius and ulna. The displacement of the humerus places the contents of the cubital fossa in jeopardy, specifically the median nerve and brachial artery. **(E) Little Leaguer's Elbow.** AP radiograph shows avulsion of the medial epicondyle (arrowhead) and soft tissue swelling on the medial side of the elbow (*).

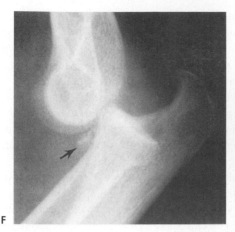
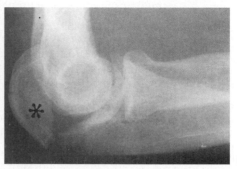

F   G

● **Figure 20-6 (Continued). (F) Posterior Dislocation of the Elbow.** Lateral radiograph shows a posterior dislocation of the elbow with a small bony fragment (arrow) arising from the tip of the coronoid process interposed between the trochlea and the base of the coronoid process. **(G) Fracture of the Olecranon.** Lateral radiograph shows comminuted fracture of the olecranon process with proximal retraction of the proximal fragments (*) caused by the unopposed action of the triceps tendon. AN = annular ligament, C = capitulum, H = humerus, HR = head of the radius, L = lateral epicondyle, M = medial epicondyle, OP = olecranon process, RC = radial collateral ligament, RT = radial tuberosity, U = ulna, UC = ulnar collateral ligament, T = trochlea.

Ⅹ   Wrist and Hand Region (Figure 20-7)

A. Wrist joint (radiocarpal joint) is the articulation of the concave distal end of the radius with the scaphoid and lunate carpal bones. The actions of flexion–extension and abduction–adduction of the hand occur at this joint. The ulnar bone plays a minor role at the wrist joint.

B. Metacarpophalangeal (MP) joint is the joint between the metacarpals and the proximal phalanx. The action of flexion at the MP joint is accomplished by the flexor digitorum superficialis, flexor digitorum profundus, and the lumbrical muscles. The action of adduction and abduction at the MP joint is accomplished by the palmar interosseus muscles (PAD acronym) and dorsal interosseus muscles (DAB acronym), respectively.

C. Proximal interphalangeal (PIP) joint is the joint between the proximal phalanx and middle phalanx. The action of flexion at the PIP joint is accomplished primarily by the flexor digitorum superficialis muscle.

D. Distal interphalangeal (DIP) joint is the joint between the middle phalanx and distal phalanx. The action of flexion at the DIP joint is accomplished primarily by the flexor digitorum profundus muscle.

E. Clinical Considerations
   1. Carpal tunnel syndrome is a tendosynovitis caused by repetitive hand movements (e.g. data entry) that compress the **median nerve** within the carpal tunnel. The flexor retinaculum (composed of the **volar carpal ligament** and the **transverse carpal ligament**) is attached to the palmar surface of the carpal bones and forms the **carpal tunnel**. The structures that pass through the carpal tunnel include **flexor digitorum superficialis tendons, flexor digitorum profundus tendons, flexor pollicis longus tendon,** and **median nerve.** No arteries pass through the carpal tunnel.

Clinical signs include sensory loss on the palmar and dorsal aspects of the index, middle, and half of the ring fingers and the palmar aspect of the thumb; flattening of thenar eminence ("ape hand"), tapping of the palmaris longus tendon produces a tingling sensation (Tinel test); and forced flexion of the wrist reproduces symptoms whereas extension of the wrist alleviates symptoms (Phalen test).

2. **Slashing of the Wrist ("suicide cuts").** A deep laceration on the radial side of the wrist may cut the following structures: **radial artery, median nerve, flexor carpi radialis tendon,** and the **palmaris longus tendon.** A deep laceration on the ulnar side of the wrist may cut the following structures: **ulnar artery, ulnar nerve,** and **flexor carpi ulnaris tendon.**

3. **Dupuytren contracture** is a thickening and contracture of the palmar aponeurosis that results in the progressive flexion of the fingers (usually more pronounced in the ring finger and little finger). This is highly correlated with coronary artery disease possibly as a result of vasospasm caused by sympathetic innervation of the vasculature within the T1 component of the ulnar nerve.

4. **Volkmann ischemic contracture** is a contracture of the forearm muscles commonly caused by a supracondylar fracture of the humerus in which the brachial artery goes into spasm thereby reducing the blood flow. This may also occur as a result of an overly tight cast or compartment syndrome in which muscles are subjected to increased pressure because of edema or hemorrhage.

5. **Fracture of the Scaphoid.** The scaphoid bone is the most commonly fractured carpal bone. The scaphoid bone articulates with the distal end of the radius at the radiocarpal joint. A fracture of the scaphoid is associated with **osteonecrosis** of the scaphoid bone (proximal fragment) because the blood supply to the scaphoid bone flows from distal to proximal. Clinical signs include tenderness in the "**anatomical snuff box**" (formed by the tendons of the extensor pollicis longus, extensor pollicis brevis, and abductor pollicis longus) because the scaphoid lies in the floor of the snuff box; radiograph may be negative for several weeks until bone resorption occurs.

6. **Colles' fracture** is a fracture of the distal portion of the radius in which the distal fragment of the radius is displaced posteriorly ("dinner fork deformity"). This occurs when a person falls on an outstretched hand with the wrist extended. A Colles' fracture is commonly accompanied by a fracture of the ulnar styloid process.

7. **Gamekeeper's thumb** is a disruption of the ulnar collateral ligament of the MP joint of the thumb often associated with an avulsion fracture at the base of the proximal phalanx of the thumb. This occurs in skiing falls in which the thumb gets entangled with the ski pole.

8. **Boxer fracture** is a fracture at the head of the fifth metacarpal (i.e. little finger). This occurs when a closed fist is used to hit something hard. Clinical signs include pain on the ulnar side of the hand, depression of the head of the fifth metacarpal, and pain when attempts to flex the little finger are made.

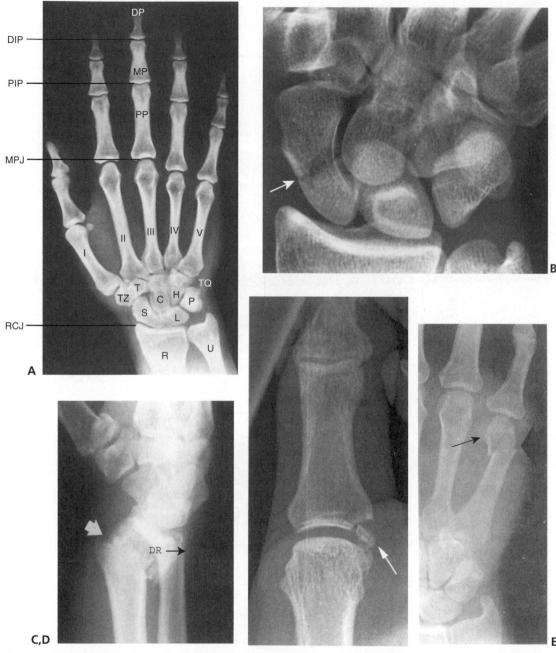

● **Figure 20-7 (A) AP Radiograph of the Hand and Wrist Region. (B) Scaphoid Fracture.** Radiograph shows a scaphoid fracture (arrow). Note that the proximal part of the scaphoid is prone to osteonecrosis. **(C) Colles' Fracture.** Lateral radiograph shows a Colles' fracture (large arrow). Note that the distal fragment of the radius (DR) is displaced posteriorly (small arrow), rotated, and impacted in the typical "dinner fork deformity." **(D) Gamekeeper's Thumb.** Radiograph shows a gamekeeper's thumb with an avulsion fracture (arrow) at the base of the proximal phalanx of the thumb associated with the ulnar collateral ligament. **(E) Boxer Fracture.** Radiograph shows a fracture at the head of the fifth metacarpal (i.e. little finger; arrow). C = capitate, DP = distal phalanx, DIP = distal interphalangeal joint, H = hamate, L = lunate, MP = middle phalanx, MPJ = metacarpophalangeal (MP) joint, P = pisiform, PIP = proximal interphalangeal joint, PP = proximal phalanx, R = radius, RCJ = radiocarpal joint, S = scaphoid, T = trapezoid, TQ = triquetrum, TZ = trapezium, U = ulna, I = first metacarpal, II = second metacarpal, III = third metacarpal, IV = fourth metacarpal, V = fifth metacarpal.

XI   Cross-Sectional Anatomy of Right Arm and Right Forearm (Figure 20-8)

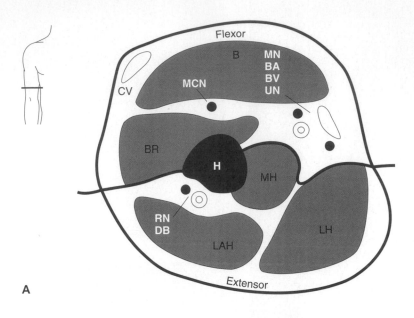

A

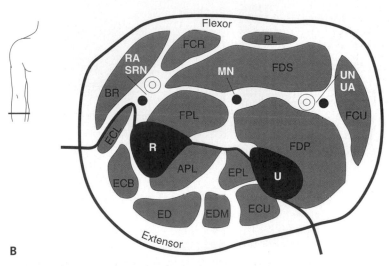

B

● **Figure 20.8 (A) Cross-Section Through the Right Brachium (Arm).** Black line divides the flexor (anterior) compartment from the extensor (posterior) compartment. Note the radial nerve (RN) within the extensor compartment traveling with the deep brachial artery (DB). Note the median nerve (MN) traveling with the brachial artery (BA). Note the ulnar nerve (UN) near the basilic vein (BV). **(B) Cross-Section Through the Right Antebrachium (Forearm).** Black line divides the flexor (anterior) compartment from the extensor (posterior) compartment. Note the location of the ulnar artery (UA), ulnar nerve (UN), median nerve (MN), radial artery (RA), and the superficial branch of the radial nerve (SRN) within the flexor compartment. APL = abductor pollicis longus, B = biceps brachii, BR = brachioradialis, CV = cephalic vein, ECB = extensor carpi radialis brevis, ECL = extensor carpi radialis longus, ECU = extensor carpi ulnaris, ED = extensor digitorum, EDM = extensor digiti minimi, EPL = extensor pollicis longus, FCR = flexor carpi radialis, FCU = flexor carpi ulnaris, FDP = flexor digitorum profundus, FDS = flexor digitorum superficialis, FPL = flexor pollicis longus, LAH = lateral head of triceps, LH = long head of triceps, MH = medial head of triceps, MCN = musculocutaneous nerve, PL = palmaris longus.

Case Study 1

On a hot, humid night, the graveyard shift of a local emergency room is contacted by an emergency medical team (EMT). The EMT brings in a 32-year-old white female police officer suffering from wounds to the right upper chest and medial shoulder with bleeding from that area. The wounds appear to be deep. Although somewhat confused, the police officer is conscious and claims to have been shot from about 7 feet with a shotgun.

Physical examination reveals a slightly weak radial pulse. The brachial pulse is somewhat stronger. There is weakness as well as intense pain when the officer tries to adduct and medially rotate the upper arm (i.e. humerus). Also noted is weakness in extension of the elbow and wrist.

Radiographs reveal six spherical radiolucent objects 2 to 6 cm inferior to the coracoid process.

Explanation

The muscles that may have been injured are the pectoralis major and minor, subscapularis, deltoid, subclavius, serratus anterior, coracobrachialis, biceps brachii, latissimus dorsi, and teres major.

The vessels that may have been injured are the cephalic vein, axillary vein, axillary artery, thoracoacromial artery, subscapular artery, and lateral thoracic artery. In this case, the patient will most likely require exploratory surgery and vascular repair.

The pain and weakness in adduction and medial rotation of the humerus may be attributed to damage to the following muscles and nerves:
- Pectoralis major: medial (C8 and T1) and lateral (C5 through C7) pectoral nerves
- Subscapularis: upper and lower subscapular nerves (C5 through C7)
- Teres major: lower subscapular nerve (C6 and C7)
- Coracobrachialis: musculocutaneous nerve (C5 through C7)
- Deltoid: axillary nerve (C5 and C6)
- Latissimus dorsi: thoracodorsal nerve (C6 through C8)

The weakness in extension of the elbow and wrist can be attributed to damage to the radial nerve of the brachial plexus. The radial nerve provides motor innervation to the triceps and extensor muscles of the forearm.

Case Study 2

Tad is a 40-year-old healthy male seaman who reports having had intermittent pain for about 3 years (since age 37) in his left arm. The pain has worsened lately, since he began a new job on a large cargo container ship that requires quite a bit of upper arm movement. The patient describes a dull ache with occasional radiations into the shoulder, neck, medial arm and forearm, and medial hand, all on the left side. He also reports some numbness and tingling in the fourth and fifth digits.

Examination shows tenderness and resistance in the left supraclavicular region. During the physical examination, pulling the upper limb downward increased the pain. The left arm seems weaker, and there is wasting of the left thenar eminence. Particularly involved are muscles that move the thumb, including flexion, abduction, adduction, opposition, and to a lesser degree, extension.

The diagnosis of cervical rib was presumed and confirmed by AP roentgenogram. On surgical excision, it was found that the accessory bony prominence (rib) continued anteriorly as a fibrous band that attached to the first rib.

- Physical examination reveals a healthy, alert black male
- Height: 6'1", weight: 205 pounds
- Pulse: 68, regular rhythm, and strong bilaterally at brachial, carotid, and femoral arteries
- Blood pressure: 145/90 mm Hg
- Drinks only when on shore leave; smokes cigars only on shore leave.

Explanation

Thoracic outlet syndrome (TOS) refers to compression of the neurovascular structures at the superior aperture of the thorax. The brachial plexus, subclavian vein, and subclavian artery are affected. Neurologic symptoms occur in 95% of cases and include pain, especially in medial aspect of arm, forearm, and ulnar 1.5 digits; paresthesias, often nocturnal, awakening patient with pain or numbness; loss of dexterity; cold intolerance; supraclavicular tenderness; diminished sensation to light touch; and weakness (usually subtle) in the affected limb. Venous symptoms occur in 4% of cases and include pain, edema, cyanosis, and distended superficial veins of the shoulder and chest. Arterial symptoms occur in 1% of cases and include pain, pallor, pulselessness, coolness on the affected side, lower blood pressure in affected arm, and multiple small infarcts on hand and fingers.

There are three major causes of TOS: anatomic, trauma or repetitive activities, and neurovascular entrapment at the costoclavicular space. Anatomic causes include the scalene triangle with the anterior scalene muscle frontally, middle scalene muscle posteriorly, and upper border of the first rib inferiorly accounting for the majority of neurologic and arterial thoracic outlet syndromes. Cervical ribs are found in the majority of arterial cases, whereas congenital fibromuscular bands are found in 80% of neurologic cases. Trauma such as a motor vehicle accident hyperextension injury and repetitive activities including vigorous arm exertion can also cause TOS. Other conditions that can cause these symptoms include carpal tunnel syndrome, rotator cuff injuries, spinal cord injuries, bursitis of the shoulder, herniated disks of the cervical vertebrae, ulnar nerve compression at the elbow, and tightness in the pectoralis minor and anterior scalene muscles related to posture and repetitive overhead movements.

The nerve involved in this case is the medial cord of the brachial plexus, C8 and T1. The patient would experience pain and sensory deficit (paresthesia) in the fourth and fifth digits, the medial side of the hand, forearm, and arm up to the axilla. Pain will also be felt in the shoulder and neck areas. These coincide with the cutaneous distribution areas of the following nerves: the medial brachial cutaneous nerve, the ulnar nerve, the medial antebrachial cutaneous nerve, and the medial root of the median nerve, all composed of C8 and T1 fibers.

Chapter 21

Lower Limb

I **Bones.** The bones of the lower limb include the hip (coxal) bone formed by the fusion of the ilium, ischium, and pubis; femur; patella; tibia; fibula; tarsal bones (talus, calcaneus, navicular, cuboid, and three cuneiform bones); metatarsals; and phalanges (proximal, middle, and distal) (Figure 21-1A).

II **Muscles**

A. **Muscles of the gluteal region (abductors and rotators of the thigh)** include the gluteus maximus, gluteus medius, gluteus minimus, tensor of fascia lata, piriformis, obturator internus, superior and inferior gemelli, and quadratus femoris.

B. **Muscles of the anterior compartment of the thigh (flexors of the hip joint and extensors of the knee joint)** include the pectineus, psoas major, psoas minor, iliacus, sartorius, rectus femoris, vastus lateralis, vastus medialis, and vastus intermedius.

C. **Muscles of the medial compartment of the thigh (adductors of the thigh)** include the adductor longus, adductor brevis, adductor magnus, gracilis, and obturator externus.

D. **Muscles of the posterior compartment of the thigh (extensors of the hip joint and flexors of the knee joint)** include the semitendinosus, semimembranosus, and biceps femoris.

E. **Muscles of the anterior and lateral compartments of the leg** include the tibialis anterior, extensor digitorum longus, extensor hallucis longus, fibularis tertius, fibularis longus, and fibularis brevis.

F. **Muscles of the posterior compartment of the leg** include the gastrocnemius, soleus, plantaris, popliteus, flexor hallucis longus, flexor digitorum longus, and tibialis posterior.

G. **Muscles of the foot** include the first layer (abductor hallucis, flexor digitorum brevis, abductor digiti minimi), second layer (quadratus plantae, lumbricals), third layer (flexor hallucis brevis, adductor hallucis, flexor digiti minimi brevis), fourth layer (plantar interossei, dorsal interossei), and dorsum of the foot (extensor digitorum brevis, extensor hallucis brevis).

III Arterial Supply (Figure 21-1)

A. **Superior gluteal artery** is a branch of the internal iliac artery and enters the buttock through the greater sciatic foramen above the piriformis muscle. This artery anastomoses with the lateral circumflex, medial circumflex, and inferior gluteal artery.

B. **Inferior gluteal artery** is a branch of the internal iliac artery and enters the buttock through the greater sciatic foramen below the piriformis muscle. This artery participates in the cruciate anastomosis and also anastomoses with the superior gluteal artery, internal pudendal artery, and obturator artery.

C. **Obturator artery** is a continuation of the internal iliac artery and passes through the obturator foramen close to the femoral ring, where it may complicate surgical repair of a femoral hernia. The obturator artery gives off the following branches:
   1. **Muscular branches to the adductor muscles**
   2. **Artery of the ligamentum teres (artery to the head of the femur).** This artery is of considerable importance in *children* because it supplies the head of the femur **proximal** to the epiphyseal growth plate. After the epiphyseal growth plate closes in the adult, this artery plays an insignificant role in supplying blood to the head of the femur.

D. **Femoral artery** is a continuation of the external iliac artery distal to the inguinal ligament and enters the **femoral triangle** posterior to the inguinal ligament and midway between the anterior superior iliac spine and the symphysis pubis. At this location the **femoral pulse** can be palpated, arterial blood can be obtained for **blood gas measurements**, or **percutaneous arterial catheterization** can be performed. The femoral artery is commonly used for percutaneous arterial catheterization because it is superficial and easily palpated, and because hemostasis can be achieved by applying pressure over the head of the femur. The preferred entry site is **below the inguinal ligament** at the level of the **midfemoral head** (a site that is confirmed by fluoroscopy). If the femoral artery is punctured above the inguinal ligament or below the femoral head, control of hemostasis is difficult or impossible. The femoral artery gives off the following branches:
   1. **Superficial epigastric artery**
   2. **Superficial circumflex iliac artery**
   3. **Superficial external pudendal artery**
   4. **Deep external pudendal artery**
   5. **Descending genicular artery**
   6. **Profunda femoris (deep femoral) artery,** which branches into the:
      a. **Four perforating arteries**, which supply the adductor magnus and the hamstring muscles. The first perforating artery participates in the cruciate anastomosis with the inferior gluteal artery and the medial and lateral circumflex arteries.
      b. **Medial circumflex artery**, which participates in the cruciate anastomosis and provides main blood supply to the head and neck of the femur in the adult.
      c. **Lateral circumflex artery**, which participates in the cruciate anastomosis and also sends a **descending branch of the lateral circumflex artery** to participate in the genicular anastomosis around the knee joint.

E. **Popliteal artery** is a continuation of the femoral artery at the adductor hiatus in the adductor magnus muscle and extends through the popliteal fossa where the **popliteal**

pulse can be palpated against the popliteus muscle with the leg flexed. The popliteal artery gives off the following branches:

1. **Genicular arteries.** The genicular arteries participate in the genicular anastomosis around the knee joint and supply the capsule and ligaments of the knee joint. There are four genicular arteries: **superior lateral, inferior lateral, superior medial, and inferior medial genicular arteries.**

2. **Anterior tibial artery** descends on the anterior surface of the interosseus membrane with the **deep fibular nerve** and terminates as the dorsalis pedis artery. The anterior tibial artery gives off the following branches:
   a. **Anterior tibial recurrent artery**
   b. **Medial malleolar artery**
   c. **Lateral malleolar artery**
   d. **Dorsalis pedis artery.** The dorsalis pedis artery lies between the extensor hallucis longus and extensor digitorum longus tendons midway between the medial and lateral malleolus where the **dorsal pedal pulse** can be palpated. The dorsalis pedis artery gives off the following branches:
      i. **Lateral tarsal artery** anastomoses with the arcuate artery.
      ii. **Arcuate artery** runs laterally across the bases of the lateral four metatarsals and gives rise to the **second, third, and fourth dorsal metatarsal arteries.** The dorsal metatarsal arteries branch into two **dorsal digital arteries.**
      iii. **First dorsal metatarsal artery**
      iv. **Deep plantar artery** enters the sole of the foot and joins the lateral plantar artery to form the **plantar arch.**

3. **Posterior tibial artery** passes behind the medial malleolus with the **tibial nerve** where an ankle pulse can be palpated. The posterior tibial artery gives off the following branches:
   a. **Fibular artery** passes behind the lateral malleolus, gives rise to the **posterior lateral malleolar artery,** and ends in branches around the ankle and heel.
   b. **Medial plantar artery** gives rise to a **superficial branch,** which forms three superficial digital branches, and a **deep branch,** which supplies the big toe.
   c. **Lateral plantar artery** arches medially across the foot to form the **plantar arch** in conjunction with the deep plantar artery (from the dorsalis pedis artery). The plantar arch gives rise to four **plantar metatarsal arteries** and three **perforating branches,** which anastomose with the arcuate artery. The plantar metatarsal arteries branch into two **plantar digital arteries.**

F. **Collateral Circulation**
   1. **Around the hip joint (cruciate anastomosis)** involves the following arteries:
      a. **Inferior gluteal artery** (a branch of the internal iliac artery)
      b. **Medial femoral circumflex artery**
      c. **Lateral femoral circumflex artery**
      d. **First perforating branch of profundus femoris artery**
   2. **Around the head of the femur (trochanteric anastomosis)** involves the following arteries:
      a. **Superior gluteal artery**
      b. **Inferior gluteal artery**
      c. **Medial femoral circumflex artery**
      d. **Lateral femoral circumflex artery**
   3. **Around the knee joint (genicular anastomosis)** maintains blood supply to the leg during full flexion and involves the following arteries:

    a. Superior lateral genicular artery
    b. Inferior lateral genicular artery
    c. Superior medial genicular artery
    d. Inferior medial genicular artery
    f. Descending genicular artery (from the femoral artery)
    g. Descending branch of the lateral femoral circumflex artery
    h. Anterior tibial recurrent artery

G. Clinical Considerations

1. **Placement of Ligatures.** In emergency situations, the femoral artery can be ligated anywhere along its course in the anterior compartment of the thigh without risking total loss of blood supply to the lower limb distal to the ligature site. However, sudden occlusion of the femoral artery by ligature or embolism is usually followed by gangrene. In general, collateral circulation in the lower limb is not as robust as in the upper limb.

2. **Acute arterial occlusion** is most commonly caused by an **embolism** or **thrombosis.** This occlusion most frequently occurs where the femoral artery gives off the profunda femoris artery. Clinical signs include pain, paralysis, paresthesia, pallor, poikiloderma, and pulselessness (i.e. the six Ps). This may lead to loss of lower limb because of muscle and nerve damage (both are very sensitive to anoxia) within 4 to 8 hours if prompt treatment does not occur.

3. **Chronic arterial occlusive disease** is most commonly caused by **atherosclerosis.** This disease most frequently involves the femoral artery near the adductor hiatus and popliteal artery (i.e. femoropopliteal in 50% of the cases), or the anterior tibial artery, posterior tibial artery, and fibular artery (i.e. tibiofibular in diabetic patients). Clinical signs include **intermittent claudication,** whose key feature is profound fatigue or aching on exertion (never by sitting or standing for prolonged periods) that is relieved by short periods of rest (5 to 10 minutes), **ischemic rest pain,** which features pain across the distal foot and toes that usually occurs at night (patient awakens from sleep), and pain that is exacerbated by elevation and relieved by a dependent position (patient sleeps with leg over the side of the bed).

4. **Compartment syndrome** is an increase in the interstitial fluid pressure within an osseofascial compartment of sufficient magnitude (30 mm Hg or greater) to compromise microcirculation (ischemia) leading to muscle and nerve damage. This syndrome most frequently occurs in the anterior compartment of the thigh as a result of crush injuries (e.g. car accidents) involving the **femoral artery** and **femoral nerve,** and in the anterior compartment; of the leg as a result of tibial fractures involving the **anterior tibial artery** and **deep fibular nerve.** Clinical signs include a swollen, tense compartment; pain on passive stretching of the tendons within the compartment; pink color; warmth; and presence of a pulse over the involved compartment.

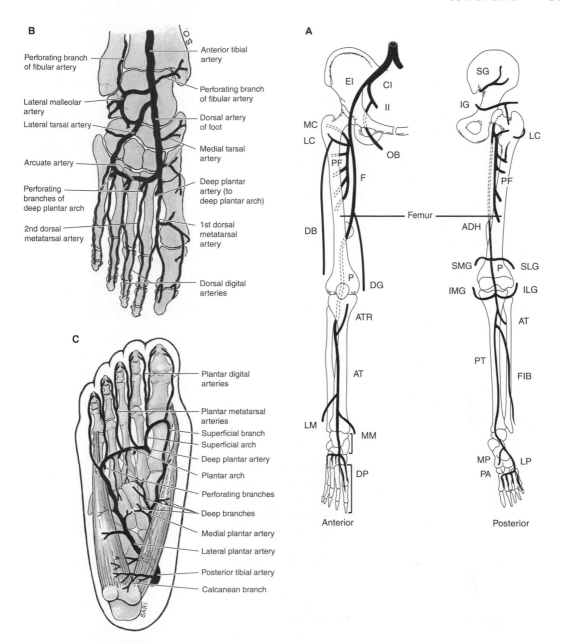

B

Perforating branch of fibular artery

Anterior tibial artery

Perforating branch of fibular artery

Lateral malleolar artery

Lateral tarsal artery

Dorsal artery of foot

Medial tarsal artery

Arcuate artery

Deep plantar artery (to deep plantar arch)

Perforating branches of deep plantar arch

2nd dorsal metatarsal artery

1st dorsal metatarsal artery

Dorsal digital arteries

C

Plantar digital arteries

Plantar metatarsal arteries

Superficial branch

Superficial arch

Deep plantar artery

Plantar arch

Perforating branches

Deep branches

Medial plantar artery

Lateral plantar artery

Posterior tibial artery

Calcanean branch

A

Anterior

Posterior

● **Figure 21-1 Bones and Arterial Supply of the Lower Limb. (A)** Anterior and posterior views. **(B)** Arterial supply of the dorsum of the foot. **(C)** Arterial supply of the sole of the foot. ADH = abductor hiatus within the adductor magnus muscle, AT = anterior tibial artery (runs with deep fibular nerve), ATR = anterior tibial recurrent artery, CI = common iliac artery, DB = descending branch of lateral femoral circumflex artery, DG = descending genicular artery, DP = dorsalis pedis artery, EI = external iliac artery, F = femoral artery (runs with femoral nerve), FIB = fibular artery, IG = inferior gluteal artery (runs with inferior gluteal nerve), II = internal iliac artery, ILG = inferior lateral genicular artery, IMG = inferior medial geniculate artery, LC = lateral femoral circumflex artery, LM = lateral malleolar artery, LP = lateral plantar artery, MC = medial femoral circumflex artery, MM = medial malleolar artery, MP = medial plantar artery, OB = obturator artery (runs with obturator nerve), P = popliteal artery (runs with sciatic nerve where it branches into tibial and common fibular nerves), PA = plantar arch, PF = profunda femoris artery, PT = posterior tibial artery (runs with tibial nerve), SG = superior gluteal artery (runs with superior gluteal nerve), SLG = superior lateral genicular artery, SMG = superior medial genicular artery.

Venous Drainage

A. Superficial Veins of the Lower Limb

1. **Great saphenous vein** (has 10 to 12 valves) is formed by the union of the dorsal vein of the big toe and the dorsal venous arch of the foot. The great saphenous vein passes anterior to the medial malleolus (travels with the **saphenous nerve**), where it is accessible for venous puncture or catheter insertion, and passes posterior to the medial condyle of the femur. The great saphenous vein anastomoses with the lesser saphenous vein. The great saphenous vein courses along the medial aspect of the leg and thigh and finally empties into the femoral vein within the femoral triangle.

2. **Small saphenous vein** is formed by the union of the dorsal vein of the little toe and the dorsal venous arch of the foot. The small saphenous vein passes posterior to the lateral malleolus (travels with the **sural nerve**). The small saphenous vein courses along the lateral border of the calcaneal tendon, ascends between the heads of the gastrocnemius muscle, and finally empties into the popliteal vein within the popliteal fossa.

B. Deep veins of the lower limb follow the arterial pattern of the leg leading finally to the **femoral vein.**

C. Communicating venous system is a network of **perforating veins** that penetrate the deep fascia and connect the superficial veins (contain valves) with the deep veins. This allows flow of blood only from the **superficial veins → deep veins** and enables muscular contractions to propel blood toward the heart against gravity. Incompetent valves allow backflow of blood into the superficial veins (superficial veins ← deep veins), causing dilation of the superficial veins leading to **varicose veins.**

D. Clinical Consideration. Deep venous thrombosis (DVT) is a blood clot (thrombus) within the deep veins of the lower limb (most commonly), which may lead to a pulmonary embolus. DVT is usually caused by venous stasis (e.g. prolonged immobilization, congestive heart failure, obesity), hypercoagulation (e.g. oral contraceptive use, pregnancy), or endothelial damage. The nidus of DVT is stagnant blood behind the cusp of a venous valve (i.e. the venous sinus). Treatment includes intravenous heparin for 5 to 7 days followed by sodium warfarin (Coumadin) for 3 months (Coumadin is contraindicated in pregnant women because it is teratogenic).

Cutaneous Nerves of the Lower Limb

A. Superior, middle, and inferior clunial nerves arise from the lumbar plexus (L1 through L3), sacral plexus (S1 through S3), and gluteal branches of the posterior femoral cutaneous nerves, respectively. They innervate the skin of the gluteal region.

B. Genitofemoral nerve arises from the lumbar plexus (L1 and L2) and innervates the skin of the lateral femoral triangle.

C. Iliohypogastric nerve arises from the lumbar plexus (L1) and innervates the skin over the superolateral quadrant of the buttock.

D. Lateral femoral cutaneous nerve arises from the lumbar plexus (L2 and L3) and innervates the skin on the anterior and lateral aspects of the thigh.

E. Posterior femoral cutaneous nerve arises from the sacral plexus (S1 through S3) and innervates the skin of the buttock, thigh, and calf.

F. Cutaneous branch of the obturator nerve arises from the obturator nerve (L2 through L4) and innervates the skin of the middle part of the medial thigh.

G. Cutaneous branch of the femoral nerve arises from the femoral nerve (L2 through L4) and innervates the skin of the anterior and medial thigh.

H. Posterior cutaneous nerve of the thigh arises from the sacral plexus (S1 through S3) and innervates the skin of the posterior thigh and popliteal fossa.

I. Saphenous nerve (travels with the great saphenous vein) arises from the femoral nerve in the femoral triangle and innervates the skin of the medial side of the leg and foot.

J. Lateral sural cutaneous nerve arises from the common fibular nerve (S1 and S2) in the popliteal fossa and innervates the skin on the posterolateral side of the leg.

K. Medial sural cutaneous nerve arises from the tibial nerve (S1 and S2) and innervates the skin of back of the leg and the lateral side of the ankle, heel, and foot.

L. Superficial fibular nerve arises from the common fibular nerve (L4 through S1) and innervates the anterolateral leg and dorsum of the foot (excluding the web between the big toe and second toe.

M. Deep fibular nerve arises from the common fibular nerve (L5) and innervates the skin of the web between the big toe and second toe.

N. Calcaneal nerves arise from the tibial nerve and sural nerve (S1 and S2) and innervate the skin of the heel.

O. Medial plantar nerve arises from the tibial nerve (L4 and L5) and innervates the skin of the medial sole of the foot and the medial three and a half toes.

P. Lateral plantar nerve arises from the tibial nerve (S1 and S2) and innervates the skin of the lateral sole of the foot and the lateral one and a half toes.

VI   Lumbosacral Plexus (Figures 21-2, 21-3). The components of the lumbosacral plexus include:

A. Rami are the L1 through L5 and S1 through S4 **ventral primary rami** of spinal nerves.

B. Divisions (anterior and posterior) are formed by rami dividing into anterior and posterior divisions.

C. Branches: The six major terminal branches are:
1. **Femoral nerve (L2 through L4)**
2. **Obturator nerve (L2 through L4)**
3. **Superior gluteal nerve (L4 through S1)**
4. **Inferior gluteal nerve (L5 through S2)**

5. **Common fibular nerve (L4 through S2)** divides into the:
   a. Superficial fibular nerve
   b. Deep fibular nerve
6. **Tibial nerve (L4 through S3):** The tibial nerve and common fibular nerve comprise the **sciatic nerve.**

D. **Clinical Considerations.** The most common condition affecting the lumbosacral plexus is the herniation of intervertebral disks.

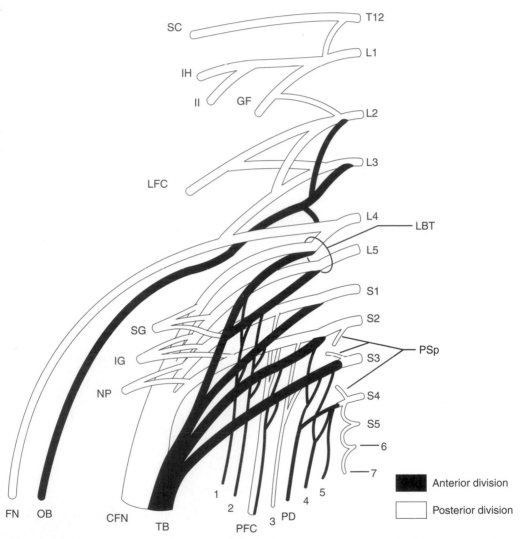

● **Figure 21-2 Lumbosacral Plexus.** Diagram of the lumbosacral plexus showing the rami, divisions, and six major terminal branches. The anterior divisions and branches are shown in black. CFN = common fibular nerve, FN = femoral nerve, GF = genitofemoral nerve, IG = inferior gluteal nerve, IH = iliohypogastric nerve, II = ilioinguinal nerve, LBT = lumbosacral trunk, LFC = lateral femoral cutaneous nerve, NP = nerve to piriformis, OB = obturator nerve, PD = pudendal nerve, PFC = posterior femoral cutaneous nerve, PSp = pelvic splanchnic nerves, SG = superior gluteal nerve, TB = tibial nerve, 1 = nerve to quadratus femoris and inferior gemellus muscles, 2 = nerve to obturator internus and superior gemellus muscles, 3 = perforating cutaneous nerve, 4 = nerve to levator ani and coccygeus muscles, 5 = perineal branch of S4 nerve, 6 = coccygeal nerve, 7 = anococcygeal nerve.

A

Psoas

Femoral nerve

Iliacus

Rectus femoris

Pectineus

Sartorius

Vastus lateralis

Vastus intermedius

Vastus medialis

Articular muscle
of knee

Obturator nerve

Obturator externus

Posterior branch

Anterior branch

Adductor brevis
Adductor longus

Adductor magnus

Gracilis

Common fibular nerve

Superficial fibular nerve

Fibularis (peroneus) longus

Fibularis (peroneus) brevis

Deep fibular nerve

Tibialis anterior

Extensor hallucis longus

Extensor digitorum longus

Fibularis (peroneus) tertius

Extensor digitorum brevis

Anterior View

B

Sciatic nerve

Semitendinosus

Biceps femoris
(long head)

Semitendinosus

Adductor magnus

Semimembranosus

Biceps femoris
(short head)

Tibial nerve

Gastrocnemius

Popliteus

Flexor digitorum
longus

Common fibular nerve

Plantaris

Gastrocnemius

Soleus

Tibialis posterior

Flexor hallucis longus

Medial plantar nerve

Abductor hallucis

Flexor digitorum brevis
Flexor hallucis brevis
Lumbrical to 2nd digit

Lateral plantar nerve

All other muscles
in sole of foot

Posterior View

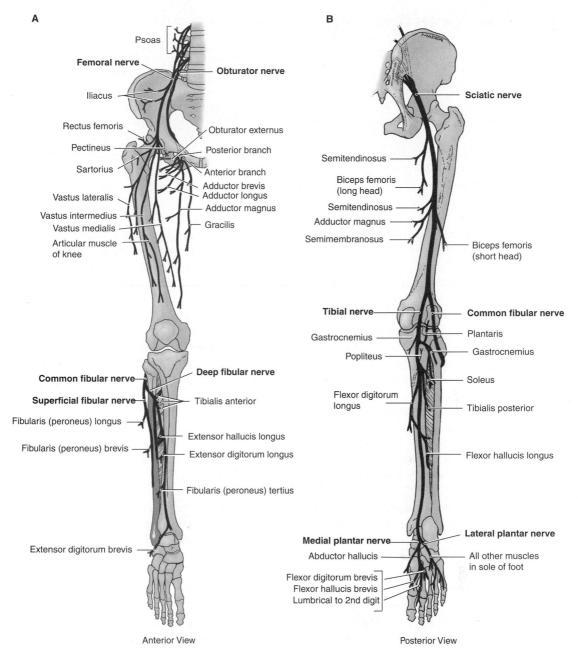

● **Figure 21-3 Innervation of the Lower Limb Muscles. (A) Anterior View.** Femoral nerve, obturator nerve, common fibular nerve, and deep fibular nerve and their branches are shown. **(B) Posterior View.** Sciatic nerve, tibial nerve, common fibular nerve, medial plantar nerve, and lateral plantar nerve and their branches are shown.

VII ## Nerve Lesions (Table 21-1)

A. Femoral nerve injury may be caused by trauma at the femoral triangle or pelvic fracture. Paralysis of the iliacus and sartorius muscles occurs so that flexion of the thigh is weakened. Paralysis of the quadriceps femoris muscles occurs so that extension of the leg is lost (i.e. loss of knee jerk reflex). Sensory loss occurs on the anterior aspect of the thigh and medial aspect of the leg.

B. Obturator nerve injury may be caused by an anterior dislocation of the hip or a radical retropubic prostatectomy. Paralysis of a portion of the adductor magnus, adductor longus, and adductor brevis muscles occurs so that adduction of the thigh is lost. Sensory loss occurs on the medial aspect of the thigh.

C. Superior gluteal nerve injury may be caused by surgery, posterior dislocation of the hip, or poliomyelitis. Paralysis of gluteus medius and gluteus minimus muscles occurs so that the ability to pull the pelvis down and abduction of the thigh is lost. Clinically, this condition is called "**gluteus medius limp,**" or "**waddling gait.**" The patient will demonstrate a **positive Trendelenburg sign**, which is tested as follows: The patient stands with his or her back to the examiner and alternately raises each foot off the ground. If the superior gluteal nerve on the <u>left</u> side is injured, then when the patient raises the right foot off the ground, the <u>right</u> pelvis will fall downward. Note that it is the side <u>contralateral</u> to the nerve injury that is affected. A Trendelenburg sign can also be observed in a patient with a hip dislocation or fracture of the neck of the femur.

D. Inferior gluteal nerve injury may be caused by surgery or posterior dislocation of the hip. Paralysis of the gluteus maximus muscle occurs so that the ability to rise from a seated position, climb stairs, or jump is lost. Clinically, the patient will be able to walk. However, the patient will lean the body trunk backward at heel strike to compensate for the loss of gluteus maximus function.

E. Common fibular nerve injury may be caused by a blow to the lateral aspect of the leg or fracture of the neck of the fibula. This is a very common type of injury. Paralysis of peroneus longus and peroneus brevis muscles (innervated by the superficial fibular nerve) occurs so that eversion of the foot is lost. Paralysis of tibialis anterior muscle (innervated by the deep fibular nerve) occurs so that dorsiflexion of the foot is lost. Paralysis of extensor digitorum longus and extensor hallucis longus muscles (innervated by the deep fibular nerve) occurs so that extension of the toes is lost. Sensory loss occurs on the anterolateral aspect of the leg and dorsum of the foot. Clinically, the patient will present with the **foot plantar flexed ("foot drop")** and **inverted.** Because of the loss of dorsiflexion, the **patient cannot stand on his or her heels.** The patient has a high-stepping gait in which the foot is raised higher than normal so that the toes do not hit the ground. In addition, the foot is brought down suddenly, which produces a "slapping" sound ("**foot slap**").

F. Tibial nerve injury (at the popliteal fossa) may be caused by trauma at the popliteal fossa. Paralysis of tibialis posterior muscle occurs so that inversion of the foot is weakened. Paralysis of the gastrocnemius, soleus, and plantaris muscles occurs so that plantar flexion of the foot is lost. Paralysis of the flexor digitorum longus and flexor hallucis longus muscles occurs so that flexion of the toes is lost. Sensory loss occurs on the sole of the foot. Clinically, the patient will present with the **foot dorsiflexed** and **everted.** Because of the loss of plantar flexion, the **patient cannot stand on his or her toes.**

TABLE 21-1	NERVE LESIONS		
Nerve Injury	**Injury Description**	**Impairments**	**Clinical Aspects**
Femoral nerve	Trauma at femoral triangle Pelvic fracture	Flexion of thigh is weakened Extension of leg is lost Sensory loss on anterior thigh and medial leg	Loss of knee jerk reflex Anesthesia on anterior thigh
Obturator nerve	Anterior hip dislocation Radical retropubic prostatectomy	Adduction of thigh is lost Sensory loss on medial thigh	
Superior gluteal nerve	Surgery Posterior hip dislocation	Gluteus medius and minimus function is lost	Gluteus medius limp or "waddling gait"
	Poliomyelitis	Ability to pull pelvis down and abduction of thigh are lost	Positive Trendelenburg sign Contralateral
Inferior gluteal nerve	Surgery Posterior hip dislocation	Gluteus maximus function is lost Ability to rise from a seated position, climb stairs, or jump is lost	Patient will lean the body trunk backward at heel strike
Common fibular nerve	Blow to lateral aspect of leg Fracture of neck of fibula	Eversion of foot is lost Dorsiflexion of foot is lost Extension of toes is lost Sensory loss on anterolateral leg and dorsum of foot	Patient will present with foot plantar flexed ("foot drop") and inverted Patient cannot stand on heels "Foot slap"
Tibial nerve at popliteal fossa	Trauma at popliteal fossa	Inversion of foot is weakened Plantar flexion of foot is lost Flexion of toes is lost Sensory loss on sole of foot	Patient will present with foot dorsiflexed and everted Patient cannot stand on toes

Hip and Gluteal Region (Figure 21-4). The piriformis muscle is the landmark of the gluteal region. The superior gluteal vessels and nerve emerge superior to the piriformis muscle, whereas the inferior gluteal vessels and nerve emerge inferior to it. Gluteal intramuscular injections can be safely made in the **superolateral portion** of the buttock.

A. **Hip joint** is the articulation of the head of the femur with the lunate surface of the acetabulum and the acetabular labrum. The hip joint is supported by the following ligaments:
   1. **Iliofemoral ligament (Y ligament of Bigelow)** is the largest ligament and reinforces the hip joint anteriorly.
   2. **Pubofemoral ligament** reinforces the hip joint inferiorly.
   3. **Ischiofemoral ligament** is the thinnest ligament and reinforces the hip joint posteriorly.
   4. **Ligamentum teres** plays only a minor role in stability but carries the **artery to the head of the femur.**

B. **Femoral Triangle.** The hip joint is related to the **femoral triangle,** whose boundaries are the inguinal ligament (superiorly), sartorius muscle (laterally), and the adductor longus muscle (medially). The floor of the femoral triangle is the pectineus and iliopsoas muscles. The roof of the femoral triangle is the fascia lata. The femoral triangle contains the following structures listed in a medial → lateral direction:
   1. **Femoral canal** (most medial structure) containing lymphatics and lymph nodes. The femoral canal is important clinically because this can be a path for herniation of abdominal contents. The femoral canal is within the femoral sheath.
   2. **Femoral vein.** The **great saphenous vein** joins the femoral vein within the femoral triangle just below and lateral to the pubic tubercle. This is an important site where a great saphenous vein cutdown can be performed. The femoral vein is within the femoral sheath.
   3. **Femoral artery.** The femoral artery is within the femoral sheath.
   4. **Femoral nerve** (most lateral structure). The femoral nerve is NOT within the femoral sheath.

C. **Clinical Considerations**
   1. **Acetabular fractures** most commonly occur in high-energy motor vehicle accidents or falls in which indirect forces are transmitted through the femoral head to the acetabulum. The acetabulum is nestled under an arch formed by the **anterior column** (iliopubic) and **posterior column** (ilioischial). Acetabular fractures may be simple or complex. Simplex fractures include fractures of the anterior rim of the acetabulum, posterior rim of the acetabulum, anterior column, posterior column, or transverse fractures through the acetabulum. Complex fractures are a combination of two or more simple fractures.
   2. **Posterior Dislocation of the Hip Joint.** The hip joint is most commonly dislocated in a posterior direction as a result of a severe trauma (e.g. car accident in which flexed knee hits the dashboard). The head of the femur comes to lie just posterior to the iliofemoral ligament, and the posterior rim of the acetabulum may also be fractured. The lower limb is **internally rotated, adducted,** and **shorter** than the normal limb. Avascular necrosis of the femoral head may occur if the medial and lateral circumflex arteries are compromised. In addition, the **sciatic nerve** may be damaged.
   3. **Anterior dislocations of the hip joint** account for the remainder of hip dislocations. The head of the femur comes to lie anterior to the iliofemoral ligament. The lower limb is **externally rotated** and **abducted.** The **femoral artery** may be damaged so that the lower limb may become cyanotic.

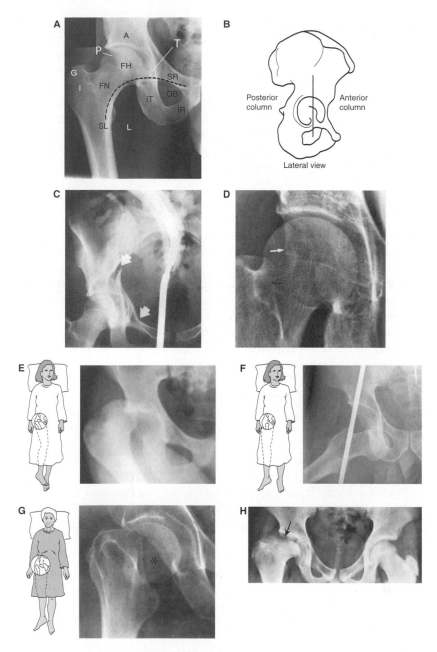

● **Figure 21-4 Hip. (A)** AP radiograph of the right hip region. FH = femoral head, FN = femoral neck, G = greater trochanter, IT = ischial tuberosity, IR = inferior ramus of the pubis, SR = superior ramus of the pubis, OB = obturator foramen, SL = Shenton's line (a radiology term describing a curved line drawn along the medial border of the femur and superior border of the obturator foramen), I = intertrochanteric crest, L = lesser trochanter, A = roof of the acetabulum, P = posterior rim of the acetabulum, T = "teardrop" appearance caused by the superimposition of structures at the inferior margin of the acetabulum. **(B–D) Acetabular Fractures. (B)** Diagram of the hip (coxal) bone showing the anterior column and posterior columns of the acetabulum. **(C)** AP radiograph shows an anterior column fracture of the acetabulum (arrows). **(D)** AP radiograph shows a posterior rim fracture of the acetabulum (arrow). **(E, F) Dislocation of Hip Joint. (E)** AP radiograph of a posterior dislocation of the hip joint. This type of dislocation is most common in car accidents whereby the lower limb is internally rotated, adducted, and shorter than the normal limb. **(F)** AP radiograph of an anterior dislocation of the hip joint. Note that the femoral head lies anterior to the obturator foramen. The lower limb is externally rotated and abducted. **(G) AP Radiograph of Femoral Neck Fracture (subcapital).** This type of fracture is most common is elderly women with osteoporosis whereby the lower limb is externally rotated and shorter than the normal limb. * = head of femur. **(H) AP Radiograph of Legg-Perthes Disease.** This 8-year-old boy complained of pain in the right hip and demonstrated a limp. Note that the femoral head on right side (arrow) is almost completely absent. Compare with normal femoral head on the left side.

4. **Femoral neck fracture** most commonly occurs in elderly women with osteoporosis just distal to the femoral head (i.e. subcapital location). The lower limb is **externally rotated** and **shorter** than the normal limb. Avascular necrosis of the femoral head may occur if the medial and lateral circumflex arteries are compromised.

5. **Legg-Perthes disease** is an idiopathic avascular necrosis of the head of the femur that possibly occurs when the medial and lateral circumflex arteries gradually replace the artery to the head of the femur as the main blood supply to the head of the femur. This disease most commonly occurs unilaterally in white boys who present with hip pain, slight external rotation, and a limp. This disease has three major phases: **initial phase**, **degenerative phase**, and **regenerative phase**.

IX Knee Region (Figure 21–5)

A. **Knee (femorotibial) joint** is the articulation of the medial and lateral condyles of the femur with the medial and lateral condyles of the tibia. The knee joint is supported by the following ligaments:

1. **Patellar ligament** is struck to elicit the knee jerk reflex. The reflex is blocked by damage to the femoral nerve, which supplies the quadriceps muscle, or damage to spinal cord segments L2 through L4.

2. **Medial (tibial) collateral ligament** extends from the medial epicondyle of the femur to the shaft of the tibia and prevents **abduction** at the knee joint. A torn medial collateral ligament can be recognized by abnormal passive abduction of the extended leg.

3. **Lateral (fibular) collateral ligament** extends from the lateral epicondyle of the femur to the head of the fibula and prevents **adduction** at the knee joint. A torn lateral collateral ligament can be recognized by the abnormal passive adduction of the extended leg.

4. **Anterior cruciate ligament** extends from the <u>anterior</u> aspect of the tibia to the lateral condyle of the femur and prevents <u>anterior</u> movement of the tibia in reference to the femur. A torn anterior cruciate ligament can be recognized by abnormal passive <u>anterior</u> displacement of the tibia called an **anterior drawer sign**. A **hyperextension injury** at the knee joint will stretch the anterior cruciate ligament.

5. **Posterior cruciate ligament** extends from the <u>posterior</u> aspect of the tibia to the medial condyle of the femur and prevents <u>posterior</u> movement of the tibia in reference to the femur. A torn posterior cruciate ligament can be recognized by abnormal passive <u>posterior</u> displacement of the tibia called a **posterior drawer sign**. A **hyperflexion injury** at the knee joint will stretch the posterior cruciate ligament.

B. The knee joints contain menisci, which include:

1. **Medial meniscus** is a C-shaped fibrocartilage that is attached to the medial collateral ligament and is easily torn because it is not very mobile.

2. **Lateral meniscus** is an O-shaped fibrocartilage. Lateral meniscus tears are most commonly associated with anterior cruciate ligament tears.

C. The knee joint is related to the popliteal fossa, which contains the following structures: **tibial nerve, common fibular nerve, popliteal artery, popliteal vein, and small saphenous vein.**

D. **Clinical Consideration. "The terrible triad of O'Donoghue"** is the result of fixation of a semiflexed leg receiving a violent blow on the lateral side (e.g. football "clip-

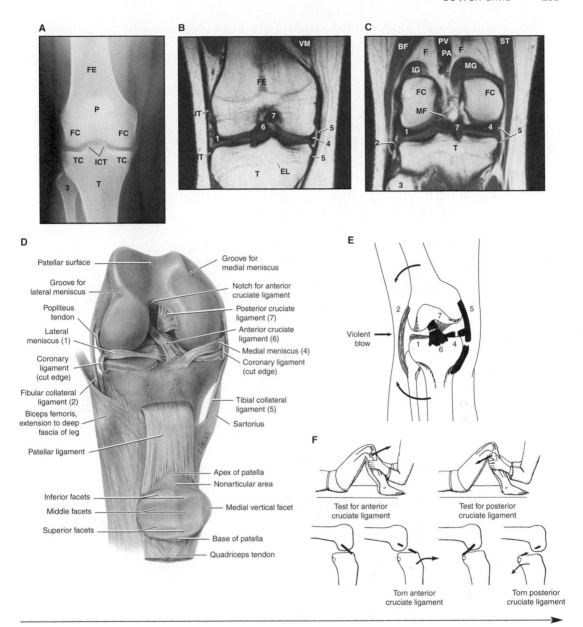

● **Figure 21-5 Knee Joint. (A)** AP radiograph of the right knee. **(B)** MRI (coronal section through the intercondylar notch). **(C)** MRI (coronal section through femoral condyles). **(D)** Diagram of the flexed knee joint with the patella reflected showing the articular surfaces and ligaments of the knee joint. **(E)** Schematic representation of the injured left knee (terrible triad) as a result of a violent blow to the lateral side of the knee (e.g. football "clipping"). The curved arrows indicate the direction of movement at the knee joint (abduction and lateral rotation). Note the torn anterior cruciate ligament (6), torn medial meniscus (4), and torn medial collateral ligament (5). **(F)** Diagram depicting the clinical tests for a torn anterior cruciate ligament (anterior drawer sign) and a torn posterior cruciate ligament (posterior drawer sign). BF = biceps femoris, EL = epiphyseal line, F = fat in popliteal fossa, FC = femoral condyle, FE = femur, ICT = intercondylar tubercles, IT = iliotibial tract, LG = lateral head of gastrocnemius, MF = meniscofemoral ligament, MG = medial head of gastrocnemius, P = patella, PA = popliteal artery, PV = popliteal vein, ST = semitendinosus, T = tibia, TC = tibial condyle, VM = vastus medialis muscle, 1 = lateral meniscus, 2 = lateral (fibular) collateral ligament, 3 = head of fibula, 4 = medial meniscus, 5 = medial (tibial) collateral ligament, 6 = anterior cruciate ligament, 7 = posterior cruciate ligament.

ping") causing abduction and lateral rotation that damages the following structures:

1. **Anterior cruciate ligament** is torn.
2. **Medial meniscus** is torn as a result of its attachment to the medial collateral ligament.
3. **Medial collateral ligament** is torn as a result of excessive abduction of the knee joint.

X   Ankle and Foot Region (Figure 21-6)

A. **Ankle (talocrural) joint** is the articulation of the inferior surface of the tibia with the trochlea of the talus where **dorsiflexion** and **plantar flexion** of the foot occur. The ankle joint is supported by the following ligaments:
   1. **Medial (deltoid) ligament** extends from the medial malleolus of the tibia to the talus, navicular, and calcaneus bones. The medial ligament consists of the **anterior tibiotalar ligament, posterior tibiotalar ligament, tibionavicular ligament**, and **tibiocalcaneal ligament**.
   2. **Lateral ligament** extends from the lateral malleolus of the fibula to the talus and calcaneus bones. The lateral ligament consists of the **anterior talofibular ligament, posterior talofibular ligament**, and **calcaneofibular ligament**.

B. The ankle joint contains the medial malleolus, which is related to the following structures:
   1. Anterior relationships include the **saphenous nerve** and **great saphenous vein** (an excellent location for a great saphenous vein cutdown).
   2. Posterior relationships include the **flexor hallucis longus tendon, flexor digitorum longus tendon, tibial posterior tendon, posterior tibial artery**, and **tibial nerve**.

C. **Subtalar joint** is the articulation of the talus and the calcaneus where **inversion** and **eversion** of the foot occur.

D. **Transverse tarsal joint (Chopart's joint)** is actually two joints: the **talonavicular joint** and the **calcaneocuboid joint**. It is the joint where **inversion** and **eversion** of the foot also occurs.

E. **Tarsometatarsal joint (Lisfranc's joint)** is the articulation of the tarsal bones with the metatarsals.

F. **Clinical Considerations (Figure 21-7)**
   1. **Inversion injury** (most common ankle injury) occurs when the foot is forcibly **inverted** and results in the following:
      a. Stretch or tear of the lateral ligament, most commonly the **anterior talofibular ligament**.
      b. Fracture of the fibula
      c. Avulsion of the tuberosity of the fifth metatarsal (called a **Jones fracture**), where the **peroneus brevis muscle** attaches (depending on the severity of the injury).
   2. **Eversion injury (Pott's fracture)** occurs when the foot is forcibly **everted** and results in the following:
      a. Avulsion of the medial malleolus (the medial ligament is so strong that instead of tearing it avulses the medial malleolus)
      b. Fracture of the fibula as a result of lateral movement of the talus.
   3. **Ski boot injury** usually results in fracture of the distal portions of the tibia and fibula.

4. **Calcaneal fracture (Lover's fracture)** occurs when a person jumps from a great height (e.g. from a second-story bedroom window, hence the name). A calcaneal fracture usually involves the **subtalar joint** and is usually associated with fractures of the **lumbar vertebrae** and **neck of the femur**.

5. **Lisfranc injury** occurs when bikers get their foot caught in the pedal clips or from high-energy trauma in a car accident. A Lisfranc injury results in fracture or dislocation at the tarsometatarsal joint (Lisfranc joint).

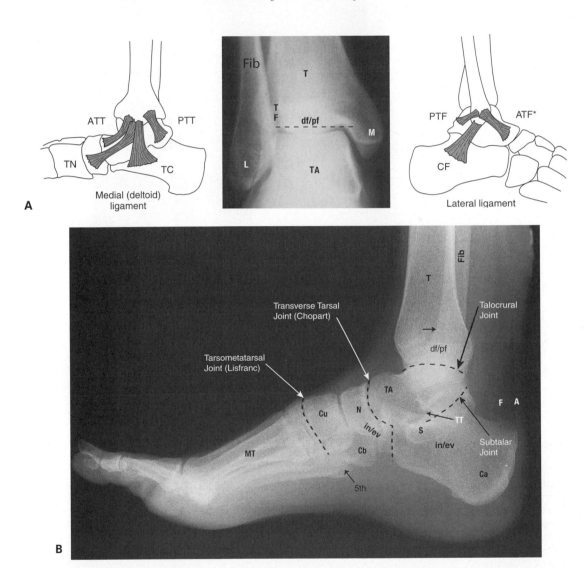

● **Figure 21-6 Ankle Joint. (A)** AP radiograph of the right ankle. The dotted line indicates the talocrural joint where dorsiflexion and plantar flexion (df/pf) occur. The diagrams show the components of the medial (deltoid) ligament and lateral ligament that provide support for the talocrural joint. The anterior talofibular ligament is most commonly injured in an ankle sprain (ATF*). **(B)** Lateral radiograph of the right ankle. The talocrural joint is shown where dorsiflexion and plantar flexion (df/pf) occur. The subtalar joint is shown where inversion and eversion (in/ev) occur. The transverse tarsal joint (Chopart joint) is shown where inversion and eversion (in/ev) also occur. The tarsometatarsal joint (Lisfranc joint) is also shown. A = Achilles tendon, ATF = anterior talofibular ligament, ATT = anterior tibiotalar ligament, Ca = calcaneus, Cb = cuboid, CF = calcaneofibular ligament, Cu = cuneiforms, F = fat, Fib = fibula, MT = metatarsals, N = navicular, PTF = posterior talofibular ligament, PTT = posterior tibiotalar ligament, S = sustentaculum tali, T = tibia, TA = talus, TC = tibiocalcaneal ligament, TN = tibionavicular ligament, TT = tarsal tunnel, 5th = fifth metatarsal (little toe), → = superimposed tibia and fibula, M = medial melleolus, L = lateral malleolus, TF = inferior tibiofibular joint.

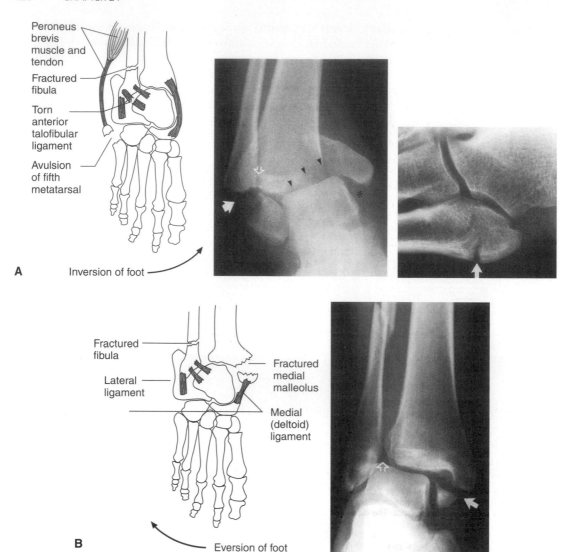

● **Figure 21-7 (A) Inversion Injury of the Right Ankle.** AP radiograph shows a bimalleolar fracture-dislocation caused by an inversion injury. The impaction force of the dislocated talus striking against the medial malleolus has resulted in an oblique fracture (arrowheads). The distance between the medial malleolus and the medial surface of the talus (asterisk) indicates that the deltoid ligament is disrupted. The force transmitted through the lateral collateral ligament has caused a fracture of the lateral malleolus (white arrow). The normal relationship between the proximal fibular fracture and tibia (open arrow) indicates that the distal tibiofibular ligaments and the interosseous membrane are intact. The lateral radiograph shows an avulsion fracture of the proximal fifth metatarsal (arrow; Jones fracture) as a result of the pull of the tendon of the peroneus brevis muscle. **(B) Eversion Injury of the Right Ankle.** AP radiograph shows an avulsion fracture of the medial malleolus (white arrow) and fracture of the fibula (black arrow). The presence of a fractured medial malleolus indicates that the medial (deltoid) ligament is intact. The widening of the tibiofibular joint (open arrow) indicates that the anterior and posterior distal tibiofibular ligaments are disrupted as well as the interosseous membrane.

XI   Cross-Sectional Anatomy of Right Thigh and Right Leg (Figure 21-8)

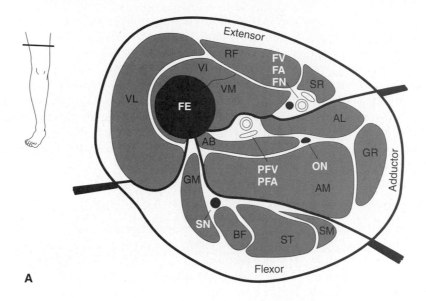

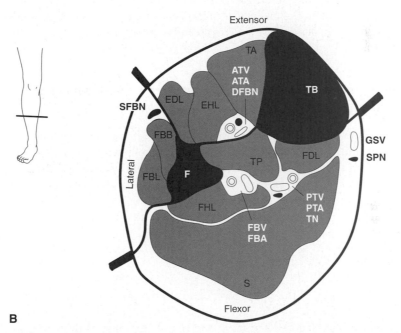

● **Figure 21-8 Thigh. (A)** A cross-section through the right thigh. Black lines divide the extensor (anterior) compartment, flexor (posterior) compartment, and adductor (medial) compartments. **(B)** A cross-section through the right leg. Black lines divide the extensor, flexor, and lateral compartments. AB = adductor brevis, AL = adductor longus, AM = adductor magnus, ATA = anterior tibial artery, ATV = anterior tibial vein, BF = biceps femoris, DFBN = deep fibular nerve, EDL = extensor digitorum longus, EHL = extensor hallucis longus, F = fibula, FA = femoral artery, FBA = fibular artery, FBB = fibularis brevis, FBL = fibularis longus, FBV = fibular vein, FDL = flexor digitorum longus, FE = femur bone, FHL = flexor hallucis longus, FN = femoral nerve, FV = femoral vein, GM = gluteus maximus, GR = gracilis, GSV = greater saphenous vein, ON = obturator nerve, PFA = profunda femoris artery, PFV = profunda femoris vein, PTA = posterior tibial artery, PTV = posterior tibial vein, RF = rectus femoris, S = soleus, SFBN = superficial fibular nerve, SM = semimembranosus, SN = sciatic nerve, SPN = saphenous nerve, SR = sartorius, ST = semitendinosus, TA = tibialis anterior, TB = tibia, TN = tibial nerve, TP = tibialis posterior, VI = vastus intermedius, VL = vastus lateralis, VM = vastus medialis.

Case Study 1

A young man who is 17 years old, 6' 5", and 270 pounds, with a promising football career, is blocked illegally from the side during the homecoming football game. His feet were firmly planted in the ground at the time he was struck by the other player. He lay on ground in pain with the knee deviated inward as a genu valgum. Attempts to move the knee were very painful, and his mother had to be called to keep him under control while being examined. He was eventually taken to the locker room, where the knee was immobilized and packed in ice. The orthopedic physician performed a Lachman stress test and during examination heard an audible click produced by the McMurray test. A visible bulge was noted over the injured knee. At the end of the physical evaluation, an MRI was ordered. After radiographic interpretation of the MRI, the physician then told the patient he was out of football for this year and he might want to hit the books because he might be out forever.

Explanation

The MRI showed that the medial meniscus, anterior cruciate ligament, and medial collateral ligament were all damaged. The history tells us the mechanism of the injury, which provides a great deal of information about the type and extent of possible injuries. In particular, information about the direction of the force and the position of his feet and legs at the time of the injury (feet firmly planted) suggest that the medial structures of the knee are the most likely to be damaged. The medial meniscus may be torn if the knee is suddenly twisted while it is flexed or if the knee receives a hard blow from the lateral side. A hard hit from the lateral side may also tear the anterior cruciate ligament and the medial (or tibial) collateral ligament. The patient's history can also tell us whether he or she may be suffering from a chronic degenerative problem.

Case Study 2

An 80-year-old man complains of severe right hip pain after an apparent slip and fall on his stairs at home leading to the basement. He heard a loud pop when he fell and could not support any weight on the injured leg after the fall. In the ER, it was noted that the right lower limb was shorter than the left, externally rotated, and very painful on passive motion test. A lateral pelvic radiograph showed a clean break between the head and neck of the right femur with the fragment still connected to the acetabulum and that the right greater trochanter was higher than the left.

Explanation

This patient is diagnosed with fracture of the right femur. The fracture occurred at the juncture of the head and neck of the right femur. The gluteus maximus, piriformis, obturator internus, superior and inferior gemelli, and quadratus femoris muscles externally rotate the distal fragment. The rectus femoris, adductor, and hamstring muscles draw the distal fragment proximal. Therefore, the lower limb presents as **externally rotated** and **shortened.**

Displaced femoral neck fractures, particularly in those who are advanced in age, are often treated with removal of the femoral head and neck and insertion of a femoral hip prosthesis. A total hip replacement, or hemiarthroplasty, would therefore be suggested for this patient.

Case Study 3

A 22-year-old man has localized swelling in the leg after being kicked very hard along the anterolateral side of the left leg during a soccer game. He attempted to keep playing, but soon had to retire because of pain. After he had showered and was beginning to dress in the locker room, he noticed that the color of his left foot was somewhat darkened. In the middle of the night of the same day, the pain was so severe that he had to go to the emergency room, where the emergency room physician noted that the anterolateral surface of the left leg was now swollen, very hard, and tender. The temperature of his left foot was noticeably less than that of his right, and the dorsalis pedis pulse was absent. The patient could not dorsiflex (i.e. extend) the toes of the left foot, and when attempting to walk, he dragged his left foot when swinging it forward (i.e. foot drop). Radiographs showed no fracture of any bone in the lower limb on either side. The physician advised him that surgical intervention was urgently needed.

Explanation

Although there was no fracture of the bone, the symptoms developed as a result of the trauma to the leg from the kick that was absorbed. This direct trauma resulted in hemorrhage and swelling inside the anterior compartment of the leg. This swelling increased pressure on the nerves, veins, and arteries inside the compartment. Without arterial circulation, muscle cells begin to die. Prolonged compression of the nerves destroys their ability to function properly. The initial numbness, severe pain, and tenderness were caused by increased pressure on the common fibular nerve. The eventual loss of dorsiflexion of the foot and the foot drop were also caused by increased pressure on the common fibular nerve. The darkened foot color and loss of dorsalis pedis pulse were caused by increased pressure on the anterior tibial artery.

This collection of symptoms is better described as anterior compartment syndrome. In the anterior compartment, the hemorrhage is from the anterior tibial artery.

Muscles and nerves can survive up to 4 hours of ischemia without irreversible damage. After 4 hours, nerves will show irreversible damage.

Compartment syndrome is treated with fasciotomy, which is used to relieve the symptoms. Two medial and lateral incisions are used to completely release all surrounding compartments. Skin incisions are left open to keep intracompartmental pressure low. Closure is performed 48 to 72 hours later. Depending on the stage of the patient's condition, debridement or amputation may be performed.

Chapter 22

Head and Neck

I **Skull.** The skull can be divided into two parts called the neurocranium and viscerocranium.

A. **Neurocranium.** The neurocranium consists of the flat bones of the skull (i.e. cranial vault) and the base of the skull, which together include the following eight bones: **frontal bone, occipital bone, ethmoid bone, sphenoid bone, paired parietal bones,** and **paired temporal bones.**

B. **Viscerocranium.** The viscerocranium consists of the bones of the face that develop from the pharyngeal arches in embryologic development, which include the following 14 bones: **mandible, vomer, paired lacrimal bones, paired nasal bones, paired palatine bones, paired inferior turbinate bones, paired maxillary bones,** and **paired zygomatic bones.**

C. **Sutures.** During fetal life and infancy, the flat bones of the skull are separated by dense connective tissue (fibrous joints) called **sutures.** There are five sutures: **frontal suture, sagittal suture, lambdoid suture, coronal suture,** and **squamous suture.** Sutures allow the flat bones of the skull to deform during childbirth (called **molding**) and to expand during childhood as the brain grows. Molding may exert considerable tension at the "obstetrical hinge" (junction of the squamous and lateral parts of the occipital bone) such that the **great cerebral vein (of Galen)** is ruptured during childbirth.

D. **Junctions of the sutures** include the following:
1. **Lambda** is the intersection of the lambdoid and sagittal sutures.
2. **Bregma** is the intersection of the sagittal and coronal sutures.
3. **Pterion** is a craniometric point at the intersection of the frontal bone, parietal bone, temporal bone, and greater wing of the sphenoid bone.
4. **Asterion** is a craniometric point at the intersection of the parietal bone, occipital bone, and mastoid part of the temporal bone.
5. **Nasion** is the intersection of the frontal bone and two nasal bones.
6. **Inion** is a craniometric point and the most prominent point of the external occipital protuberance.
7. **Vertex** is the superior point of the neurocranium.
8. **Glabella** is a smooth prominence on the frontal bones superior to the root of the nose.

E. **Fontanelles** are large fibrous areas where several sutures meet. There are six fontanelles: **anterior fontanelle, posterior fontanelle, two sphenoid fontanelles,** and **two mastoid fontanelles.** The anterior fontanelle is the largest fontanelle and readily palpable in the infant. It pulsates because of the underlying cerebral arteries and can be used to obtain a blood sample from the underlying **superior sagittal sinus**. The anterior fontanelle and the mastoid fontanelles close at about 2 years of age when the main growth of the brain ceases. The posterior fontanelle and the sphenoid fontanelles close at about 6 months of age.

F. **Foramina of the Skull (Figure 22-1).** The floor of the cranial cavity can be divided into the anterior cranial fossa, middle cranial fossa, and posterior cranial fossa, all of which contain foramina and fissures through which blood vessels and cranial nerves are transmitted. In addition, the **falx cerebri** and **tentorium cerebelli** divide the interior of the skull into compartments, which becomes clinically important when increased intracranial pressure in one compartment causes the brain to "herniate" or shift to a lower-pressure compartment.

G. **Clinical Considerations (Figure 22-2)**
  1. **Abnormalities in Skull Shape.** These may result from failure of cranial sutures to form or from premature closure of sutures (**craniosynostoses**).
     a. **Microcephaly** results from failure of the brain to grow; it is usually associated with mental retardation.
     b. **Oxycephaly (turricephaly or acrocephaly)** is a **towerlike skull** caused by premature closure of the **lambdoid and coronal sutures.** It should be differentiated from **Crouzon syndrome**, which is a dominant genetic condition with a presentation quite similar to that of oxycephaly but is accompanied by malformations of the face, teeth, and ears.
     c. **Plagiocephaly** is an asymmetric skull caused by premature closure of the **lambdoid and coronal sutures** on one side of the skull.
     d. **Brachycephaly** is a short, square-shaped skull caused by premature closure of the **coronal sutures.**
     e. **Scaphocephaly** is a long skull (in the anteroposterior plane) caused by premature closure of the **sagittal suture.**
     f. **Kleeblattschädel** is a cloverleaf skull caused by premature closure of **all sutures,** forcing brain growth through the anterior and sphenoid fontanelles.
     g. **Crouzon syndrome** is an autosomal dominant genetic disorder characterized by premature craniosynostosis, midface hypoplasia with shallow orbits, and ocular proptosis. This syndrome is caused by a mutation in the gene for fibroblast growth factor receptor 2 (*FGFR2*) located on chromosome 10q25–q26.
     h. **Apert syndrome** is an autosomal dominant genetic disorder characterized by craniosynostosis leading to turribrachycephaly; syndactyl of hands and feet; various ankyloses; progressive synostoses of the hands, feet, and cervical spine; and mental retardation. This syndrome is caused by a mutation in the gene for fibroblast growth factor receptor 2 (*FGFR2*) located on chromosome 10q25–q26, exclusively of paternal origin.
     i. **Pfeiffer syndrome** is an autosomal dominant genetic disorder characterized by craniosynostosis leading to turribrachycephaly, syndactyl of hands and feet, and broad thumbs and great toes. This syndrome is caused by a mutation in the gene for fibroblast growth factor receptor 2 (*FGFR2*) located on chromosome 10q25–q26.
  2. **Temporal Bone Formation**
     a. **Mastoid Process.** This portion of the temporal bone is absent at birth, which leaves the **facial nerve (cranial nerve [CN] VII)** relatively unprotected as it emerges from the stylomastoid foramen. In a difficult delivery, forceps may damage CN VII. The mastoid process forms by 2 years of age

b. **Petrosquamous Fissure.** The petrous and squamous portions of the temporal bone are separated by the petrosquamous fissure, which opens directly into the mastoid antrum of the middle ear. This fissure, which may remain open until 20 years of age, provides a route for the spread of infection from the middle ear to the meninges.

3. **Spheno-occipital joint** is a site of growth up to about 20 years of age.

4. **Transtentorial uncal herniation** is a very common brain herniation caused by increased intracranial pressure or tumor mass. It occurs when the parahippocampal gyrus and uncus of the cerebral hemisphere herniate from the supratentorial compartment through the tentorial incisure and into the infratentorial compartment. This results in stretching of CN III and compression of cerebral peduncles. Clinical signs include CN III paralysis with droopy upper eyelid as a result of paralysis of levator palpebrae muscle, eye "looks down and out" as a result of paralysis of superior rectus muscle, medial rectus muscle, inferior rectus muscle, and inferior oblique muscle and the unopposed action of the superior oblique muscle (CN IV) and lateral rectus muscle (CN VI); double vision (diplopia); fixed and dilated pupil as a result of paralysis of sphincter pupillae muscle; lack of accommodation (cycloplegia) as a result of paralysis of the ciliary muscle; and contralateral hemiparesis as a result of compression of the cerebral peduncles.

5. **Foramen magnum herniation (or Arnold-Chiari malformation)** is a congenital malformation and occurs when the cerebellar vermis, cerebellar tonsils, and medulla herniate through the foramen magnum along with cerebral aqueductal stenosis and breaking of the tectal plate. This results in stretching of CN IX, CN X, and CN XII and compression of the medulla. Clinical signs include spastic dysphonia, difficulty in swallowing, laryngeal stridor (vibrating sound heard during respiration as a result of obstructed airway), diminished gag reflex, apnea, vocal cord paralysis, and hydrocephalus as a result of aqueductal stenosis.

6. **LeFort I fracture** is a horizontal fracture of the maxillae bones that passes superior to the maxillary alveolar process (i.e. root of the teeth).

7. **LeFort II fracture** passes from the posterolateral parts of the maxillary sinus superomedially through the infraorbital foramina, lacrimal bones, and ethmoid bones to the bridge of the nose. This effectively separates the entire central part of the face from the rest of the cranium.

8. **LeFort III fracture** is a horizontal fracture that passes through the superior orbital fissures, ethmoid bones, and nasal bones to extend laterally through the greater wings of the sphenoid bone and the frontozygomatic sutures. If the zygomatic arches are concurrently fractured, this effectively separates the maxillae and zygomatic bones from the rest of the cranium.

9. **Fracture of the pterion** may result in a rupture of the anterior branches of the middle meningeal artery and result in a life-threatening epidural hemorrhage.

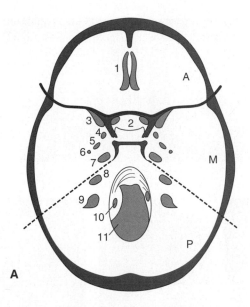

A

Foramen	Structures Transmitted
Anterior Cranial Fossa	
1. Cribriform plate	CN I; Discharge of CSF from the nose **(rhinorrhea)** will result from fracture of cribriform plate and dural tear
Foramen cecum	Emissary vein
Anterior and posterior Ethmoidal foramina	Anterior and posterior ethmoidal nerves and arteries
Middle Cranial Fossa	
2. Optic canal	CN II, ophthalmic artery, central artery and vein of retina
3. Superior orbital fissure	CN III, CN IV, CN V_1, CN VI, ophthalmic veins
4. Foramen rotundum	CN V_2
5. Foramen ovale	CN V_3, lesser petrosal nerve, accessory meningeal artery
6. Foramen spinosum	Middle meningeal artery; **epidural hemorrhage** will result from a fracture in this area
7. Foramen lacerum	Empty
Carotid canal	Internal carotid artery and sympathetic carotid plexus
Hiatus of facial canal	Greater petrosal nerve
Posterior Cranial Fossa	
8. Internal acoustic meatus	CN VII, CN VIII, labyrinthine artery; discharge of CSF from *external* acoustic meatus **(otorrhea)** will result from fracture of mastoid process and dural tear
9. Jugular foramen	CN IX, CN X, CN XI, sigmoid sinus; **mass in jugular foramen** will result in difficulty in swallowing (dysphagia) and speaking (dysarthria), uvula paralysis, and inability to shrug shoulders
10. Hypoglossal canal	CN XII
11. Foramen magnum	Medulla of the brainstem, CN XI, vertebral arteries
Condyloid foramen	Emissary vein
Mastoid foramen	Branch of occipital artery to the dura, emissary vein

CSF = cerebrospinal fluid.

B

● **Figure 22-1 Base of the Skull (Interior Aspect). (A)** The various foramina within the anterior (A), middle (M), and posterior (P) cranial fossae are numbered. In a clinical vignette question, first identify the clinical features mentioned in the question, then match the features with the appropriate structures transmitted and foramen and finally identify the foramen in the figure. Common clinical situations are indicated (e.g. rhinorrhea, epidural hemorrhage, otorrhea, and mass in jugular foramen). **(B)** Table foramen and structures.

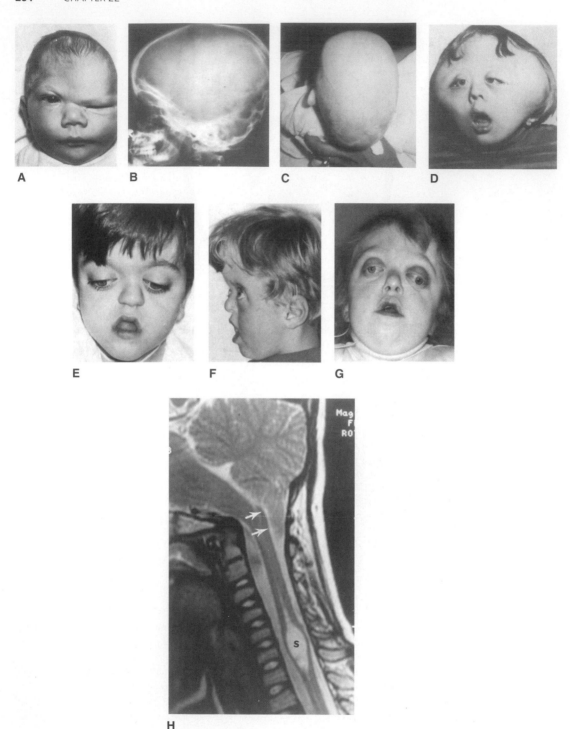

● **Figure 22-2 (A) Plagiocephaly. (B) Brachiocephaly. (C) Scaphocephaly. (D) Kleeblattschädel. (E) Crouzon Syndrome. (F) Apert Syndrome. (G) Pfeiffer Syndrome. (H) MRI of the Arnold-Chiari Malformation.** Note the herniation of the brainstem and cerebellum (arrows) through the foramen magnum. Note the presence of a syrinx (S) in the cervical spinal cord.

II **Scalp.** The scalp is composed of five layers. The first three layers constitute the **scalp proper**, which moves as a unit. The five layers include the following:

A. **Skin.** The thin skin has many sweat glands, sebaceous glands, and hair follicles.

B. **Connective Tissue.** The connective tissue forms a thick, vascularized subcutaneous layer.

C. **Aponeurosis.** The aponeurosis is a broad, strong tendinous sheet that covers the calvaria and serves as the attachment for the occipitofrontalis muscle, temporoparietalis muscle, and superior auricular muscle. These structures collectively constitute the musculoaponeurotic **epicranius**.

D. **Loose Areolar Tissue.** The loose areolar tissue allows free movement of the scalp proper over the cranium.

E. **Pericranium.** The pericranium forms the **periosteum** of the neurocranium.

III **Meninges**

A. **Dura Mater.** The cranial dura mater is a two-layered membrane consisting of the **external periosteal layer** (i.e. the **endosteum** of the neurocranium) and the **internal meningeal layer**, which is continuous with the dura of the vertebral canal and forms dural infoldings or reflections that divide the cranial cavity into compartments.
  1. **Dural Infolding or Reflections**
     a. **Falx cerebri** extends between the cerebral hemispheres and contains the **inferior sagittal sinus** and **superior sagittal sinus**.
     b. **Falx cerebelli** extends between the cerebellar hemispheres.
     c. **Tentorium cerebelli** supports the occipital lobes of the cerebral hemispheres and covers the cerebellum. It encloses the **transverse sinus** and the **superior petrosal sinus**.
     d. **Diaphragma sellae** forms the roof of the sella turcica covering the hypophysis.
  2. **Vasculature of the Dura.** The arterial supply of the dura mater is by the **middle meningeal artery** (a branch of the maxillary artery), which branches into an anterior branch and posterior branch. The venous drainage of the dura mater is by the **middle meningeal veins**, which drain into the **pterygoid plexus**.
  3. **Innervation of the Dura.** The innervation of the dura mater is by meningeal branches from CN V_1, CN V_2, and CN V_3, and sensory nerve fibers that travel with CN X and CN XII.

B. **Arachnoid.** The arachnoid is a filmy, transparent layer that is connected to the pia mater by **arachnoid trabeculae**. The arachnoid is separated from the pia mater by the **subarachnoid space**, which contains cerebrospinal fluid (CSF) and enlarges at several locations to form **subarachnoid cisterns**. The arachnoid projects **arachnoid villi** (collections of which are called **arachnoid granulations**) into the cranial venous sinuses, which serve as sites where CSF diffuses into the venous blood.

C. **Pia Mater.** The pia mater is a shiny, delicate layer that is closely applied to the brain and follows all the contours of the brain. The cerebral arteries that run in the subarachnoid space penetrate the pia mater as they enter the brain, whereby the pia mater is reflected onto the surface of the cerebral artery continuous with the tunica adventitia.

D. Clinical Considerations

1. **Headaches.** The dura mater is sensitive to pain. If the dura is irritated or stretched (e.g. after a lumbar puncture to remove CSF), a headache results where pain is referred to regions supplied by CN V.

2. **Bacterial Meningitis.** Meningitis is inflammation of the pia-arachnoid area of the brain, spinal cord, or both. Bacterial meningitis is caused by group B streptococci (e.g. *Streptococcus agalactiae*), *Escherichia coli,* and *Listeria monocytogenes* in newborns (<1 month); *Streptococcus pneumoniae* in older infants and young children (1 to 23 months); *Neisseria meningitidis* in young adults (2 to 18 years); and *S. pneumoniae* in older adults (19 years and older). CSF findings include numerous neutrophils, decreased glucose levels, and increased protein levels. Clinical findings include fever, headache, nuchal rigidity, and Kernig sign.

3. **Viral Meningitis (aseptic meningitis).** Viral meningitis is caused by mumps, echovirus, coxsackie virus, Epstein-Barr virus, and herpes simplex type 2. CSF findings include numerous lymphocytes, normal glucose levels, and moderately increased protein levels. Clinical findings include fever, headache, nuchal rigidity, and Kernig sign.

IV   Muscles of the Head and Neck

A. Muscles of the face and scalp include the occipitofrontalis, orbicularis oculi, corrugator supercilii, procerus, levator labii superioris alaeque nasi, orbicularis oris, levator labii superioris, zygomaticus minor, buccinator, zygomaticus major, levator anguli oris, risorius, depressor anguli oris, depressor labii inferioris, mentalis, and platysma. All these muscles are innervated by CN VII.

B. Muscles of mastication include the temporal, masseter, lateral pterygoid, and medial pterygoid.

C. Muscles of the soft palate include the tensor veli palatini, levator veli palatini, palatoglossus, palatopharyngeus, and musculus uvulae.

D. Muscles of the tongue include the genioglossus, hyoglossus, styloglossus, and palatoglossus.

E. Muscles of the superficial neck include the platysma, sternocleidomastoid, and trapezius.

F. Muscles of the anterior cervical region include the mylohyoid, geniohyoid, stylohyoid, digastric, sternohyoid, omohyoid, sternothyroid, and thyrohyoid.

G. Muscles of the prevertebral area include the longus colli, longus capitis, rectus capitis anterior, anterior scalene, rectus capitis lateralis, splenius capitis, levator scapulae, middle scalene, and posterior scalene.

H. Muscles of the larynx include the cricothyroid, thyroarytenoid, posterior cricoarytenoid, lateral cricoarytenoid, transverse and oblique arytenoids, and vocalis.

I. Muscles of the pharynx include the superior constrictor, middle constrictor, inferior constrictor, palatopharyngeus, salpingopharyngeus, and stylopharyngeus.

Ⓥ Arterial Supply (Figures 22-3, 22-5)

A. Branches of the Arch of the Aorta (see Chapter 5 and Figure 5-8)
   1. Brachiocephalic artery
      a. Right subclavian artery, which gives rise to the right vertebral artery
      b. Right common carotid artery
   2. Left common carotid artery
   3. Left subclavian artery, which gives rise to the left vertebral artery

B. External carotid artery (Figure 22-3) has eight branches in the neck, the more important of which include the **superior thyroid artery, lingual artery, facial artery, occipital artery, maxillary artery,** and **superficial temporal artery.** The maxillary artery enters the infratemporal fossa by passing posterior to the neck of the mandible and branches into the:
   1. **Middle meningeal artery,** which supplies the periosteal **dura mater** in the cranium. Skull fractures in the area of the **pterion** (junction of the parietal, frontal, temporal, and sphenoid bones) may sever the middle meningeal artery, resulting in an **epidural hemorrhage.**
   2. **Inferior alveolar artery**

C. Internal carotid artery (Figure 22-4, 22-5) has no branches in the neck and forms the anterior circulation of the circle of Willis. The internal carotid artery has a number of important branches, which include:
   1. **Ophthalmic artery** enters the orbit with the optic nerve (CN II) and branches into the **central artery of the retina.** Occlusion results in **monocular blindness.**
   2. **Anterior cerebral artery (ACA)** supplies the motor cortex and sensory cortex for the leg. Occlusion results in **contralateral paralysis and contralateral anesthesia of the leg.**
   3. **Middle Cerebral Artery (MCA).** Occlusion of the main stem of the MCA results in **contralateral hemiplegia, contralateral hemianesthesia, homonymous hemianopia,** and **aphasia** if the dominant hemisphere is involved.
      a. **Outer cortical branches** supply the motor cortex and sensory cortex for the face and arm. Occlusion results in **contralateral paralysis and contralateral anesthesia of the face and arm.**
      b. **Lenticulostriate arteries (deep branches or lateral striate)** supply the basal ganglia and the internal capsule. Occlusion results in the **classic "paralytic stroke"** with primarily a **contralateral hemiplegia** caused by destruction of descending motor fibers in the posterior limb of the internal capsule; **contralateral hemianesthesia** may occur if ascending sensory thalamocortical fibers in the internal capsule are also destroyed. The lenticulostriate arteries are prone to **hemorrhagic infarction** as a result of hypertension or atherosclerotic occlusion. Because these arteries branch at right angles, they are not likely sites for an embolus to lodge causing an embolic infarction.
   4. **Anterior communicating artery** connects the two anterior cerebral arteries. It is the most common site of an **aneurysm** (e.g. congenital berry aneurysm), the rupture of which will result in a **subarachnoid hemorrhage** and possibly **bitemporal lower quadrantanopia** because of its close proximity to the optic chiasm.
   5. **Posterior communicating artery** connects the anterior circulation of the circle of Willis with the posterior circulation of the circle of Willis. It is the second most common site of an **aneurysm** (e.g. congenital berry aneurysm), the rupture of which will result in a **subarachnoid hemorrhage** and possibly **oculomotor nerve**

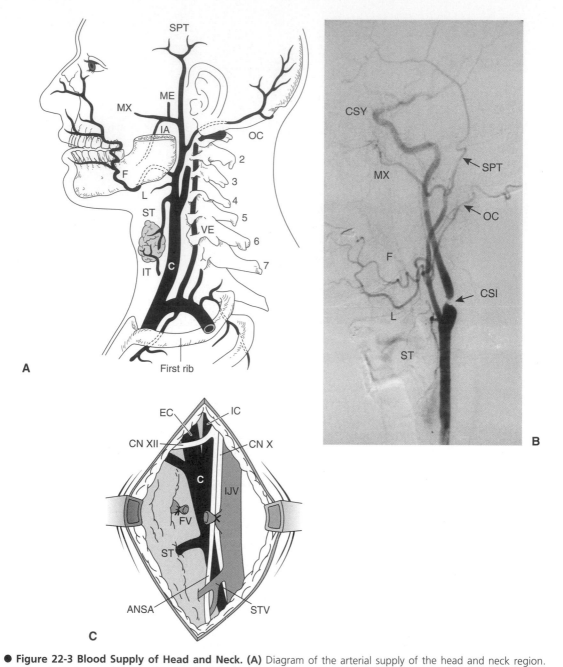

● **Figure 22-3 Blood Supply of Head and Neck. (A)** Diagram of the arterial supply of the head and neck region. **(B)** Lateral arteriogram (digital subtraction) of the head and neck region with a blocked internal carotid artery (arrow). The most common location of atherosclerosis in the carotid artery system is at the **bifurcation of the common carotid artery.** Carotid artery plaques are usually ulcerated plaques. **(C)** Diagram of the surgical exposure used in a carotid endarterectomy within the anterior (carotid) triangle of the neck. Note the anatomic structures in this area that may be put in jeopardy during this procedure. In this procedure, the incision is made along the anterior border of the sternocleidomastoid muscle, and the facial vein is ligated and cut to better expose the carotid bifurcation. **Carotid endarterectomy** is a surgical procedure to remove blockages of the internal carotid artery. This procedure can reduce the risk of stroke in patients who have emboli or plaques that cause **transient monocular blindness (amaurosis fugax).** Transient monocular blindness is the classic ocular symptom of a **transient ischemic attack (TIA)** that should not be ignored because it involves emboli to the **central artery of the retina,** a terminal branch of the internal carotid artery (internal carotid artery → ophthalmic artery → central artery of retina). **Hollenhorst cholesterol plaques** are observed during a retinal examination. Contralateral hemiplegia and contralateral hemianesthesia may also occur as a result of insufficient blood flow to the middle cerebral artery. ANSA = nerves of the ansa cervicalis, C = common carotid artery, CN X = vagus nerve, CN XII = hypoglossal nerve, CSI = carotid sinus, CSY = carotid siphon, EC = external carotid artery, F = facial artery, FV = facial vein (cut), IA = inferior alveolar artery, IC = internal carotid artery, IJV = internal jugular vein, IT = inferior thyroid artery, L = lingual artery, ME = middle meningeal artery, MX = maxillary artery, OC = occipital artery, SPT = superficial temporal artery, ST = superior thyroid artery, STV = superior thyroid vein, VE = vertebral artery.

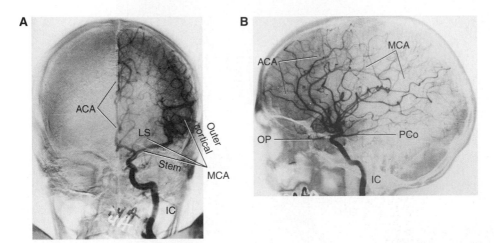

Occluded Artery	Neurologic Deficit of Stroke
Ophthalmic	Monocular blindness (transient)
ACA	Contralateral paralysis and contralateral anesthesia of leg
MCA	
At stem	Contralateral hemiplegia, contralateral hemianesthesia, homonymous hemianopia, and aphasia
Lenticulostriate	Classic "paralytic stroke" Contralateral hemiplegia, possibly contralateral hemianesthesia
Outer cortical	Contralateral paralysis and contralateral anesthesia of face and arm
PCA	Contralateral sensory loss of all modalities with concomitant severe pain (i.e., thalamic syndrome of Dejerine and Roussy) Homonymous hemianopia with macular sparing

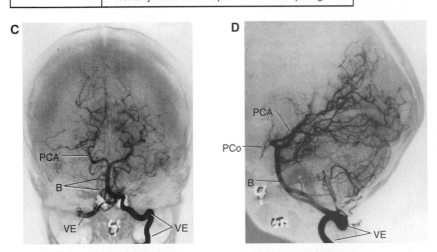

● **Figure 22-4 Blood Supply to Brain. (A)** AP arteriogram (digital subtraction) of the internal carotid artery. **(B)** Lateral arteriogram (digital subtraction) of the internal carotid artery. **(C)** AP arteriogram (digital subtraction) of the vertebral artery. **(D)** Lateral arteriogram (digital subtraction) of the vertebral artery. **(E)** CT scan shows a large left middle cerebral artery (MCA) territory stroke with edema and mass effect. No visible hemorrhage is apparent because most strokes are caused by thrombosis or embolism. 1 = ischemic brain parenchyma, 2 = midline shift to the right, 3 = right frontal horn of the lateral ventricle. **Cerebrovascular disorders ("strokes")** are most commonly cerebral infarcts caused by occlusion of cerebral vessels by thrombosis or embolism, not by hemorrhage. Strokes are characterized by a relatively abrupt onset of a focal neurologic deficit. The appropriate way to use this figure is to identify the neurologic deficit of stroke in the clinical vignette question on the USMLE, match the deficit to the occluded artery in the table, and then identify that artery on the arteriogram. ACA = anterior cerebral artery, B = basilar artery, IC = internal carotid artery, LS = lenticulostriate arteries of MCA, OP = ophthalmic artery, PCA = posterior cerebral artery, PCo = posterior communicating artery, VE = vertebral artery, MCA = middle cerebral artery (stem and outer cortical branches).

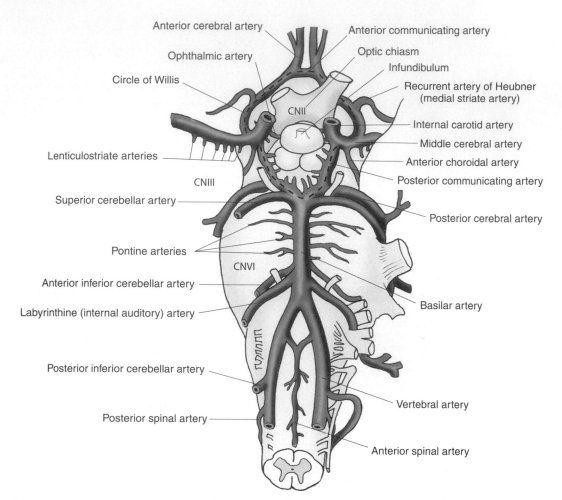

● **Figure 22-5 Internal Carotid Artery and Vertebrobasilar System.** The basilar artery is formed by the confluence of the two vertebral arteries. Note the cerebral arterial circle (circle of Willis; marked by the thick dashed black line). Note the close relationship of CN II, CN III, and CN VI to the vasculature.

(CN III) paralysis (droopy upper eyelid, eye "looks down and out," diplopia, fixed and dilated pupil, and lack of accommodation).

D. The **right vertebral artery** (a branch of the right subclavian artery) and the **left vertebral artery** (a branch of the left subclavian artery) both pass through the transverse foramina of C1 through C6 vertebrae (and foramen magnum) and form the posterior circulation of the circle of Willis.

1. The **basilar artery** is formed by the union of the right and left vertebral arteries. The basilar artery gives off a number of branches that includes the posterior cerebral artery (PCA).
2. The **posterior cerebral artery (PCA)** supplies the midbrain, thalamus, and occipital lobe with the visual cortex. Occlusion results in **contralateral sensory loss of all modalities with concomitant severe pain** (i.e. **thalamic syndrome of Dejerine and Roussy**) as a result of damage to the thalamus and **contralateral hemianopia with macular sparing**.

VI Venous Drainage (Figure 22-6)

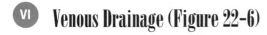

A. Facial and Scalp Areas

1. The **facial vein** (no valves) provides the major venous drainage of the face and drains into the **internal jugular vein**. The facial vein makes clinically important connections with the **cavernous sinus** via the **superior ophthalmic vein, inferior ophthalmic vein,** and **pterygoid plexus of veins**. This connection with the cavernous sinus provides a potential route of infection from the superficial face ("**danger zone of the face**") to the dural venous sinuses within the cranium.
2. **Diploic veins** (no valves) run within the flat bones of the skull.
3. **Emissary veins** (no valves) form an anastomosis between the superficial veins on the outside of the skull and the dural venous sinuses.

B. Dural venous sinuses (no valves) form between the external periosteal layer and the internal meningeal layer of the dura mater. The dural venous sinuses consist of the following:

1. **Superior sagittal sinus** is located along the superior aspect of the falx cerebri. **Arachnoid granulations**, which transmit cerebrospinal fluid (CSF) from the subarachnoid space to the dural venous sinuses, protrude into its wall.
2. **Inferior sagittal sinus** is located along the inferior aspect (free edge) of the falx cerebri.
3. **Straight sinus** is formed by the union of the inferior sagittal sinus and the **great vein of Galen** (drains venous blood from deep areas of the brain).
4. **Occipital sinus** is located in the attached border of the tentorium cerebelli.
5. **Confluence of sinuses** is formed by the union of the superior sagittal sinus, straight sinus, and occipital sinus.
6. **Transverse sinus** drains venous blood from the confluence of sinuses to the sigmoid sinus.
7. **Sigmoid sinus** drains into the internal jugular vein.
8. **Cavernous sinuses** are located on either side of the sphenoid bone and receive venous blood from the facial vein, superior ophthalmic vein, inferior ophthalmic vein, pterygoid plexus of veins, central vein of the retina, and each other via the **intercavernous sinuses** that pass anterior and posterior to the hypophyseal stalk. They drain venous blood into the superior petrosal sinus → transverse sinus and the inferior petrosal sinus → internal jugular vein. They are anatomically related

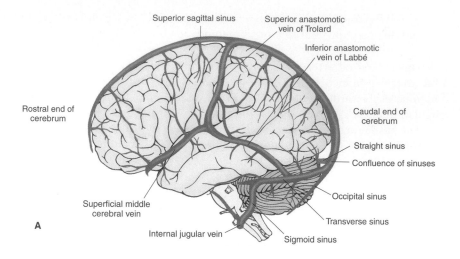

A

Superior sagittal sinus

Superior anastomotic vein of Trolard

Inferior anastomotic vein of Labbé

Rostral end of cerebrum

Caudal end of cerebrum

Straight sinus

Confluence of sinuses

Occipital sinus

Transverse sinus

Sigmoid sinus

Superficial middle cerebral vein

Internal jugular vein

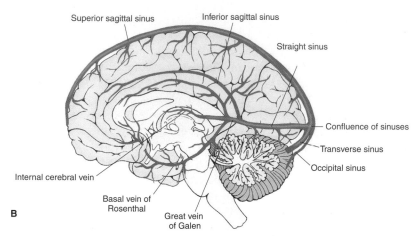

B

Superior sagittal sinus

Inferior sagittal sinus

Straight sinus

Confluence of sinuses

Transverse sinus

Occipital sinus

Internal cerebral vein

Basal vein of Rosenthal

Great vein of Galen

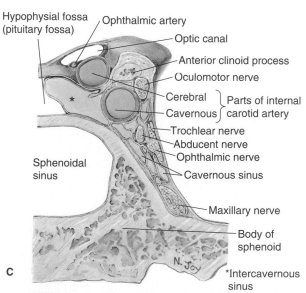

C

Hypophysial fossa (pituitary fossa)

Ophthalmic artery

Optic canal

Anterior clinoid process

Oculomotor nerve

Cerebral

Cavernous

Parts of internal carotid artery

Trochlear nerve

Abducent nerve

Ophthalmic nerve

Cavernous sinus

Maxillary nerve

Body of sphenoid

Sphenoidal sinus

N. Joy

*Intercavernous sinus

Posterior view of coronal section of right cavernous sinus

● **Figure 22-6 (A, B) Major Dural Sinuses and Veins. (C) Cavernous Sinus.** Coronal section.

to the **internal carotid artery** (carotid siphon), postganglionic sympathetic nerves, and CN III, CN IV, CN VI, CN V_1, and CN V_2. **The cavernous sinuses** are the most clinically significant sinuses. For example, in infections of the superficial face (see above), **thrombophlebitis** can result in poor drainage and enlargement involving CN III, CN IV, CN VI, CN V_1, and CN V_2, thereby producing ocular signs; infections can spread from one side to the other through the intercavernous sinuses; poor drainage may result in exophthalmus and edema of the eyelids and conjunctiva; and carotid artery–cavernous sinus fistula can result in a headache, orbital pain, diplopia, arterialization of the conjunctiva, and ocular bruit.

(VII) Clinical Consideration. Hemorrhages (Figure 22-7) within the head area include **epidural hemorrhage**, **subdural hemorrhage**, **subarachnoid hemorrhage**, and **extracranial hemorrhage**.

(VIII) Cervical Plexus (Figure 22-8A). The cervical plexus is formed by the ventral primary rami of C1 through C4 and has both sensory and motor branches.

A. **Sensory Nerves**
1. **Lesser occipital nerve** ascends along the sternocleidomastoid muscle and innervates the skin of the scalp behind the auricle.
2. **Great auricular nerve** ascends on the sternocleidomastoid muscle and innervates the skin behind the auricle and on the parotid gland.
3. **Transverse cervical nerve** turns around the posterior border of the sternocleidomastoid muscle and innervates the skin of the anterior cervical triangle.
4. **Supraclavicular nerve** emerges as a common trunk from under the sternocleidomastoid muscle and divides into the anterior branch, middle branch, and lateral branch to innervate the skin over the clavicle and the shoulder.

B. **Motor Nerves**
1. **Ansa cervicalis** is a nerve loop formed by the descendens hypoglossi (C1) and the descendens cervicalis (C2 and C3). The ansa cervicalis innervates the infrahyoid muscles (except the thyrohyoid).
2. **Phrenic nerve** is formed by C3, C4, and C5 cervical nerves and innervates the diaphragm (motor and sensory).

(IX) Cranial Nerves (Figure 22-8B, C)

(X) Cervical Triangles of the Neck (Figure 22-9)

A. **General Features.** The sternocleidomastoid muscle divides the neck into the **anterior triangle** and the **posterior triangle**, both of which are further subdivided into the **carotid triangle** and the **occipital triangle**, respectively. The carotid triangle and occipital triangle contain important anatomic structures as indicated in Figure 22-9.

B. **Clinical Considerations**
1. **Anterior (carotid) Triangle**
   a. The **platysma muscle** lies in the superficial fascia above the anterior triangle and is innervated by the **facial nerve**. Accidental damage during surgery of the facial nerve in this area can result in **distortion of the shape of the mouth**.

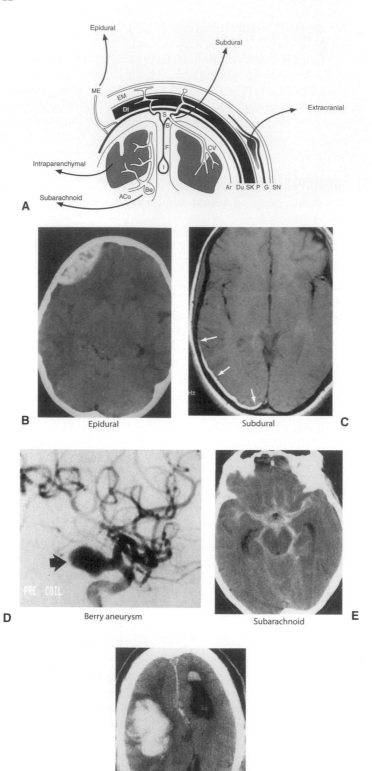

A

B Epidural

C Subdural

D Berry aneurysm

E Subarachnoid

F Intraparenchymal

EPIDURAL, EPIDURAL SUBDURAL, SUBARACHNOID, INTRAPARENCHYMAL, AND EXTRACRANIAL HEMORRHAGES

Hemorrhage	Injury	Blood Vessel	Clinical Features
Epidural (B)	Skull fracture near pterion or greater wing of sphenoid Middle cranial fossa A medical emergency	Middle meningeal artery	CT scan shows lens-shaped (biconvex) hyperdensity adjacent to bone; arterial blood located between skull and dura Lucid interval for a few hours followed by death ("talk and die syndrome") May cause a transtentorial herniation that compresses (1) CN III, causing ipsilateral dilated pupil, and (2) cerebral peduncles, causing contralateral hemiparesis No blood in the CSF after lumbar puncture
Subdural (C)	Violent shaking of head (e.g. child abuse or car accident) Common in alcoholics and elderly	Superior cerebral veins ("bridging veins")	CT scan shows a thin, crescent-shaped hyperdensity that hugs contours of brain; venous blood located between dura and arachnoid Blood accumulates slowly (days to weeks after trauma) No blood in CSF after lumbar puncture
Subarachnoid (D, E)	Contusion or laceration injury to brain Berry aneurysm	Cerebral artery Anterior or posterior communicating artery	CT scan shows hyperdensity in the cisterns, fissures, and sulci; thickening of falx cerebri; arterial blood within subarachnoid space Irritation of meninges causes sudden onset of the "worst headache of my life," stiff neck, nausea, vomiting and decreased mentation; earlier "herald headaches" may occur Blood within the CSF after lumbar puncture
Intraparenchymal (F)	Hemorrhage Trauma	Intraparenchymal cerebral artery	CT scan shows hyperdensity within the substance of the brain
Extracranial	Depressed cranial fracture Normal childbirth	Emissary veins Branches of superficial temporal and occipital arteries	Venous and arterial blood located between galea aponeurotica and skull (subaponeurotic space) Lumpy clot, "black eye" No blood in CSF after lumbar puncture

CSF = cerebrospinal fluid

● **Figure 22-7 Hemorrhages. (A)** Diagram depicting epidural, subdural, subarachnoid, intraparenchymal, and extracranial hemorrhages. EM = emissary vein, DI = diploic vein, ME = middle meningeal artery, ACo = anterior communicating artery (most common site for a berry aneurysm), Be = berry (congenital aneurysm), I = inferior sagittal sinus, S = superior sagittal sinus, B = bridging vein, CV = cerebral vein, F = falx cerebri, Ar = arachnoid, Du = dura mater. **(B)** Epidural hemorrhage. **(C)** Subdural hemorrhage, SN = skin, G = galea aponeurotica, SK = skull, P = periosteum. **(D)** Berry aneurysm. **(E)** Subarachnoid hemorrhage. **(F)** Intraparenchymal hemorrhage.

b. The **carotid pulse** is easily palpated at the anterior border of the sternocleido-mastoid muscle at the level of the superior border of the thyroid cartilage (C5).

c. The **bifurcation of the common carotid artery** into the internal carotid artery and external carotid artery occurs in the anterior triangle of the neck at the level of C4. At the bifurcation, the **carotid body** and **carotid sinus** can be found.

The carotid body is an **oxygen chemoreceptor.** Its sensory information is carried to the central nervous system by **CN IX** and **CN X.** The carotid sinus is a **pressure receptor.** Its sensory information is carried to the central nervous system by **CN IX** and **CN X.**

d. A **carotid enterectomy** is performed in the anterior (carotid) triangle.

e. **Internal Jugular Vein Catheterization.** The most commonly used approach is on the right side, above the level of the thyroid cartilage (C5; high approach) and medial to the sternocleidomastoid muscle within the anterior (carotid) triangle (see Figure 5-5).

f. **Stellate Ganglion Nerve Block.** The stellate ganglion is the lowest of the three ganglia of the cervical sympathetic trunk. The term "stellate ganglion nerve block" is not strictly correct because injection of anesthetic is made above the stellate ganglion and enough anesthetic is injected to spread up and down. The needle is inserted between the trachea medially and the sternocleidomastoid muscle and the common carotid artery laterally using the **cricoid cartilage (C6)** and the **transverse process of C6 vertebra** as landmarks. A successful block results in **vasodilation** of the blood vessels of the head, neck, and upper limb and **Horner's syndrome** in which **miosis** (constriction of the pupil because of paralysis of the dilator pupillae muscle), **ptosis** (drooping of the eyelid because of paralysis of superior tarsal muscle), and **hemianhydrosis** (loss of sweating on one side) occurs. A stellate ganglion nerve block is used in Raynaud's phenomenon and to relieve vasoconstriction after frostbite or microsurgery of the hand.

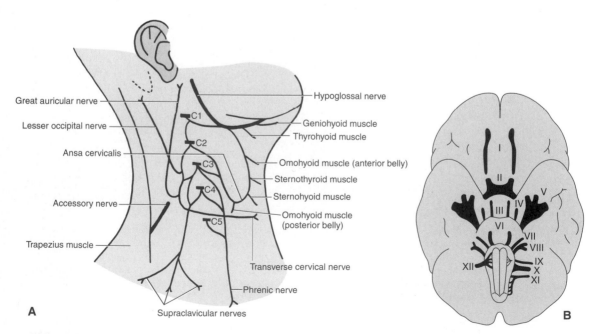

● **Figure 22-8 Cervical Plexus and Cranial Nerves. (A)** Cervical plexus. **(B)** Diagram of the base of the brain showing the location of the cranial nerves.

Cranial Nerve	Clinical Aspects
I Olfactory	Mediates the sense of smell (olfaction)
II Optic	Mediates the sense of sight (vision)
III Oculomotor	CN III lesion (e.g. **transtentorial [uncal] herniation)** results in droopy upper eyelid as a result of paralysis of levator palpebrae muscle; eye "looks down and out" as a result of paralysis of superior rectus muscle, medial rectus muscle, inferior rectus muscle, and inferior oblique muscle and the unopposed action of the superior oblique muscle (CN IV) and lateral rectus muscle (CN VI); double vision (diplopia) when patient looks in direction of paretic muscle; fixed and dilated pupil as a result of paralysis of sphincter pupillae muscle; lack of accommodation (cycloplegia) as a result of paralysis of the ciliary muscle; CN III lesions are associated with diabetes; an aneurysm of the posterior cerebral artery or superior cerebellar artery may exert pressure on CN III as it passes between these vessels
IV Trochlear	Innervates the superior oblique muscle CN IV lesion results in extortion of the eye, vertical diplopia that increases when looking down (e.g. reading a book), head tilting to compensate for extorsion
V Trigeminal	Provides sensory innervation to the face and motor innervation to the muscles of mastication CN V lesion results in hemianesthesia of the face, loss of afferent limb of corneal reflex, loss of afferent limb of oculocardiac reflex, paralysis of muscle of mastication, deviation of jaw to the injured side, hypoacusis as a result of paralysis of tensor tympani muscle, and tic douloureux (recurrent, stabbing pain)
VI Abducens	Innervates the lateral rectus muscle CN VI lesion results in convergent strabismus, inability to abduct the eye, horizontal diplopia when patient looks toward paretic muscle; an aneurysm of the labyrinthine artery or anterior inferior cerebellar artery may exert pressure on CN VI as it passes between these vessels
VII Facial	Provides motor innervation to the muscles of facial expression; mediates taste, salivation, and lacrimation CN VII lesion results in paralysis of muscle of facial expression (upper and lower face; called Bell's palsy), loss of efferent limb of corneal reflex, hyperacusis as a result of paralysis of stapedius muscle, and **crocodile tears syndrome** (tearing during eating) as a result of aberrant regeneration after trauma
VIII Vestibulocochlear	Mediates equilibrium and balance (vestibular) and hearing (cochlear) CN VIII (vestibular) lesion results in disequilibrium, vertigo, and nystagmus CN VIII (cochlear) lesion (e.g. **acoustic neuroma**) results in hearing loss and tinnitus
IX Glossopharyngeal	Mediates taste, salivation, swallowing, and input from the carotid sinus and carotid body CN IX lesion results in loss of afferent limb of gag reflex, loss of taste from posterior one third of tongue, loss of sensation from pharynx, tonsils, fauces, and back of tongue
X Vagus	Mediates speech and swallowing; innervates viscera in thorax and abdomen CN X lesion results in paralysis of pharynx and larynx, uvula deviates to **opposite side** of injured nerve, loss of efferent limb of gag reflex, and loss of efferent limb of oculocardiac reflex
XI Spinal Accessory	Innervates the sternocleidomastoid and trapezius muscle CN XI lesion results in inability to turn head to **opposite side** of injured nerve, inability to shrug shoulder
XII Hypoglossal	Innervates intrinsic and extrinsic muscles of the tongue CN XII lesion results in tongue deviation to the **same side** of injured nerve

C

● **Figure 22-8** (continued)   **(C)** Table of the clinical aspects of the cranial nerves. The appropriate way to use this figure and table is to identify the clinical aspect in the clinical vignette question on the USMLE, match the clinical aspect to the appropriate cranial nerve, and then identify the cranial nerve in the figure.

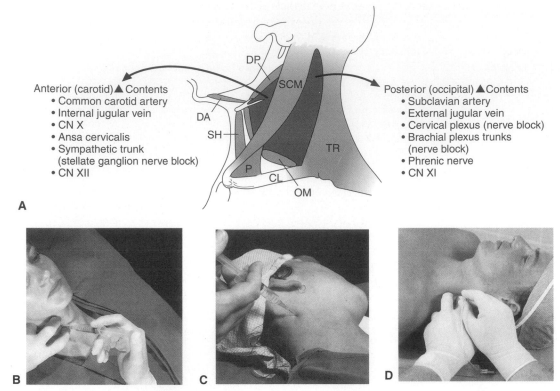

Anterior (carotid)▲Contents
- Common carotid artery
- Internal jugular vein
- CN X
- Ansa cervicalis
- Sympathetic trunk
  (stellate ganglion nerve block)
- CN XII

Posterior (occipital)▲Contents
- Subclavian artery
- External jugular vein
- Cervical plexus (nerve block)
- Brachial plexus trunks
  (nerve block)
- Phrenic nerve
- CN XI

● **Figure 22-9 Cervical Triangles and Nerve Blocks. (A)** Diagram of the lateral aspect of the neck showing the cervical triangles and their contents. Note that the common carotid artery, internal jugular vein, and CN X all lie within the **carotid sheath. (B–D)** Photographs of various nerve blocks are shown. **(B)** Stellate ganglion nerve block. **(C)** Cervical plexus nerve block. **(D)** Brachial plexus nerve block. CL = clavicle, DA = digastric muscle (anterior belly), DP = digastric muscle (posterior belly), OM = omohyoid muscle (inferior belly), P = platysma, SCM = sternocleidomastoid muscle, SH = sternohyoid muscle, TR = trapezius muscle.

2. **Posterior (occipital) Triangle**
    a. **Injury to CN XI** within the posterior (occipital) triangle as a result of surgery or a penetrating wound will cause paralysis of the **trapezius muscle** so that **abduction of the arm *past* the horizontal position** is compromised.
    b. **Injuries to the trunks of the brachial plexus,** which lie in the posterior (occipital) triangle, will result in **Erb-Duchenne** or **Klumpke** syndromes (see Chapter 20).
    c. **Severe upper limb hemorrhage** may be stopped by compressing the subclavian artery against the first rib by applying downward and posterior pressure. The brachial plexus and subclavian artery enter the posterior (occipital) triangle in an area bounded anteriorly by the **anterior scalene muscle,** posteriorly by the **middle scalene muscle,** and inferiorly by the **first rib.**
    d. **Enlarged supraclavicular lymph nodes** as a result of upper gastrointestinal or lung cancer may be palpated in the posterior (occipital) triangle.
    e. **Cervical Plexus Nerve Block.** The needle is inserted at **vertebral level C3** along a landmark line connecting the mastoid process to the transverse process of C6, and enough anesthetic is injected to spread up and down. A cervical plexus nerve block is used in superficial surgery on the neck or thyroid gland and pain management.

f.   **Brachial Plexus Nerve Block.** The needle is inserted at **vertebral level C6** into the interscalene groove (between the anterior and middle scalene muscles), using the cricoid cartilage (C6) and sternocleidomastoid muscle as landmarks.

XI Larynx (Figure 22-10)

A.   General Features. The larynx consists of five major cartilages, which include the **cricoid, thyroid, epiglottis,** and two **arytenoid** cartilages. The **ventricle** of the larynx is bounded superiorly by the **vestibular folds (false vocal cords)** and inferiorly by the **vocal folds (true vocal cords).** All intrinsic muscles of the larynx are innervated by the **inferior laryngeal nerve of CN X** (a continuation of the **recurrent laryngeal nerve**), except the **cricothyroid muscle**, which is innervated by the **external branch of the superior laryngeal nerve of CN X.** The intrinsic muscles of the larynx include the:

1.   **Posterior cricoarytenoid muscle** *abducts* the vocal folds and opens the airway during respiration. This is the *only* muscle that abducts the vocal folds.
2.   **Lateral cricoarytenoid muscle** adducts the vocal folds.
3.   **Arytenoideus muscle** adducts the vocal folds.
4.   **Thyroarytenoid muscle** relaxes the vocal folds.
5.   **Vocalis muscle** alters the vocal folds for speaking and singing.
6.   **Transverse and oblique arytenoid muscles** close the laryngeal aditus (sphincter function).
7.   **Cricothyroid muscle** stretches and tenses the vocal folds.

B.   Clinical Considerations

1.   **Unilateral damage to the recurrent laryngeal nerve** can result from dissection around the ligament of Berry or ligation of the inferior thyroid artery during thyroidectomy. It will result in a hoarse voice, inability to speak for long periods, and movement of the vocal fold on the affected side toward the midline.
2.   **Bilateral damage to the recurrent laryngeal nerve** can result from dissection around the ligament of Berry or ligation of the inferior thyroid artery during thyroidectomy. It will result in acute breathlessness (dyspnea) because both vocal folds move toward the midline and close off the air passage.
3.   **Damage to the superior laryngeal nerve** can result when ligating the superior thyroid artery during thyroidectomy. This can be avoided by ligating the superior thyroid artery at its entrance into the thyroid gland. It will result in a weak voice with loss of projection, and the vocal cord on the affected side appears flaccid.
4.   **Cricothyroidotomy** is a procedure in which a tube is inserted between the cricoid and thyroid cartilages for emergency airway management. The incision made for this procedure will pass through the following structures: skin → superficial fascia and platysma muscle (avoiding the anterior jugular veins) → deep cervical fascia → pretracheal fascia (avoiding the sternohyoid muscle) → cricothyroid ligament (avoiding the cricothyroid muscle). This procedure may be complicated by a **pyramidal lobe** of the thyroid gland in the midline (present in 75% of the population).
5.   **Tracheotomy** is a procedure in which a tube is inserted between the **second and third tracheal cartilage rings** when long-term ventilation support is necessary as it reduces the incidence of vocal cord paralysis or subglottic stenosis. The incision made for this procedure will pass through the following structures: skin → superficial fascia and platysma muscle (avoiding the anterior jugular veins) → deep cervical fascia → pretracheal fascia → cartilage rings. The following structures are

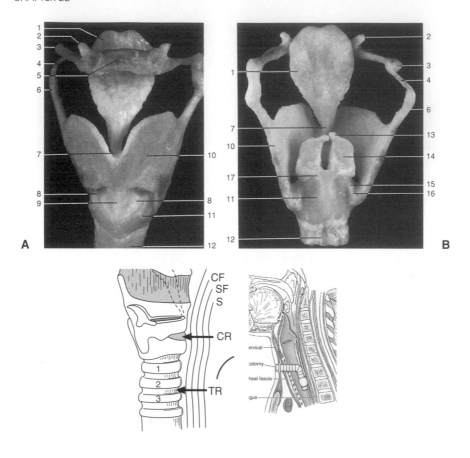

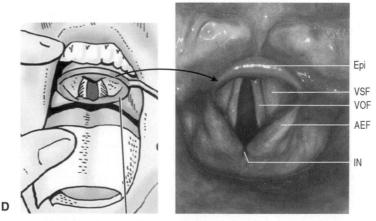

● **Figure 22-10 Laryngeal Cartilages. (A)** Anterior view of the laryngeal cartilages. **(B)** Posterior view of the laryngeal cartilages. **(C)** Lateral view of the laryngeal cartilages showing the location for a cricothyroidotomy (CR) and a tracheotomy (TR). Note the anatomic layers that must be penetrated. **(D)** Photograph depicting the structures observed during inspection of the vocal folds using a laryngeal mirror. 1 = epiglottis, 2 = lesser cornu of hyoid bone, 3 = greater cornu of hyoid bone, 4 = lateral thyrohyoid ligament, 5 = body of hyoid bone, 6 = superior cornu of thyroid cartilage, 7 = thyroepiglottic ligament, 8 = conus elasticus, 9 = cricothyroid ligament, 10 = thyroid cartilage, 11 = cricoid cartilage, 12 = trachea, 13 = corniculate cartilage, 14 = arytenoid cartilage, 15 = posterior cricoarytenoid ligament, 16 = cricothyroid joint, 17 = cricoarytenoid joint, AEF = aryepiglottic fold, CF = deep cervical fascia, Epi = epiglottis, IN = interarytenoid notch, PF = pretracheal fascia, S = skin, SF = superficial fascia, VOF = vocal fold, VSF = vestibular fold.

put in jeopardy of injury: **inferior thyroid veins**, which form a plexus anterior to the trachea, the **thyroid ima artery** (present in 10% of people), which supplies the inferior border of the isthmus of the thyroid gland, and the **thymus gland** in infants. This procedure can be complicated by massive hemorrhage 1 to 2 weeks after placement of the tube as a result of erosion of the **brachiocephalic (innominate) artery**.

XII Thyroid Gland

A. General Features. The arterial supply of the thyroid gland is from the external carotid artery via the **superior thyroid artery**, the subclavian artery–thyrocervical trunk via the **inferior thyroid artery**, and sometimes the arch of the aorta via the **thyroid ima artery** (present in about 10% of the population). The venous drainage is to the **superior thyroid veins, middle thyroid veins**, and **inferior thyroid veins**, all of which empty into the internal jugular vein. The **right recurrent laryngeal nerve** (which recurs around the subclavian artery) and **left recurrent laryngeal nerve** (which recurs around the arch of the aorta at the ligamentum arteriosum) run in the tracheoesophageal groove along the posterior surface of the thyroid gland. **The ligament of Berry** is the superior suspensory ligament of the thyroid gland located adjacent to the cricoid cartilage on the posterior surface of the thyroid gland.

B. Clinical Considerations
1. **Complications of a thyroidectomy** include thyroid storm (hyperpyrexia and tachyarrhythmias), hypoparathyroidism (develops within 24 hours as a result of low serum calcium), and recurrent laryngeal nerve or superior laryngeal nerve damage.
2. **Aberrant thyroid tissue** may occur anywhere along the path of its embryologic descent; that is, from the base of the tongue (foramen cecum), where it is called a **lingual cyst**, to the superior mediastinum.
3. **Thyroglossal duct cyst** is a cystic remnant of the descent of the thyroid during embryologic development.

XIII Parathyroid Gland

A. General Features. The parathyroid glands are yellowish-brown masses ($2 \times 3 \times 5$ mm in size; 40 g in weight). Most people have four parathyroid glands, but five, six, or seven glands are possible. These glands are rarely embedded within the thyroid gland. The **superior parathyroid glands** are consistently located on the posterior surface of the upper thyroid lobes near the inferior thyroid artery. The **inferior parathyroid glands** are usually located on the lateral surface of the lower thyroid lobes (are more variable in location than the superior parathyroid glands). The arterial supply of the superior and inferior parathyroid glands is from the inferior thyroid artery.

B. Clinical Considerations
1. **Primary hyperparathyroidism** results from autonomous secretion of parathyroid hormone (PTH) as a result of glandular hyperplasia, adenoma, or rarely carcinoma. The clinical sign is persistent hypercalcemia. Surgical removal of the hyperfunctioning glands results in a 90% cure rate.
2. **Injury to the parathyroid glands** most commonly results during a thyroidectomy because of disruption of the blood supply from the inferior thyroid artery.

Parotid Gland

A. **General Features.** The parotid gland secretes a serous saliva that enters the mouth via the **parotid duct of Stensen.** The facial nerve (CN VII) enters the substance of the parotid gland after emerging from the stylomastoid foramen and branches into the temporal, zygomatic, buccal, mandibular, and cervical branches, which innervate the muscles of facial expression (Note: CN VII has no function in the parotid gland). The arterial supply is from branches of the external carotid artery. The venous drainage is to the retromandibular vein → external jugular vein. The parotid gland is innervated by postganglionic sympathetic axons from the superior cervical ganglion that reach the parotid gland with the arteries to stimulate a thick mucous secretion and vasoconstriction causing a dry mouth. The parotid gland is also innervated by preganglionic parasympathetic axons with cell bodies in the **inferior salivatory nucleus of the glossopharyngeal nerve (CN IX).** These axons travel within the **tympanic nerve** and the **lesser petrosal nerve** to synapse on cell bodies within the otic ganglion. Postganglionic parasympathetic axons leave the otic ganglion and are distributed with the **auriculotemporal nerve** of the trigeminal nerve (CN V) to the parotid gland to stimulate a watery secretion.

B. **Clinical Considerations**

1. **Surgery on the parotid gland** may damage the **auriculotemporal nerve of CN V** and cause loss of sensation in the auriculotemporal area of the head. Because the auriculotemporal nerve also carries postganglionic sympathetic nerve fibers to sweat glands of the head and postganglionic parasympathetic nerve fibers to the parotid gland for salivation, if this nerve is severed aberrant regeneration may result in a person sweating during eating (**Frey's syndrome**).

2. **Surgery on the Parotid Gland or Bell's Palsy.** Both of these conditions cause a lower motor neuron lesion of the facial nerve (CN VIII). This results in an **ipsilateral paralysis** of muscles of facial expression of the **upper and lower face,** loss of corneal reflex (efferent limb), loss of taste from the anterior two thirds of the tongue, and hyperacusis (increased acuity to sound). Clinical signs include inability to blink eye or raise eyebrow (upper face deficit involving orbicularis oculi and frontalis muscles, respectively) and inability to seal lips or smile properly (lower face deficit involving orbicularis oris muscle) on the affected side.

3. **Stroke.** A stroke within the internal capsule affecting the corticobulbar tract causes an upper motor neuron lesion of the facial nerve (CN VII). This results in a **contralateral paralysis** of the **lower face** but spares the upper face. Clinical signs include inability to seal the lips or smile properly (lower face deficit involving orbicularis oris muscle) on contralateral side.

4. **Facial Laceration.** A facial laceration near the anterior border of the masseter muscle will cut the **parotid duct of Stensen** and the **buccal branch of CN VII.**

Chapter 23

Eye

Ⅰ Bony Orbit (Figure 23-1)

A. General Features. The bony orbit is a pyramid-shaped cavity surrounded by a shell of bone to protect the eyeball. The roof of the orbit is formed by the **frontal bone** and the **lesser wing of the sphenoid bone**. The medial wall is formed by the **ethmoid bone** and the **lacrimal bone**. The lateral wall is formed by the **zygomatic bone** and the **greater wing of the sphenoid bone**. The floor of the orbit is formed by the **maxilla bone** and the **palatine bone**.

B. Fissures, Foramina, and Canals
1. **Superior Orbital Fissure.** The superior orbital fissure is formed by a gap between the greater and lesser wings of the sphenoid bone and communicates with the middle cranial fossa. This fissure transmits the following: **oculomotor nerve (cranial nerve [CN] III), trochlear nerve (CN IV), ophthalmic nerves (branches of the ophthalmic division of trigeminal nerve [CN V$_1$]), abducens nerve (CN VI), and ophthalmic vein.**
2. **Inferior Orbital Fissure.** The inferior orbital fissure is formed by a gap between the greater wing of the sphenoid bone and the maxillary bone and communicates with the infratemporal fossa and pterygopalatine fossa. This fissure transmits the following: **infraorbital nerve (a branch of the maxillary division of CN V$_2$), infraorbital artery, and inferior ophthalmic vein.**
3. **Infraorbital Foramen and Groove.** This foramen and groove transmit the following: infraorbital nerve, infraorbital artery, and **inferior ophthalmic vein.**
4. **Supraorbital Foramen (or notch).** This foramen transmits the following: **supraorbital nerve, supraorbital artery, and superior ophthalmic vein.**
5. **Anterior Ethmoidal Foramen.** This foramen transmits the following: anterior ethmoidal nerve and anterior ethmoidal artery.
6. **Posterior Ethmoidal Foramen.** This foramen transmits the following: posterior ethmoidal nerve and posterior ethmoidal artery.
7. **Optic Canal.** This canal is formed by an opening through the lesser wing of the sphenoid bone and communicates with the middle cranial fossa. This canal transmits the following: **optic nerve (CN II) and ophthalmic artery** (a branch of the internal carotid artery).
8. **Nasolacrimal Canal.** This canal is formed by the maxilla bone, lacrimal bone, and inferior nasal concha. This canal transmits the following: nasolacrimal duct from the lacrimal sac to the inferior nasal meatus.

ⅠⅠ Eyelids and Lacrimal Apparatus (Figure 23-1A, B)

A. **Eyelids.** The eyelids cover the globe anteriorly and serve as a barrier to excessive light and debris and maintain cornea moisture by spreading lacrimal secretions. The exterior surface of the eyelid is typical **thin skin.** The interior surface of the eyelid is a mucous membrane called the **palpebral conjunctiva.** The palpebral conjunctiva is reflected onto the eyeball, where it is then called the **bulbar conjunctiva.** The bulbar conjunctiva is continuous with the corneal epithelium. The palpebral and bulbar conjunctiva enclose a space called the **conjunctival sac.** Within the upper and lower eyelids, there is a dense plate of collagen called the **superior tarsal plate** and **inferior tarsal plate,** respectively. The superior and inferior tarsal plates merge on either side of the eye to form the **medial** and **lateral palpebral ligaments.** The tarsal plate contains **tarsal glands,** which are specialized sebaceous glands opening via a duct onto the edge of the eyelid. A number of **eyelashes** and their associated sebaceous glands called **ciliary glands** are found at the margin of each eyelid. The **medial** and **lateral palpebral commissures** are formed where the upper and lower eyelids come together, thus defining the **angles of the eye.** There are three important muscles associated with the eyelid, which include:

1. **Levator Palpebrae Superioris Muscle.** This **skeletal muscle** is located in the upper eyelid and attaches to the skin of the upper eyelid and anterior surface of the superior tarsal plate. This muscle is innervated by **CN III,** and its function is **to keep the eye open (main player).**

2. **Superior Tarsal Muscle.** This **smooth muscle** is located in the upper eyelid and attaches to the superior tarsal plate. This muscle is innervated by **postganglionic sympathetic neurons** that follow the carotid arterial system into the head and neck, and its function is **to keep the eye open (minor player).**

3. **Orbicularis Oculi Muscle (palpebral portion).** This **skeletal muscle** is located in the upper and lower eyelid and lies superficial to the tarsal plates. This muscle in innervated by **CN VII,** and its function is **to close the eye.**

B. **Lacrimal Apparatus (Figure 23-1C). Lacrimal glands** are located in the superior lateral aspect of each orbit and secrete a **lacrimal fluid (or tears).** Lacrimal fluid contains **lysozyme** (an antibacterial enzyme), **lactoferrin** (sequesters iron necessary for bacteria metabolism), and **IgA.** Lacrimal fluid, mucous secretion from the palpebral and bulbar conjunctiva, and sebaceous secretions from the tarsal glands all contribute to form the **tear film** on the surface of the eye. The tear film spreads over the conjunctiva and cornea where it lubricates and protects the outer surface of the eyeball and provides nutrients and dissolved oxygen to the cornea. Lacrimal fluid follows this pathway: lacrimal gland → excretory ducts → conjunctival sac → medial angle of the eye → lacrimal canaliculi opening on the lacrimal papilla → lacrimal sac (the superior dilated portion of the nasolacrimal duct) → nasolacrimal duct → inferior nasal meatus. Lacrimation is stimulated by the parasympathetic nervous system. The preganglionic neuronal cell bodies are located in the **superior salivatory nucleus and lacrimal nucleus.** Preganglionic axons from the superior salivatory nucleus and the lacrimal nucleus run with **CN VII** (by way of the **nervus intermedius, greater petrosal nerve, and the nerve of the pterygoid canal**) and enter the **pterygopalatine ganglion** where they synapse with postganglionic neurons. Postganglionic axons leave the pterygopalatine ganglion and run with the **zygomaticofacial branch of CN V₂** and the **lacrimal branch of CN V₁** to innervate the lacrimal gland.

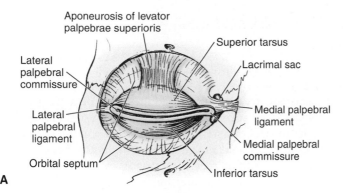

A

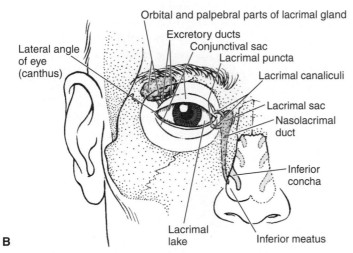

B

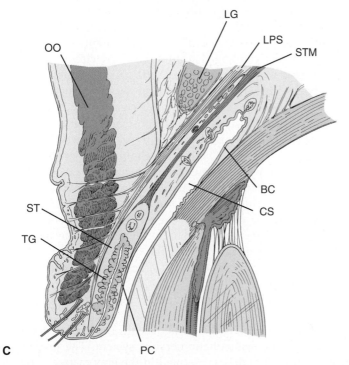

C

● **Figure 23-1 (A) Skeleton of the Eyelid. (B) Lacrimal Apparatus. (C) Upper Eyelid.** BC = bulbar conjunctiva, CS = conjunctival sac, LG = lacrimal gland, LPS = levator palpebrae superioris muscle, OO = orbicularis oculi muscle, PC = palpebral conjunctiva, ST = superior tarsal plate, STM = superior tarsal muscle, TG = tarsal gland.

III **The Globe or Eyeball.** The globe of the eye consists of three concentric tunics that make up the wall of the eye as indicated below.

A. Corneoscleral Tunic. This is the outermost fibrous tunic and consists of the **cornea, sclera,** and **corneoscleral junction (limbus).**

1. **Cornea.** The cornea is a transparent structure composed histologically of five layers (corneal epithelium, Bowman layer, stroma, Descemet membrane, and corneal endothelium) and makes up the anterior one sixth of the globe. The central portion of the cornea receives nutrients from the aqueous humor within the anterior chamber of the eye, whereas the peripheral portion receives nutrients from blood vessels of the limbus. The cornea is an avascular structure but is highly innervated by **branches of CN V$_1$ (ophthalmic division of trigeminal nerve).**

2. **Sclera.** The sclera is a white, opaque structure composed histologically of collagen and elastic fibers and makes up the posterior five sixths of the globe. The sclera gives the globe its shape and provides attachments for the extraocular eye muscles.

3. **Corneoscleral Junction (limbus).** The limbus is the junction of the transparent cornea and the opaque sclera. The limbus contains a **trabecular network** and the **canals of Schlemm,** which are involved in the flow of aqueous humor. The flow of aqueous humor follows this route: **posterior chamber → anterior chamber → trabecular network → canal of Schlemm → aqueous veins → episcleral veins.** The drainage rate of aqueous humor is balanced by the secretion rate of aqueous humor from the ciliary epithelium, thus maintaining a constant **intraocular pressure of 23 mm Hg.** An obstruction of aqueous humor flow will increase intraocular pressure, causing a condition called **glaucoma.**

B. Uveal Tunic. This is the middle vascular tunic and consists of the **choroid, stroma of the ciliary body,** and the **stroma of the iris.**

1. **Choroid.** The choroid is a pigmented vascular bed that lies immediately deep to the corneoscleral tunic. The profound vascularity of the choroid is responsible for the "red eye" that occurs with flash photography.

2. **Stroma of the Ciliary Body.** The stroma of the ciliary body contains the **ciliary muscle.** The ciliary muscle is circularly arranged around the entire circumference of the ciliary body and is innervated by the parasympathetic nervous system. The preganglionic neuronal cell bodies are located in the **Edinger-Westphal nucleus of CN III.** Preganglionic axons from the Edinger-Westphal nucleus travel with CN III and enter the **ciliary ganglion** where they synapse with postganglionic neurons. Postganglionic axons leave the ciliary ganglion where they travel with the **short ciliary nerves** to innervate the ciliary muscle. The postganglionic parasympathetic neurons release **acetylcholine (ACh),** which stimulates contraction (i.e. **accommodation**) via **muscarinic acetylcholine receptors (mAChR).** Accommodation is the process by which the lens becomes rounder to focus a nearby object or flatter to focus a distant object. For **close vision** (e.g. reading), the ciliary muscle contracts, which reduces tension on the zonular fibers attached to the lens and thereby allows the lens to take a rounded shape. **For distant vision,** the ciliary muscle relaxes, which increases tension on the zonular fibers attached to the lens and thereby allows the lens to take a flattened shape.

3. **Stroma of the Iris.** The stroma contains the **dilator pupillae muscle** and **sphincter pupillae muscle.**

   a. **Dilator pupillae muscle** is radially arranged around the entire circumference of the iris and is innervated by the sympathetic nervous system. The preganglionic sympathetic neuronal cell bodies are located in the gray matter of the

T1 through L2 or L3 spinal cord. Preganglionic axons project from this area, enter the paravertebral chain ganglia, and ascend to the **superior cervical ganglion** where they synapse with postganglionic neurons. Postganglionic axons leave the superior cervical ganglion and follow the carotid arterial system into the head and neck where they travel with the **long ciliary nerves** to innervate the dilator pupillae muscle. The postganglionic sympathetic neurons release **norepinephrine**, which stimulates contraction (i.e. pupil dilation or mydriasis) via α-**adrenergic receptors**. Any pathology that compromises this sympathetic pathway will result in **Horner's syndrome.**

   b. **Sphincter pupillae muscle** is circularly arranged around the entire circumference of the iris and is innervated by the parasympathetic nervous system. The preganglionic parasympathetic neuronal cell bodies are located in the **Edinger-Westphal nucleus of CN III**. Preganglionic axons from the Edinger-Westphal nucleus enter the **ciliary ganglion** where they synapse with postganglionic neurons. Postganglionic axons leave the ciliary ganglion where they travel with the **short ciliary nerves** to innervate the sphincter pupillae muscle. The postganglionic parasympathetic neurons release **ACh**, which stimulates contraction (i.e. **pupil constriction or miosis**) via **mAChR**. Lesions involving **CN III** will result in a **fixed and dilated pupil.**

C. **Retinal Tunic.** This is the innermost tunic, which develops embryologically from two layers of simple columnar epithelium (i.e. the outer pigment epithelium layer and the inner neural layer) that form as a result of the invagination of the optic vesicle to form a two-layered optic cup that persists in the adult. In the adult, the retinal tunic consists of the outer **pigment epithelium** and the inner **neural retina (posteriorly)** and the **epithelium of the ciliary body and epithelium of the iris (anteriorly).**
   1. **Pigment Epithelium and Neural Retina.** The outer pigment epithelium and the inner neural retina together constitute the **retina.** The **intraretinal space** separates the outer pigment epithelium from the inner neural retina. Although the intraretinal space is obliterated in the adult, it remains a weakened area prone to **retinal detachment.** The posterior two-thirds of the retina is a light-sensitive area (**pars optica**) and the anterior one-third is a light-insensitive area (**par ciliaris and irides**). These two areas are separated by the **ora serrata.** The retina is composed histologically of 10 layers. The retina has a number of specialized areas, which include the following:
      a. **Optic Disc.** The optic disc is the site where axons of the ganglion cells converge to form the optic nerve (CN II) by penetrating the sclera, forming the **lamina cribrosa.** The optic disc lacks rods and cones and is therefore a **blind spot.** The central artery and vein of the retina pass through the optic disc.
      b. **Fovea.** The fovea is a shallow depression of the retina located 3 mm lateral (temporal side) to the optic disc along the visual axis. The **fovea centralis** is located at the center of the fovea and is the area of highest visual acuity and color vision. The fovea centralis contains **only cones (no rods or capillaries)**, which are arranged **at an angle** so that light directly impinges on the cones without passing through other layers of the retina and are linked to a single ganglion, both of which contribute to visual acuity. The **macula lutea** is a yellowish area (owing to xanthophyll pigment accumulation in ganglion cells) surrounding the fovea centralis.
   2. **Epithelium of the Ciliary Body.** The ciliary body is lined by two layers of simple columnar epithelium called the **ciliary epithelium.** The outer layer of epithelium is pigmented and continuous with the pigmented epithelium of the retina. The inner

layer of epithelium is nonpigmented and continuous with the neural retina. The ciliary epithelium **secretes aqueous humor** and **produces the zonular fibers** that attached to the lens.

3. **Epithelium of the Iris.** The iris is lined by a two layers of simple columnar epithelium. The outer layer of epithelium is pigmented and continuous with the pigmented epithelium of the retina. The inner layer of epithelium is pigmented and continuous with the neural retina.

D. Contents of the Globe. The globe is divided by the lens into two cavities called the **anterior cavity** and **posterior cavity**.

1. The **anterior cavity** consists of the **anterior chamber** (the area between the cornea and iris) and the **posterior chamber** (the area between the iris and lens). These chambers are filled with the watery **aqueous humor**, which is secreted by the epithelium of the ciliary body.

2. The **posterior cavity** consists of the **vitreous chamber** (the area between the lens and retina). The vitreous chamber is filled with the **vitreous body** (a jellylike substance) and **vitreous humor** (a watery fluid), which hold the retina in place and support the lens.

3. Between the anterior cavity and posterior cavity is the **lens** of the eye. The lens is a biconvex, transparent, and avascular structure that receives its nutrients from the aqueous humor. It consists of the following components:
   a. **Lens capsule** is a thick basement membrane that completely surrounds the lens.
   b. **Lens epithelium** is a simple cuboidal epithelium located beneath the lens capsule only on the anterior surface (i.e. no epithelium is found on the posterior surface). The lens epithelium is mitotically active and migrates to the equatorial region of the lens where the cells elongate and rotate so that they are parallel to the lens surface.
   c. **Lens fibers** are prismatic remnants of the elongated lens epithelium that lose their nuclei and organelles. They are filled with cytoskeletal proteins called **filensin** and **α,β,γ-crystallin**, which maintain the conformation and transparency of the lens. The older lens fibers are displaced to the center of the lens, whereas the newer lens fibers are found at the periphery.

IV Extraocular Musculature (Figure 23-2, Table 23-1). There are seven extraocular muscles of the orbit, which include the **levator palpebrae superioris muscle, superior rectus muscle, inferior rectus muscle, lateral rectus muscle, medial rectus muscle, superior oblique muscle,** and **inferior oblique muscle.** The four rectus muscles arise from the **common tendinous ring** at the apex of the orbit and extend anteriorly to insert in the sclera of the globe. Although individual rectus muscles exert unique forces on the globe, they rarely act independently. The **superior oblique muscle** originates from the sphenoid bone, extends superomedially (its tendon passes through a trochlea attached to the frontal bone), reverses direction, and inserts into the posterolateral superior quadrant of the globe. The **inferior oblique muscle** originates from the anterior part of the medial orbit floor, extends posterolaterally, and inserts into the posterolateral inferior quadrant of the globe. The innervation to the extraocular muscles can be remembered by the chemical formula $LR_6SO_4AO_3$ (lateral rectus, CN VI; superior oblique, CN IV; all others, CN III).

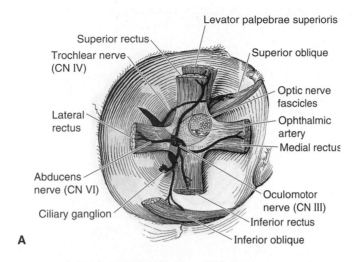

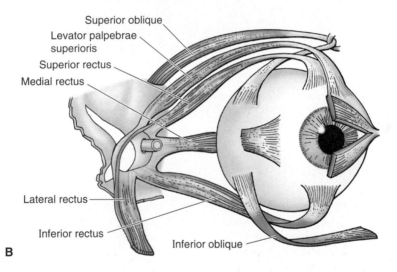

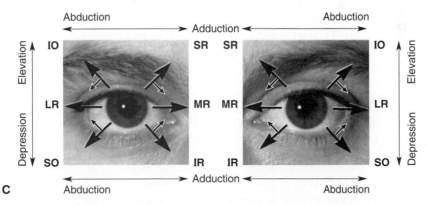

● **Figure 23-2 (A) Nerves of the Orbit After Excision of the Eyeball. (B) Extraocular Muscles (anterolateral view from the right). (C) Eye Movements.** Large arrows indicate the direction of eye movements caused by the various extraocular muscles. Small arrows indicate either intorsion (medial rotation of the superior pole of the eyeball) or extorsion (lateral rotation of the superior pole of the eyeball). IO = inferior oblique, LR = lateral rectus, SO = superior oblique, MR = medial rectus, IR = inferior rectus. See Table 23-1.

TABLE 23-1	TESTING MUSCLES AND NERVES OF THE EYE	
Muscle	Nerve	Clinical Test[a]
Levator palpebrae	CN III	Keeps eye open
Superior rectus	CN III	Patient is asked to look to the side and then to look up
Medial rectus	CN III	Patient is asked to look to the nose (medially)
Inferior rectus	CN III	Patient is asked to look to the side and then to look down
Inferior oblique	CN III	Patient is asked to look to the nose and then to look up **"up and in" toward bridge of the nose**
Superior oblique	CN IV	Patient is asked to look to the nose and then to look **"down and in" toward the tip of the nose**
Lateral rectus	CN VI	Patient is asked to look to the side (laterally)
Orbicularis oculi	CN VII	Closes the eye; efferent limb of corneal reflex
Dilator pupillae	Postganglionic sympathetic	Dilates the pupil
Superior tarsal	Postganglionic sympathetic	Keeps eye open
Sphincter pupillae	Postganglionic parasympathetic	Constricts the pupil
Ciliary muscle	Postganglionic parasympathetic	Performs accommodation

[a]Because the actions of the superior rectus, inferior rectus, superior oblique, and inferior oblique are complicated, the physician tests eye movements with the eye placed in a position where a single action of the muscle predominates.

 Nerves of the Orbit

A. **Optic Nerve (CN II).** CN II forms as a collection of axons derived from ganglion cells of the retina. CN II passes through the optic canal in association with the **central artery and vein of the retina.** The visual pathway originates at the retina and terminates in Brodmann's area 17, the **visual cortex.**

B. **Oculomotor Nerve (CN III).** The superior division of CN III innervates the levator palpebrae superioris muscle, superior rectus muscle, and inferior rectus muscle. The inferior division of CN III innervates the inferior rectus muscle and inferior oblique muscle. CN III also contains preganglionic parasympathetic axons from the Edinger-Westphal nucleus on their way to the ciliary ganglion.

C. **Trochlear Nerve (CN IV).** CN IV innervates the superior oblique muscle.

D. **Abducens Nerve (CN VI).** CN VI innervates the lateral rectus muscle.

E. **Ophthalmic Division of the Trigeminal Nerve (CN V₁).** CN V_1 conveys sensory information from the orbital areas. The primary branches are as follows:
   1. The **lacrimal nerve** conveys sensory information from the lateral eyelids and palpebral conjunctiva. The lacrimal nerve also carries postganglionic parasympathetic axons from the pterygopalatine ganglion via the zygomaticofacial branch of CN V_2 to innervate the lacrimal gland.
   2. The **frontal nerve** bifurcates into the:
      a. **Supraorbital nerve.** The supraorbital nerve conveys sensory information from the eyelid, forehead, and scalp.

b. **Supratrochlear nerve.** The supratrochlear nerve conveys sensory information from the medial portions of the eyelids and center of the forehead.

3. The **nasociliary nerve** branches into the:

a. **Anterior ethmoidal nerve.** The anterior ethmoidal nerve conveys sensory information from the anterior ethmoidal air cells, nasal septum, lateral walls of the nasal cavity, and tip of the nose.

b. **Posterior ethmoidal nerve.** The posterior ethmoidal nerve conveys sensory information from the sphenoid sinus and posterior ethmoidal air cells.

c. **Infratrochlear nerve.** The infratrochlear nerve conveys sensory information from the eyelids, conjunctiva, nose, and lacrimal sac.

d. **Long ciliary nerves.** The long ciliary nerves convey sensory information from the iris and cornea. The long ciliary nerves also carry postganglionic sympathetic axons from the superior cervical ganglion to innervate the dilator pupillae muscle.

e. **Sensory ramus.** The sensory ramus connects with the ciliary ganglion. The sensory ramus conveys sensory information from the iris and cornea via the **short ciliary nerves** (considered to be part of CN V_1), which connect with the ciliary ganglion also. The short ciliary nerves also carry postganglionic parasympathetic axons from the ciliary ganglion to innervate the ciliary muscle and sphincter pupillae muscle. The short ciliary nerves also carry postganglionic sympathetic axons from the superior cervical ganglion.

Vasculature of the Orbit

A. **Arterial Supply.** The **ophthalmic artery** is a branch of the **internal carotid artery** and is the primary arterial supply to the orbit. The ophthalmic artery enters the orbit via the optic canal and gives off various branches, which include:

1. **Central artery of the retina** runs in the dural sheath of CN II and pierces CN II near the eyeball and then appears at the center of the optic disc. This artery supplies a portion of the retina.

2. **Supraorbital artery** passes superiorly and posteriorly after leaving the supraorbital foramen. This artery supplies the forehead and scalp.

3. **Supratrochlear artery** passes from the supraorbital margin. This artery supplies the forehead and scalp.

4. **Lacrimal artery** passes along the superior border of the superior rectus muscle. This artery supplies the lacrimal gland, conjunctiva, and eyelids.

5. **Dorsal nasal artery** passes along the dorsal aspect of the nose. This artery supplies the surface of the nose.

6. **Short posterior ciliary arteries** pierce the sclera at the periphery of CN II. These arteries supply the choroid, which in turn supplies a portion of the retina.

7. **Long posterior ciliary arteries** pierce the sclera. These arteries supply the ciliary body and iris.

8. **Anterior ethmoidal artery** passes through the anterior ethmoidal foramen to enter the anterior cranial fossa. This artery supplies the anterior and middle ethmoidal air cells, frontal sinus, nasal cavity, and skin of the dorsum of the nose.

9. **Posterior ethmoidal artery** passes through the posterior ethmoidal foramen. This artery supplies the posterior ethmoidal air cells.

10. **Anterior ciliary artery** pierces the sclera near the attachments of the rectus muscles. This artery supplies the ciliary body and iris.

11. **Infraorbital artery** (a branch of the third part of the maxillary artery) passes along the infraorbital groove and through the infraorbital foramen. This artery supplies the face.

B. Venous Drainage

1. **Superior Ophthalmic Vein.** The superior ophthalmic vein is formed by the union of the supraorbital vein, supratrochlear vein, and angular vein. The veins that run with the branches of the ophthalmic artery and the inferior ophthalmic vein empty into the superior ophthalmic vein, which ultimately drains into the **cavernous sinus.**

2. **Inferior Ophthalmic Vein.** The inferior ophthalmic vein is formed by the union of small veins in the floor of the orbit. This vein communicates with the pterygoid venous plexus and empties into the superior ophthalmic vein.

3. **Central Vein of the Retina.** The central vein of the retina most often drains into the cavernous sinus directly but may join the superior or inferior ophthalmic vein.

4. **Vorticose Veins.** The vorticose veins from the choroid layer of the globe drain into the inferior ophthalmic vein.

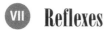 **Reflexes**

A. Pupillary Light Reflex. This reflex is mediated by CN II (afferent limb) and CN III (efferent limb). The pupillary light reflex is the constriction of the pupil in response to light stimulation. Light shined into one eye causes both pupils to constrict. The response in the stimulated eye is called the direct pupillary light reflex. The response in the opposite eye is called the consensual pupillary light reflex. It includes the following structures:

1. **Ganglion cells of the retina,** which project bilaterally to the pretectal nuclei.

2. **Pretectal nucleus of the midbrain,** which projects (through the posterior commissure) crossed and uncrossed fibers to the Edinger-Westphal nucleus.

3. **Edinger-Westphal nucleus of CN III,** which houses preganglionic parasympathetic neuronal cell bodies. Preganglionic axons run with CN III and enter the **ciliary ganglion,** where they synapse with postganglionic neurons. Postganglionic axons leave the ciliary ganglion, where they travel with the short ciliary nerves to innervate the sphincter pupillae muscle.

B. Pupillary Dilation Pathway. This pathway is mediated by the sympathetic nervous system. If this sympathetic pathway is interrupted at any level, ipsilateral Horner syndrome results. It includes the following structures:

1. **Hypothalamus.** The hypothalamic neurons of the paraventricular nucleus project directly to the ciliospinal center of Budge (T1 and T2) of the intermediolateral cell column of the spinal cord.

2. **Ciliospinal center of Budge (T1 and T2)** projects preganglionic sympathetic axons through the paravertebral chain ganglia to the superior cervical ganglion.

3. **Superior cervical ganglion** projects postganglionic sympathetic axons that follow the carotid arterial system into the head and neck where they travel with the long ciliary nerves to innervate the dilator pupillae muscle.

C. The Near Reflex and Accommodation Pathway. This reflex and pathway is mediated by CN III. Accommodation is the adjustment of the eye to focus on a near object. It includes the following structures:

1. **Cortical visual pathway** projects from the primary visual cortex (Brodmann area 7) to the visual association cortex (Brodmann area 19).

2. **Visual association cortex (Brodmann area 19)** projects through the corticotectal tract to the superior colliculus and pretectal nucleus.

3. **Superior colliculus and pretectal nucleus** project to the oculomotor complex of the midbrain. This complex includes the following structures:
   a. **Rostral Edinger-Westphal nucleus**, which mediates contraction of the sphincter pupillae muscle.
   b. **Caudal Edinger-Westphal nucleus**, which mediates contraction of the ciliary muscle.
   c. **Medial rectus subnucleus of CN III**, which mediates convergence.

D. **Corneal (Blink) Reflex.** This reflex is mediated by CN V_1 (afferent limb) and CN VII (efferent limb). During a neurologic examination, the physician touches the cornea with a wisp of cotton. The normal response is a blink.

 # Clinical Considerations

A. **Orbital Fractures.** A direct impact to the face (e.g. being punched in the eye) is transmitted to the walls of the bony orbit. A portion of the **ethmoid bone** known as the **lamina papyracea** (as the name implies, a "paper-thin" bone) is the weakest segment of the medial wall and is thus prone to fracture. This fracture results in direct communication between the orbit and the nasal cavity by way of the ethmoid sinuses. The **infraorbital canal** (which contains the infraorbital branch of the maxillary nerve) is the weakest portion of the orbital floor and is also prone to fracture. This fracture results in direct communication between the orbit and nasal cavity by way of the maxillary sinus.

B. **Sty.** A sty is a painful, erythematous, suppurative swelling of the eyelid that results from an obstructed and infected ciliary gland found at the margin of the eyelid. When a sebaceous gland of the eyelid becomes obstructed and forms a cyst, this is known as a **chalazia**. Obstruction of the tarsal glands produces inflammation known as a **tarsal chalazion**.

C. **Dry eye** is caused by a disruption in the production of tears or damage to the eyelid. This may lead to ulceration, perforation, loss of aqueous humor, and blindness.

D. **Red eye** is caused most commonly by conjunctivitis (i.e. inflammation of the conjunctiva). A purulent discharge indicates bacterial infection. A watery discharge indicates a viral infection.

E. **Bogorad Syndrome (crocodile tears).** This syndrome is the spontaneous lacrimation during eating caused by a lesion of CN VII proximal to the geniculate ganglion. This syndrome occurs after facial paralysis and is caused by the misdirection of regenerating preganglionic parasympathetic axons (that formerly innervated the salivary glands) to the lacrimal glands.

F. **Hyperopia, Myopia, and Astigmatism.** Abnormalities in the refractive capacity of the cornea that cannot be corrected by the lens result in improper localization of the focal point. When there is insufficient corneal refraction, the focal point falls behind the retina and results in **farsightedness or hyperopia**. When there is excessive corneal refraction, the focal point falls in front of the retina and results in **nearsightedness or myopia**. When there are irregularities in corneal shape, the focal point falls outside of the vertical plane in front of or behind the retina and results in **astigmatism**.

G. Glaucoma is the obstruction of aqueous humor flow that results in an increased intraocular pressure. This increased pressure causes impaired retinal blood flow, producing retinal ischemia, degeneration of retinal cells particularly at the optic disc, defects in the visual field, and blindness. There are two types of glaucoma:

1. **Open-angle glaucoma** (most common) occurs when the trabecular network is open but the canal of Schlemm is obstructed.

2. **Closed-angle glaucoma** occurs when the trabecular network is closed, usually as a result of an inflammatory process of the uvea (uveitis; e.g. infection by cytomegalovirus).

H. Cataracts are an opacity (milky white) of the lens or the lens capsule as a result of changes in the solubility of the lens proteins filensin and α,β,γ-crystallin. This results in reduced light reaching the retina, with blurred images and poor vision. The most common cause of blindness is **cataracts**.

I. Presbyopia is a condition in which the power of accommodation is reduced as a result of the loss of elasticity of the lens with advancing age. This is corrected with bifocal glasses (i.e. reading glasses).

J. Obstruction of the central artery of the retina is generally caused by an embolus and leads to retinal ischemia with instantaneous complete blindness. The blindness is often described as a dark curtain coming down over the eye, and when the attack is brief it is called **amaurosis fugax.** These events are most often monocular and may last only a few seconds or can result in permanent blindness.

K. Cavernous Sinus Thrombosis. The anastomoses between the angular vein of the face and the inferior ophthalmic vein can result in spread of infectious agents from periorbital and paranasal areas to the cavernous sinus, resulting in thrombosis. This thrombosis prevents retinal drainage, eventually leading to retinal ischemia and blindness.

L. Papilledema (choked disc) is a noninflammatory edema of the optic disc (papilla) as a result of increased intracranial pressure, usually caused by brain tumors, subdural hematoma, or hydrocephalus. It usually does not alter visual acuity, but may cause bilateral **enlarged blind spots.**

M. Retinal detachment may result from head trauma or may be congenital. The site of detachment is between the outer pigment epithelium and the inner neural retina (i.e. outer segment layer of the rods and cones of the neural retina).

N. Retinitis pigmentosa (RP) is a genetic disease characterized by degeneration of rods, night blindness (nyctalopia), and "gun barrel" vision. RP may be caused by abetalipoproteinemia (Bassen-Kornzweig syndrome) and may be arrested by massive doses of vitamin A. In RP, blood supply to the retina is reduced and a pigment is observed on the surface of the retina (hence the name). The family of RP genes is located on chromosomes X, 3, and 6. Interestingly, the gene for rhodopsin also maps to chromosome 3.

O. Diabetic Retinopathy. In patients with diabetes, retinal blood vessels frequently become leaky and exude fluid into the retina (particularly in the fovea), leading to loss of visual acuity. It is the leading cause of blindness in the developed world and may be reduced by strict regulation of blood glucose levels.

P. Night blindness (nyctalopia) is a condition in which vision in poor illumination is defective because of vitamin A (retinol) deficiency. An aldehyde of vitamin A (retinol) called **retinal** is the chromophore component of rhodopsin.

Q. Retinoblastoma (Rb) is a tumor of the retina that occurs in childhood and develops from precursor cells in the immature retina. The Rb gene is located on chromosome 13 and encodes for Rb protein, which binds to a gene regulatory protein and causes suppression of the cell cycle (i.e. the Rb gene is a tumor-suppressor gene (also called an anti-oncogene]). A mutation in the Rb gene encodes an abnormal Rb protein such that there is no suppression of the cell cycle. This leads to the formation of retinoblastoma. Hereditary retinoblastoma causes multiple tumors in both eyes. Nonhereditary retinoblastoma causes one tumor in one eye.

R. Strabismus (crossed eye) is caused by damage to CN III that results in weakness or paralysis of the extraocular eye muscles. Strabismus is a visual disorder in which the visual axes do not meet the desired objective point (or the eyes are misaligned and point in different directions because of the uncoordinated action of the extraocular eye muscles. The affected eye may turn inward, outward, upward, or downward, leading to decreased vision and misaligned eyes.

S. Diplopia (double vision) is caused by paralysis of one or more extraocular muscles, resulting from injury of the nerves supplying them.

T. Ocular Motor Palsies and Pupillary Syndromes (Figure 23-3)
1. **CN III Palsy**
2. **CN III Palsy with Ptosis**
3. **CN IV Palsy**
4. **CN VI Palsy**
5. **Marcus Gunn Pupil.** The Marcus Gunn pupil has a paradoxic dilation of both pupils during the swinging flashlight test as a result of a CN II nerve lesion in one eye. During the swinging flashlight test, the light is moved quickly back and forth from one eye to the other. When light is shined on the normal eye, both pupils constrict (i.e. direct and consensual reflexes). When the light is shined on the eye with the CN II lesion, a lesser signal reaches the Edinger-Westphal nucleus, which senses the lesser light intensity and shuts off the parasympathetic response to the light stimulus, causing a paradoxic dilation of both pupils.
6. **Argyll Robertson Pupil.** The Argyll Robertson pupil has no constriction of the pupil in response to light (no pupillary light reflex) but does constrict as a component of the accommodation reflex. The pupillary light reflex is absent because the pretectal area of the brain is damaged. However, the pretectal area is not necessary to elicit the accommodation reflex. Argyll Robertson pupil occurs in syphilis and diabetes.
7. **Horner syndrome** is caused by injury to the cervical sympathetic nerves and results in **miosis** (constriction of pupil as a result of paralysis of dilator pupillae muscle), **ptosis** (drooping of eyelid as a result of paralysis of superior tarsal muscle), **hemianhidrosis** (loss of sweating on one side), **enophthalmos** (retraction of the eyeball into the orbit as a result of paralysis of the orbitalis muscle), and **flushing** (vasodilation and increased blood flow to the head and neck). Horner syndrome may be caused by brainstem stroke, tuberculosis, Pancoast tumor, trauma, and injury to the carotid arteries.

8. **Medial longitudinal fasciculus (MLF) syndrome (internuclear ophthalmoplegia)** is caused by demyelination of the MLF between CN III and CN VI nuclei and results in medial rectus muscle palsy on attempted lateral conjugate gaze and monocular horizontal nystagmus in the abducting eye, but convergence is normal. This syndrome is most commonly seen in multiple sclerosis.

9. **Parinaud syndrome** is caused by lesions in the pretectal area and results in paralysis of upward gaze and convergence, a large pupil, and retraction of the eyelids.

10. **Lesion of Right Frontal Eye Field (e.g. a comatose patient)**

11. **Adie Pupil.** The Adie pupil has a sluggish constriction of the pupil in response to light as a result of pathologic changes in the ciliary ganglion.

U. Visual Field Defects (Figure 23-4)

V. Common Ophthalmoscopic Disorders (Figure 23-5)

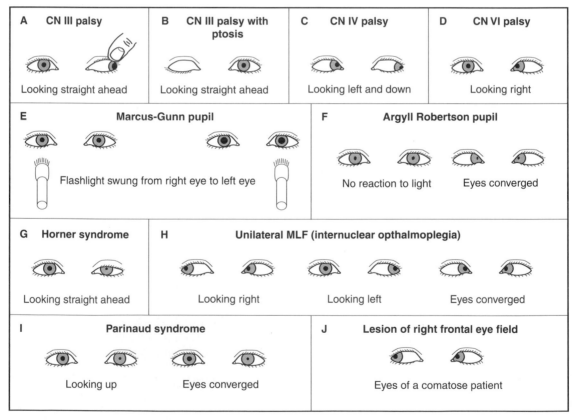

● **Figure 23-3 Ocular Motor Palsies and Pupillary Syndromes. (A)** CN III palsy. **(B)** CN III palsy with ptosis. **(C)** CN IV palsy. **(D)** CN VI palsy. **(E)** Marcus-Gunn pupil. **(F)** Argyll Robertson pupil. **(G)** Horner syndrome. **(H)** Unilateral medial longitudinal fasciculus (MLF) syndrome (internuclear ophthalmoplegia). **(I)** Parinaud syndrome. **(J)** Lesion of the right frontal eye field (e.g. a comatose patient).

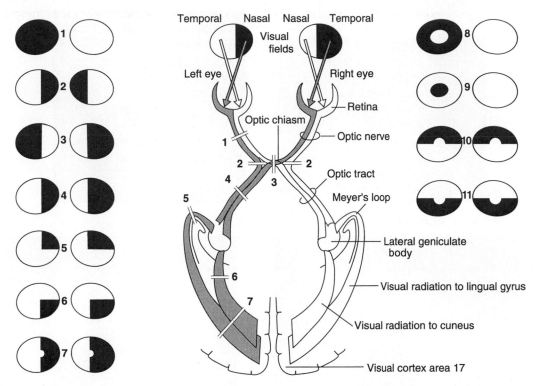

● **Figure 23-4 Visual Field Defects.** (1) Ipsilateral blindness. (2) Binasal hemianopia. (3) Bitemporal hemianopia. (4) Right hemianopia. (5) Right upper quadrantanopia. (6) Right lower quadrantanopia. (7) Right hemianopia with macular sparing. (8) Left constricted field as a result of end-stage glaucoma. (9) Left central scotoma as seen in optic (retrobulbar) neuritis in multiple sclerosis. (10) Upper altitudinal hemianopia as a result of bilateral destruction of the lingual gyri. (11) Lower altitudinal hemianopia as a result of bilateral destruction of the cunei.

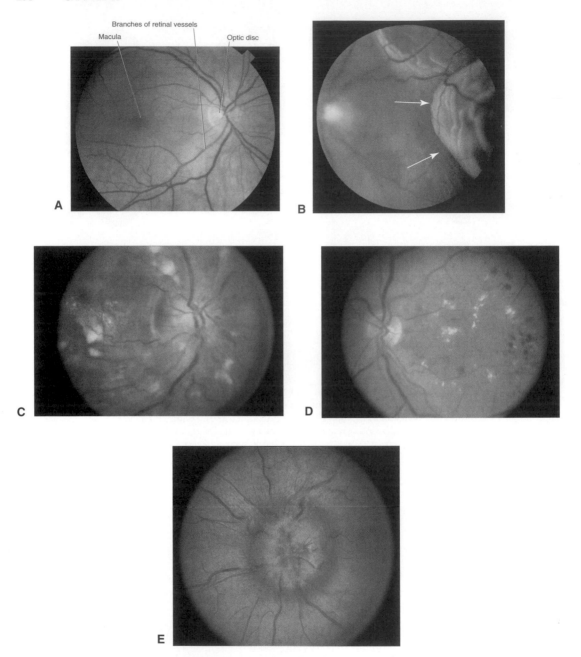

● **Figure 23-5 Common Ophthalmoscopic Disorders. (A)** Normal fundus. **(B)** Detached retina (arrows). **(C)** Hypertensive retinopathy. The optic nerve head is edematous and the retina contains numerous exudates and "cotton-wool" spots. **(D)** Diabetic retinopathy. The retina contains several yellowish "hard" exudates that are rich in lipids and several relatively small retinal hemorrhages. **(E)** Chronic papilledema. The optic nerve head is congested and protrudes anteriorly toward the interior of the eye. The optic disc has blurred margins, and the blood vessels within it are poorly seen.

Chapter 24

Ear

I **General Features.** The ear is the organ of hearing and balance. The ear consists of the external ear, middle ear, and inner ear.

II **External Ear (Figure 24-1)** consists of the following:

A. **Auricle** (known as "the ear" by lay people) is supported by elastic cartilage and covered by skin. The auricle develops from **six auricular hillocks** that surround pharyngeal groove 1. The auricle is innervated by **cranial nerve (CN) V₃, CN VII, CN IX, and CN X**, and **cervical nerves C2 and C3.**

B. **External auditory meatus** is an air-filled tubular space. The lateral portion is supported by cartilage and lined by skin that contains hair follicles, sebaceous glands, and ceruminous glands (produce ear wax). The medial portion is supported by the temporal bone and is lined by thinner skin. The external auditory meatus develops from **pharyngeal groove 1**, which becomes filled with ectodermal cells, forming a temporary **meatal plug** that disappears before birth. The external auditory meatus is innervated by **CN V₃** and **CN IX.**

C. **Tympanic membrane (eardrum)** develops from **pharyngeal membrane 1.** The tympanic membrane separates the middle ear from the external auditory meatus of the external ear. The tympanic membrane consists of three layers: keratinized stratified squamous epithelium covers the external surface; connective tissue, which is vascularized and innervated, constitutes the middle layer; and simple squamous epithelium covers the internal surface. The external (lateral) concave surface is innervated (sensory) by the **auriculotemporal branch of CN V₃** and the **auricular branch of CN X.** The internal (medial) surface is innervated by the **tympanic branch of CN IX.** The **pars flaccida** is a small triangular portion between the anterior and posterior malleolar folds; the remainder of the tympanic membrane is called the **pars tensa.** The **cone of light** is a triangular reflection of light seen in the anterior-inferior quadrant. The **umbo** is the most depressed center point of the tympanic membrane concavity.

III **Middle Ear (Figure 24-2).** The middle ear is an air-filled chamber lined by a mucosa that is innervated (sensory) by the **tympanic nerve of CN IX**, which forms the **tympanic plexus** with caroticotympanic nerves from the arterial carotid sympathetic plexus. The middle ear consists of the following:

A. **Tympanic (middle ear) Cavity.** The **tympanic cavity proper** is a space internal to the tympanic membrane. The **epitympanic recess** is a space superior to the tympanic membrane that contains the head of the malleus and body of the incus. The tympanic cavity communicates with the nasopharynx via the auditory (eustachian) tube and the mastoid air cells and mastoid antrum. The roof of the tympanic cavity is the **tegmen tympani**. The floor is the **jugular fossa**. The anterior wall is the **carotid canal**. The posterior wall is the **mastoid air cells** and **mastoid antrum**. The lateral wall is the **tympanic membrane**. The medial wall is a **promontory** formed by the basal turn of the cochlea, **oval window**, and **round window**.

B. **Ossicles.** The ossicles function as amplifiers to overcome the impedance mismatch at the air–fluid interface between the tympanic cavity (air) and the inner ear (fluid).

1. **Malleus (hammer)** develops from cartilage of **pharyngeal arch 1** (Meckel's cartilage). The malleus consists of a **head, neck**, and **handle** along with **anterior** and **lateral processes**. The head articulates with the body of the incus in the epitympanic recess. The handle is fused to the internal (medial) surface of the tympanic membrane and is moved by the **tensor tympani muscle**, which is innervated by CN V_3.

2. **Incus (anvil)** develops from the cartilage of **pharyngeal arch 1** (Meckel's cartilage). The incus consists of a **body**, a **short process**, and a **long process**. The body of the incus articulates with the head of the malleus. The short process extends horizontally backward and attaches to the ligament of the incus. The long process descends vertically and articulates with the stapes.

3. **Stapes (stirrup)** develops from the cartilage of **pharyngeal arch 2** (Reichert's cartilage). The stapes consists of a **head, neck, two processes**, and a **footplate**. The stapes is moved by the **stapedius** muscle, which is innervated by CN VII. The footplate is attached to the **oval window** of the vestibule.

C. **Muscles**

1. **Tensor tympani muscle** inserts on the handle of the malleus. The tensor tympani muscle draws the tympanic membrane medially and tightens it in response to a loud noise, thereby reducing the vibration of the tympanic membrane. This muscle is innervated by CN V_3.

2. **Stapedius muscle** inserts on the neck of the stapes. The stapedius muscle pulls the stapes posteriorly and reduces excessive oscillation, thereby protecting the inner ear from injury from a loud noise. This muscle is innervated by CN VII.

D. **Oval window (fenestra vestibuli)** is pushed back and forth by the footplate of the stapes and transmits sonic vibrations of the ossicles to the perilymph of the scala vestibuli of the inner ear.

E. **Round window (fenestra cochlea)** is closed by the mucous membrane of the middle ear and accommodates pressure waves transmitted to the perilymph of the scala tympani.

F. **Auditory (Eustachian) Tube.** The auditory tube connects the middle ear to the nasopharynx. It allows air to enter or leave the tympanic cavity, thereby balancing the air pressure of the tympanic cavity with the atmospheric pressure. This allows free movement of the tympanic membrane. The auditory tube can be opened by contraction of the tensor veli palatini and the salpingopharyngeus muscles.

IV   **Inner Ear (Figure 24-3).** The inner ear consists of the semicircular ducts, utricle, saccule, and cochlear duct, all of which are referred to as the **membranous labyrinth** containing **endolymph**. The membranous labyrinth is initially surrounded by mesoderm that later becomes cartilaginous and ossifies to become the **bony labyrinth** of the temporal bone. The mesoderm closest to the membranous labyrinth degenerates, thus forming the **perilymphatic space** containing **perilymph**. Consequently, the membranous labyrinth is suspended within the bony labyrinth by perilymph. Perilymph, which is similar in composition to **cerebrospinal fluid (CSF)**, communicates with the subarachnoid space via the **perilymphatic duct**.

A. Semicircular Ducts (kinetic labyrinth). The semicircular ducts consist of the **anterior (superior)**, **lateral**, and **posterior ducts** along with their dilated ends called **ampullae**. **Type I** and **type II hair cells** that cover the **cristae ampullaris** (a prominent ridge within the ampulla) have numerous stereocilia and a single **kinocilium** on their apical border. These cells synapse with bipolar neurons of the vestibular ganglion of CN VIII. The kinetic labyrinth also contains **supporting cells**. Hair cells and supporting cells are covered by a gelatinous mass called **cupula**. The semicircular ducts respond to **angular acceleration** and **deceleration of the head**.

B. Utricle and Saccule (static labyrinth). The utricle and saccule are dilated membranous sacs that contain specialized receptors called **maculae**. The macula of the utricle has a horizontal orientation and the macula of the saccule has a vertical orientation. **Type I** and **type II hair cells** within the **maculae** have stereocilia and a single **kinocilium** on their apical border. These cells synapse with bipolar neurons of the vestibular ganglion of CN VIII. The static labyrinth also contains **supporting cells**. Hair cells and supporting cells are covered by a gelatinous mass called the **otolithic membrane**, which contains $CaCO_3$ crystals (**otoliths**). The utricle and saccule respond to the position of the head with respect to **linear acceleration** and the **pull of gravity**.

C. Cochlear Duct. The cochlear duct is a triangular duct wedged between the scala vestibuli and scala tympani. The cochlear duct consists of a **vestibular membrane** (roof), **basilar membrane** (floor), and **stria vascularis** (lateral wall). The stria vascularis participates in the formation of endolymph. The cochlear duct contains the **organ of Corti**. The organ of Corti contains a single row of **inner hair cells** and three rows of **outer hair cells** that have stereocilia (but no kinocilium) on their apical border and synapse with bipolar neurons of the cochlear (spiral) ganglion of CN VIII (90% of these bipolar neurons synapse with inner hair cells). It also contains **pillar** and **phalangeal supporting cells**. The outer hair cells are in contact with a gelatinous mass called the **tectorial membrane** (contains α- and β-tectorin protein). The organ of Corti responds to **sound**. High-frequency sounds cause maximum displacement of the basilar membrane and stimulation of hair cells at the **base of the cochlea**. Low-frequency sounds cause maximum displacement of the basilar membrane and stimulation of hair cells at the **apex of the cochlea**.

V Clinical Considerations

A. Rubella Virus. The organ of Corti may be damaged by exposure to rubella virus during week 7 and week 8 of embryologic development.

B. Ménière disease is caused by an increase in endolymph. Clinical findings include vertigo (the illusion of rotational movement), nausea, positional nystagmus (involuntary rhythmic oscillations of the eye), vomiting, and tinnitus (ringing of the ears).

C. Waardenburg syndrome is an autosomal dominant congenital deafness associated with pigment abnormalities resulting from abnormal neural crest cell migration.

D. Otitis media is a middle ear infection that may spread from the nasopharynx through the auditory tube. This may cause temporary or permanent deafness.

E. Hyperacusis is caused by a lesion of CN VIII, which results in the paralysis of the stapedius muscle. This results in increased sensitivity to loud sounds as a result of the uninhibited movements of the stapes.

F. Conductive hearing loss results from an interference of sound transmission through the external ear or middle ear. This is most commonly caused by **otitis media** in children or **otosclerosis** (abnormal bone formation around the stapes) in adults.

G. Sensorineural hearing loss results from a loss of hair cells in the organ of Corti or a lesion of the cochlear part of CN VIII or a central nervous system auditory pathway.

H. Presbycusis is caused by a progressive loss of hair cells at the base of the organ of Corti, which results in high-frequency hearing loss in the elderly.

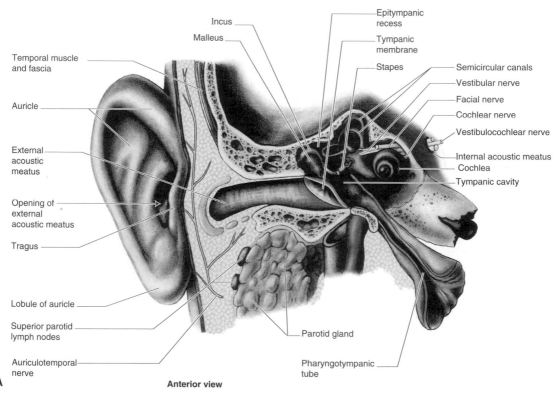

Anterior view

● **Figure 24-1 Anatomy of Ear. (A)** Coronal section of the ear.

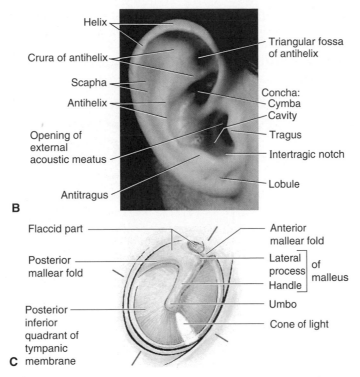

Helix

Triangular fossa
of antihelix

Crura of antihelix

Scapha

Concha:
Cymba
Cavity

Antihelix

Opening of
external
acoustic meatus

Tragus

Intertragic notch

Lobule

Antitragus

B

Flaccid part

Anterior
mallear fold

Posterior
mallear fold

Lateral
process ⎤ of
Handle ⎦ malleus

Posterior
inferior
quadrant of
tympanic
membrane

Umbo

Cone of light

C

● **Figure 24-1 (*continued*).**   **(B)** External ear. **(C)** Otoscopic view of the right tympanic membrane.

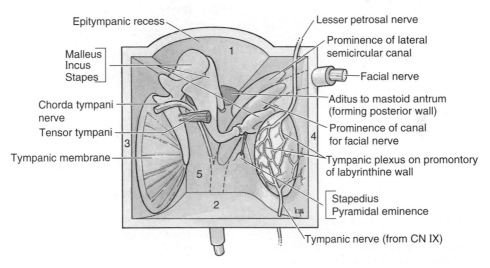

Epitympanic recess

Lesser petrosal nerve

Prominence of lateral
semicircular canal

Malleus
Incus
Stapes

Facial nerve

Chorda tympani
nerve

Aditus to mastoid antrum
(forming posterior wall)

Tensor tympani

Prominence of canal
for facial nerve

Tympanic membrane

Tympanic plexus on promontory
of labyrinthine wall

Stapedius
Pyramidal eminence

Tympanic nerve (from CN IX)

● **Figure 24-2 View of the Tympanic Cavity.** The anterior wall (carotid canal) has been removed. 1 = tegmen tympani, 2 = jugular fossa, 3 = lateral wall (tympanic membrane), 4 = medial wall (promontory, oval window, round window), 5 = posterior wall (mastoid air cells and mastoid antrum).

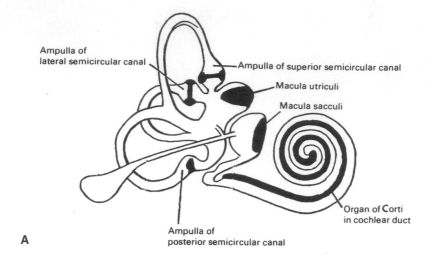

A

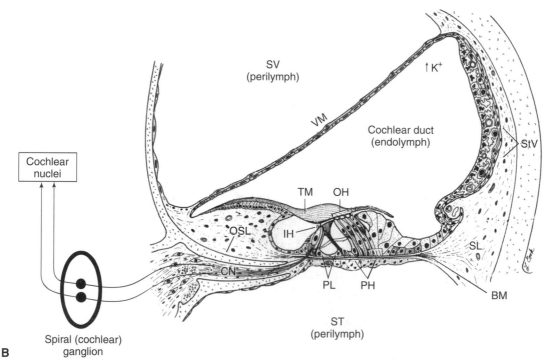

B

● **Figure 24-3 Anatomy of Inner Ear. (A)** Diagram of the membranous labyrinth. Note the location of the specialized sensory areas (black) for angular acceleration (cristae ampullaris), linear acceleration (maculae), and hearing (organ of Corti). **(B)** Organ of Corti of the cochlear duct. The organ of Corti responds to sound. The hearing process begins when airborne sound waves cause vibration of the tympanic membrane, which moves the stapes against the oval window. This produces waves of perilymph within the scala vestibuli (SV) and scala tympani (ST). The waves of perilymph cause an upward displacement of the basilar membrane (BM) such that the stereocilia of the hair cells hit the tectorial membrane (TM). As a result, potassium ion channels open, hair cells are depolarized, and afferent nerve fibers are stimulated. Note that the endolymph has a high potassium concentration, which is maintained by the stria vascularis (StV). The basilar membrane extends between the osseous spiral lamina (OSL) and the spiral ligament (SL). IH = one row of inner hair cells, NF = nerve fibers, OH = three rows of outer hair cells, PH = outer phalangeal cells, PL = pillar cells, VM = vestibular membrane.

Credits

Figure 1-1: A1, A2, and A3: From Moore KL, Dalley AF. Clinically Oriented Anatomy, 5th ed. Lippincott Williams & Wilkins, Baltimore, 2006, page 479, Figure 4.1 A, B, C. **B:** From Moore KL, Dalley AF. Clinically Oriented Anatomy, 5th ed. Lippincott Williams & Wilkins, Baltimore, 2006, page 514, Figure 4.17. **C:** From Moore KL, Dalley AF. Clinically Oriented Anatomy, 5th ed. Lippincott Williams & Wilkins, Baltimore, 2006, page 515, Figure B4.16.

Figure 1-2: From Moore KL, Dalley AF. Clinically Oriented Anatomy, 5th ed. Lippincott Williams & Wilkins, Baltimore, 2006, page 507, Figure 4.14A.

Figure 1-3: A: From Daffner RH. Clinical Radiology: The Essentials, 2nd ed. Lippincott Williams & Wilkins, Baltimore, 1999, page 544, Figure 13-7.

Figure 1-4: A and B: From Chew FS. Musculoskeletal Imaging: The Core Curriculum. Lippincott Williams & Wilkins, Baltimore, 2003, page 163, Figure 5.26A, B. **C:** From Dudek RW. High Yield Gross Anatomy, 2nd ed. Lippincott Williams & Wilkins, Baltimore, 2002, page 12, Figure 1-7A, B. **D:** From Osborn AG. Head Trauma. In: Eisenberg RL, Amberg JR (eds). Critical Pathways in Radiology. Lippincott Williams & Wilkins, Philadelphia, 1981. **E:** From Daffner RH. Clinical Radiology: The Essentials, 2nd ed. Lippincott Williams & Wilkins, Baltimore, 1999, page 556, Figure 13.20.

Figure 1-5A: From Agur AMR, Dalley AF. Grant's Atlas of Anatomy, 11th ed. Lippincott Williams & Wilkins, Baltimore, 2005, page 789, Figure 8.41B.

Figure 1-5B: From Esses SI. Textbook of Spinal Disorders. Lippincott Williams & Wilkins, Baltimore, 1995, page 85, Figure 4-7.

Figure 1-6A: From Esses SI. Textbook of Spinal Disorders. Lippincott Williams & Wilkins, Baltimore, 1995, page 88, Figure 4-10.

Figure 1-6B: From Esses SI. Textbook of Spinal Disorders. Lippincott Williams & Wilkins, Baltimore, 1995, page 89, Figure 4-11.

Figure 1-7: A: From Chew FS. Musculoskeletal Imaging: The Core Curriculum. Lippincott Williams & Wilkins, Baltimore, 2003, page 88, Figure 3.14A. **B:** From Harris JH, Harris WH. The Radiology of Emergency Medicine, 4th ed. Lippincott Williams & Wilkins, Baltimore, 2000, page 253, Figure 206D. **C:** From Chew FS. Musculoskeletal Imaging: The Core Curriculum. Lippincott Williams & Wilkins, Baltimore, 2003, page 90, Figure 3.17A. **D:** From Daffner RH. Clinical Radiology: The Essentials, 2nd ed. Lippincott Williams & Wilkins, Baltimore, 1999, page 563, Figure 13.26B.

Figure 2-1: A: From Moore KL, Dalley AF. Clinically Oriented Anatomy, 5th ed. Lippincott Williams & Wilkins, Baltimore, 2006, page 523, Figure 4.24. **B:** From Dudek RW. High Yield Gross Anatomy, 2nd ed. Lippincott Williams & Wilkins, Baltimore, 2002, page 14, Figure 2-1B.

Figure 2-2: A: From Moore KL, Dalley AF. Clinically Oriented Anatomy, 5th ed. Lippincott Williams & Wilkins, Baltimore, 2006, page 49, Figure 1.28. **B:** From Dudek RW. High Yield Gross Anatomy, 2nd ed. Lippincott Williams & Wilkins, Baltimore, 2002, page 15, Figure 2-2.

Figure 2-3: From Dudek RW. High Yield Gross Anatomy, 2nd ed. Lippincott Williams & Wilkins, Baltimore, 2002, page 17, Figure 2-3.

Figure 2-4: From Dudek RW. High Yield Gross Anatomy, 2nd ed. Lippincott Williams & Wilkins, Baltimore, 2002, page 20, Figure 2-4. **Inset:** From Scott DB. Techniques of Regional Anaesthesia. Appleton and Lange, East Norwalk, CT, 1989, page 169, Figure 169.5.

Figure 2-5: A: From Eisenberg RL. Clinical Imaging: An Atlas of Differential Diagnosis, 4th ed. Lippincott Williams & Wilkins, Baltimore, 2003, page 1007, Figure SP18-2. Courtesy of M. Smith, MD, Nashville, TN. With permission from Neuroradiology Companion, M. Castillo, Lippincott-Raven. **B, C and D:** From Runge VM. Contrast Media in Magnetic Resonance Imaging: A Clinical Approach. Lippincott Williams & Wilkins, Baltimore, 1992, page 97–99.

Figure 5-1: From Moore KL, Dalley AF. Clinically Oriented Anatomy, 5th ed. Lippincott Williams & Wilkins, Baltimore, 2006, page 75, Figure 1.1A.

Figure 5-2: From Dudek RW. High Yield Lung, 1st ed. Lippincott Williams & Wilkins, Baltimore, 2006, page 18, Figure 2-1. Original sources **A:** From Dudek RW. High Yield Gross Anatomy, 2nd ed. Lippincott Williams & Wilkins, Baltimore, 2002, page 24, Figure 3-1A. **B:** From Brandt WE, Helms CA. Fundamentals of Diagnostic Radiology, 2nd ed. Lippincott Williams & Wilkins, Baltimore, 1999, page 496, Figure 21.4. **C.** From Daffner RH. Clinical Radiology: The Essentials, 2nd ed. Lippincott Williams & Wilkins, Baltimore, 1999, page 243, Figure 6.6. **D:** From Daffner RH. Clinical Radiology: The Essentials, 2nd ed. Lippincott Williams & Wilkins, Baltimore, 1999, page 245, Figure 6.9.

Figure 5-3: B: From Swischuck LE. Imaging of the Newborn, Infant, and Young Child, 5th ed. Lippincott Williams & Wilkins, Baltimore, 2004, page 288, Figure 3.98A. **C:** From Brandt WE, Helms CA. Fundamentals of Diagnostic Radiology, 2nd ed. Lippincott Williams & Wilkins, Baltimore, 1999, page 579, Figure 24.6C. **D:** From Brandt WE, Helms CA. Fundamentals of Diagnostic Radiology, 2nd ed. Lippincott Williams & Wilkins, Baltimore, 1999, page 582, Figure 24.9B. **E:** From Brandt WE, Helms CA. Fundamentals of Diagnostic Radiology, 2nd ed. Lippincott Williams & Wilkins, Baltimore, 1999, page 596, Figure 24.27B.

Figure 5-4: Diagram A: Adapted from Moore KL. Clinically Oriented Anatomy, 5th ed. Lippincott Williams & Wilkins, Baltimore, 1992, page 102, Figure B1.4. **B:** From Chen H, Sonneday CJ, Lillemoe KD, eds. Manual of Common Bedside Surgical Procedures, 2nd ed. Lippincott Williams & Wilkins, Baltimore, 2000, page 123, Figure 4.9. **C:** From Scott DB. Techniques of Regional Anaesthesia. Appleton and Lange, East Norwalk, CT, 1889, page 147, Figure 147.4.

Figure 5-5A: Adapted from Moore KL. Clinically Oriented Anatomy, 5th ed. Lippincott Williams & Wilkins, Baltimore, 1992, page 317, Figure SA2.5.

Figure 5-5C: From Freundlich IM, Bragg DG. A Radiologic Approach to Diseases of the Chest, 2nd ed. Lippincott Williams & Wilkins, Baltimore, 1997, page 610.

Figure 5-6: From Collins J, Stern EJ. Chest Radiology: The Essentials. Lippincott Williams & Wilkins, Philadelphia, 1999, page 3, Figure 1-1A.

Figure 5-7: From Collins J, Stern EJ. Chest Radiology: The Essentials. Lippincott Williams & Wilkins, Philadelphia, 1999, page 4, Figure 1-1B.

Figure 5-8: From Moore KL, Dalley AF. Clinically Oriented Anatomy, 5th ed. Lippincott Williams & Wilkins, Baltimore, 2006, page 187, Figure 1.69. Courtesy of Dr. E.L. Lansdown, Professor of Medical Imaging, University of Toronto, Ontario, Canada.

Figure 6-1: **A:** From Brandt WE, Helms CA. Fundamentals of Diagnostic Radiology, 2nd ed. Lippincott Williams & Wilkins, Baltimore, 1999, page 463, Figure 20.6. **B:** Adapted from Freundlich IM, Bragg DG. A Radiologic Approach to Diseases of the Chest, 2nd ed. Lippincott Williams & Wilkins, Baltimore, 1997, page 270, Figure 16-15.

Figure 6-2: **A:** Modified from Rohen JW, Yokochi C, Lutjen-Drecoll E. Color Atlas of Anatomy. 4th ed; Lippincott Williams & Wilkins, Baltimore, 1998, page 235. **B and C:** Adapted from Collins J, Stern EJ. Chest Radiology: The Essentials. Lippincott Williams & Wilkins, Philadelphia, 1999, page 10, Figure 1-8A, and page 11, Figure 1-8B. **D:** From Moore KL, Dalley AF. Clinically Oriented Anatomy, 5th ed. Lippincott Williams & Wilkins, Baltimore, 2006, page 127, Figure 1.29.

Figure 6-3: **A:** From Collins J, Stern EJ. Chest Radiology: The Essentials. Lippincott Williams & Wilkins, Philadelphia, 1999, page 171, Figure 11-3A. **B:** From Collins J, Stern EJ. Chest Radiology: The Essentials. Lippincott Williams & Wilkins, Philadelphia, 1999, page 50, Figure 4-2A. **C:** From Collins J, Stern EJ. Chest Radiology: The Essentials. Lippincott Williams & Wilkins, Philadelphia, 1999, page 183, Figure 12-7. **D:** From Daffner RH. Radiology: The Essentials. Lippincott Williams & Wilkins, Baltimore, 1999, page 158, Figure 4.95. **E:** From Collins J, Stern EJ. Chest Radiology: The Essentials. Lippincott Williams & Wilkins, Philadelphia, 1999, page 195, Figure 13-5. **F:** From Freundlich IM, Bragg DG. A Radiologic Approach to Diseases of the Chest, 2nd ed. Lippincott Williams & Wilkins, Baltimore, 1997, page 716, Figure 38-6B.

Figure 6-4: **A:** From Daffner RH. Clinical Radiology: The Essentials, 2nd ed. Lippincott Williams & Wilkins, Baltimore, 1999, page 146, Figure 4.83. **B:** From Damjanov I. Histopathology: A Color Atlas and Textbook, 1996, Lippincott Williams & Wilkins, Baltimore, page 141, Figure 6.14. **C:** From Rubin E, Farber JL. Pathology, 3rd ed. Lippincott Williams & Wilkins, Baltimore, 1999, page 629, Figure 12-49B. **D:** From Damjanov I. Histopathology: A Color Atlas and Textbook, 1996, Lippincott Williams & Wilkins, Baltimore, page 144, Figure 6.22.A.

Figure 6-5: **A:** From Daffner RH. Clinical Radiology: The Essentials, 2nd ed. Lippincott Williams & Wilkins, Baltimore, 1999, page 152, Figure 4.89A. **B:** From Sternberg SS. Diagnostic Surgical Pathology, Vol 1, 3rd ed. Lippincott Williams & Wilkins, Baltimore, 1999, page 1013, Figure 1. **C:** From Rubin E, Farber JL. Pathology, 3rd ed. Lippincott Williams & Wilkins, Baltimore, 1999, page 637, Figure 12-56. **D:** From Damjanov I. Histopathology: A Color Atlas and Textbook. Lippincott Williams & Wilkins, Baltimore, 1996, page 143, Figure 6.21A, B. **E:** From Rubin E, Farber JL. Pathology, 3rd ed. Lippincott Williams & Wilkins, Baltimore, 1999, page 636, Figure 12-54. **F:** From Damjanov I. Histopathology: A Color Atlas and Textbook. Lippincott Williams & Wilkins, Baltimore, 1996, page 143, Figure 6.20A, B. **G:** From Sternberg SS. Histology for

Pathologists, 2nd ed. Lippincott Williams & Wilkins, Baltimore, 1997, page 452, Figure 26B.

Figure 6-6: **A:** From Freundlich IM, Bragg DG. A Radiologic Approach to Diseases of the Chest, 2nd ed. Lippincott Williams & Wilkins, Baltimore, 1997, page 309, Figure 18-16. **B:** From Dudek RW. High Yield Histology, 2nd ed. Lippincott Williams & Wilkins, Baltimore, 2000, page 135, Figure18-3C. **C:** From Collins J, Stern EJ. Chest Radiology: The Essentials. Lippincott Williams & Wilkins, Philadelphia, 1999, page 94, Figure 7-4A. **D:** From Collins J, Stern EJ. Chest Radiology: The Essentials. Lippincott Williams & Wilkins, Philadelphia, 1999, page 94, Figure 7-4B.

Figure 6-7: From Slaby F, Jacobs ER. Radiography Anatomy, NMS Series, Harwal, Philadelphia, 1990, page 108, Figure 3-5.

Figure 6-8: **A:** From Slaby F, Jacobs ER. Radiography Anatomy, NMS Series, Harwal, Philadelphia, 1990, page 110, Figure 3-6. **B:** From Barret CP, Andersen LD, Holder LE, Pliakoff SJ. Primer of Sectional Anatomy with MRI and CT Correlation, 2nd ed. Lippincott Williams & Wilkins, Baltimore, 1994, page 54, Plate 27.

Figure 6-9: **A:** From Slaby F, Jacobs ER. Radiography Anatomy, NMS Series, Harwal, Philadelphia, 1990, page 112, Figure 3-7. **B:** From Barret CP, Andersen LD, Holder LE, Pliakoff SJ. Primer of Sectional Anatomy with MRI and CT Correlation, 2nd ed. Lippincott Williams & Wilkins, Baltimore, 1994, page 56, Plate 28.

Figure 6-10: From Slaby F, Jacobs ER. Radiography Anatomy, NMS Series, Harwal, Philadelphia, 1990, page 116, Figure 3-8.

Figure 7-1: **A:** From Allen HD, et al., eds. Moss and Adam's Heart Disease in Infants, Children, and Adolescents, vol I, 6th ed. Lippincott Williams & Wilkins, Baltimore, 2001, page 86, Figure 6.6A. **B:** From Allen HD, et al., eds. Moss and Adam's Heart Disease in Infants, Children, and Adolescents, vol I, 6th ed. Lippincott Williams & Wilkins, Baltimore, 2001, page 86, Figure 6.6B. **C:** From Moore KL, Dalley AF. Clinically Oriented Anatomy, 5th ed. Lippincott Williams & Wilkins, Baltimore, 2006 page 168, Figure SA1.7.

Figure 7-2: From Dudek RW. High Yield Heart. Lippincott Williams & Wilkins, Baltimore, 2006, Figure 2-5.

Figure 7-3: Modified from Dudek RW. High Yield Histology, 3rd ed. Lippincott Williams & Wilkins, Baltimore, 2004, page 99, Figure 10-3.

Figure 7-4: **A:** From Brandt WE, Helms CA. Fundamentals of Diagnostic Radiology, 2nd ed. Lippincott Williams & Wilkins, Baltimore, 1999, page 374, Figure 15.11A. **B:** From Collins J, Stern EJ. Chest Radiology: The Essentials. Lippincott Williams & Wilkins, Philadelphia, 1999, page 263, Figure 17-21B. **B:** From Brandt WE, Helms CA. Fundamentals of Diagnostic Radiology, 2nd ed. Lippincott Williams & Wilkins, Baltimore, 1999, page 364, Figure 15.2. **D:** From Brandt WE, Helms CA. Fundamentals of Diagnostic Radiology, 2nd ed. Lippincott Williams & Wilkins, Baltimore, 1999, page 532, Figure 22.11.

Figure 7-5: **A:** From Pohost GM, et al. Imaging in Cardiovascular Disease. Lippincott Williams & Wilkins, Baltimore, 2000, page 355, Figure 10D. **B:** From Pohost GM, et al. Imaging in Cardiovascular Disease. Lippincott Williams & Wilkins, Baltimore, 2000, page 355, Figure 10E. **C:** From Pohost GM, et al. Imaging in Cardiovascular Disease. Lippincott Williams & Wilkins, Baltimore, 2000, page 354, Figure 10A. **D:** From Pohost GM, et al. Imaging in Cardiovascular Disease. Lippincott Williams & Wilkins, Baltimore, 2000, page 354, Figure 10B.

Figure 7-6, 7-7, 7-8: Barrett CP, Anderson LD, Holder LE, et al. Primer of Sectional Anatomy with MRI and CT Correlation, 2nd ed. Williams & Wilkins, Baltimore, 1994, pages 53, 54, Plate 27; pages 59, 60, Plate 30; pages 69, 70, Plate 35.

Figure 8-2 B: From Moore KL, Dalley AF. Clinically Oriented Anatomy, 5th ed. Lippincott Williams & Wilkins, Baltimore, 2006 page 216, Figure 2.12A.

Figure 10-1: B: From Erkonen WE, Smith WL. Radiology 101: The Basics and Fundamentals of Imaging, 2nd ed. Lippincott Williams & Wilkins, Baltimore, 2005, page 111, Figure 3-46. **C:** From Moore KL, Dalley AF. Clinically Oriented Anatomy, 5th ed. Lippincott Williams & Wilkins, Baltimore, 2006, page 338, Figure B2.28A. **D:** From Moore KL, Dalley AF. Clinically Oriented Anatomy, 5th ed. Lippincott Williams & Wilkins, Baltimore, 2006, page 338, Figure B2.28B.

Figure 11-1: A: From Sternberg SS. Histology for Pathologists, 2nd ed. Lippincott Williams & Wilkins, Baltimore, 1997, page 463, Figure 5. **B:** From Sternberg SS. Histology for Pathologists, 2nd ed. Lippincott Williams & Wilkins, Baltimore, 1997, page 467, Figure 10B. **C:** From Ross MH, Kaye GI, Pawlina W. Histology: A Text and Atlas, 4th ed. Lippincott Williams & Wilkins, Baltimore, 2003, page 513, Plate 51, Figure 1. **D:** From Sternberg SS. Histology for Pathologists, 2nd ed. Lippincott Williams & Wilkins, Baltimore, 1997, page 475, Figure 22. **E:** From Sternberg SS. Histology for Pathologists, 2nd ed. Lippincott Williams & Wilkins, Baltimore, 1997, page 476, Figure 23A.

Figure 11-2: A: From Cormack DH. Clinically Integrated Histology. Lippincott Williams & Wilkins, Baltimore, 1998, page 193, Figure 8-9. **B:** From Erkonen WE, Smith WL. Radiology 101: The Basics and Fundamentals of Imaging, 2nd ed. Lippincott Williams & Wilkins, Baltimore, 2005, page 91, Figure 3-20B.

Figure 11-3: A: From Erkonen WE, Smith WL. Radiology 101: The Basics and Fundamentals of Imaging, 2nd ed. Lippincott Williams & Wilkins, Baltimore, 2005, page 113, Figure 3-51. **B:** From Erkonen WE, Smith WL. Radiology 101: The Basics and Fundamentals of Imaging, 2nd ed. Lippincott Williams & Wilkins, Baltimore, 2005, page 113, Figure 3-52.

Figure 11-4: A: From Yamada T, et al. Atlas of Gastroenterology, 2nd ed. Lippincott Williams & Wilkins, Philadelphia, 1999, page 334, Figure 36-10. **B:** From Erkonen WE, Smith WL. Radiology 101: The Basics and Fundamentals of Imaging, 2nd ed. Lippincott Williams & Wilkins, Baltimore, 2005, page 114, Figure 3-54. **C:** From Rubin E, Farber JL. Pathology, 3rd ed. Lippincott Williams & Wilkins, Baltimore, 1999, page 731, Figure 11-45. **D:** From Erkonen WE, Smith WL. Radiology 101: The Basics and Fundamentals of Imaging, 2nd ed. Lippincott Williams & Wilkins, Baltimore, 2005, page 115, Figure 3-56.

Figure 11-5: B: From Moore KL, Dalley AF. Clinically Oriented Anatomy, 5th ed. Lippincott Williams & Wilkins, Baltimore, 2006 page 346, Figure 2.82B. **C:** From Yamada T, et al. Atlas of Gastroenterology, 2nd ed. Lippincott Williams & Wilkins, Philadelphia, 1999, page 474, Figure 52-1B. **D:** From Yamada T, et al. Atlas of Gastroenterology, 2nd ed. Lippincott Williams & Wilkins, Philadelphia, 1999, page 475, Figure 52-4. **E:** From Erkonen WE, Smith WL. Radiology 101: The Basics and Fundamentals of Imaging, 2nd ed. Lippincott Williams & Wilkins, Baltimore, 2005, page 138, Figure 3-105. **F:** From Erkonen WE, Smith WL. Radiology 101: The Basics and Fundamentals of Imaging, 2nd ed. Lippincott Williams & Wilkins, Baltimore, 2005, page 350, Figure 9-10 (third row, third from the left). **G:** From Erkonen WE, Smith WL. Radiology 101: The Basics and Fundamentals of Imaging, 2nd ed. Lippincott Williams & Wilkins, Baltimore, 2005, page 352, Figure 9-12B (top row, third from the left).

Figure 11-6: D: From Yamada T, et al. Atlas of Gastroenterology, 2nd ed. Lippincott Williams & Wilkins, Philadelphia, 1999, page 490, Figure 53-16.

Figure 11-7: A: From Sternberg SS. Histology for Pathologists, 2nd ed. Lippincott Williams & Wilkins, Baltimore, 1997, page 614, Figure 2. **B:** From Cubilla AL, Fitzgerald PJ. Tumors of the exocrine pancreas. In: Hartmann WH, Sobin LH, eds. Atlas of Tumor Pathology, 2nd series, fascicle 19. Armed Forces Institute of Pathology, Washington, DC, 1984. **C:** From Dudek RW, Fix J. BRS Embryology, 3rd ed. Lippincott Williams & Wilkins, Baltimore, 2005, page 107, Figure 10-5D. **D:** From Yamada T, et al.Textbook of Gastroenterology, Vol 2, 3rd ed. Lippincott Williams & Wilkins, Philadelphia, 1999, page 2118, Figure 92-9. Courtesy of Peter B. Cotton, Durham, NC. **E:** From Misiewicz JJ, Bartram CI. Atlas of Clinical Gastroenterology. Gower Medical Publishing, London, 1987.

Figure 11-8: From Barrett CP, Anderson LD, Holder LE, et al. Primer of Sectional Anatomy with MRI and CR Correlation, 2nd ed. Lippincott Williams & Wilkins, Baltimore, 1994, pages 75, 76, Plate 38.

Figure 11-9: From Barrett CP, Anderson LD, Holder LE, et al. Primer of Sectional Anatomy with MRI and CR Correlation, 2nd ed. Lippincott Williams & Wilkins, Baltimore, 1994, pages 79, 80, Plate 40.

Figure11-10: From Barrett CP, Anderson LD, Holder LE, et al. Primer of Sectional Anatomy with MRI and CR Correlation, 2nd ed. Lippincott Williams & Wilkins, Baltimore, 1994, pages 81, 82, Plate 41.

Figure 11-11: A: From Erkonen WE, Smith WL. Radiology 101: The Basics and Fundamentals of Imaging, 2nd ed. Lippincott Williams & Wilkins, Baltimore, 2005, page 92, Figure 3-21. **B:** From Moore KL, Dalley AF. Clinically Oriented Anatomy, 5th ed. Lippincott Williams & Wilkins, Baltimore, 2006 page 345, Figure 2.81A.

Figure 12-1: A: From Dudek RW. High Yield Gross Anatomy, 2nd ed. Lippincott Williams & Wilkins, Baltimore, 2002, page 85, Figure 10-1A. **B:** From Yamada T, et al. Textbook of Gastroenterology, Vol 2, 3rd ed. Lippincott Williams & Wilkins, Baltimore, 1999, page 2959, Figure 133-24A. **C:** From Yamada T, et al. Textbook of Gastroenterology, Vol 2, 3rd ed. Lippincott Williams & Wilkins, Baltimore, 1999, page 2956, Figure 133-20B.

Figure 12-3: A: From Brandt WE, Helms CA. Fundamentals of Diagnostic Radiology, 2nd ed. Lippincott Williams & Wilkins, Baltimore, 1999, page 1168, Figure 52.20. **B:** From Daffner RH. Clinical Radiology: The Essentials, 2nd ed. Lippincott Williams & Wilkins, Baltimore, 1999, page 309, Figure 8.27.

Figure 14-1: Original sources A: From Dudek RW. High Yield Kidney. Lippincott Williams & Wilkins, Baltimore, 2005, page 12, Figure 2-1. **B:** Adapted from Moore KL. Clinically Oriented Anatomy, 3rd ed. Lippincott Williams & Wilkins, Baltimore, 1992, page 174, Figure 2-46. **C:** Adapted from Moore KL. Clinically Oriented Anatomy, 3rd ed. Lippincott Williams & Wilkins, Baltimore, 1992, page 213, Figure 2-86. **H:** From Moore KL. Clinically Oriented Anatomy, 3rd ed. Lippincott Williams & Wilkins, Baltimore, 1992, page 215, Figure 2-88B.

Figure 14-2: From Dudek RW. High Yield Kidney. Lippincott Williams & Wilkins, Baltimore, 2005, page 14, Figure 2-2.

Figure 14-3: From Dudek RW. High Yield Kidney. Lippincott Williams & Wilkins, Baltimore, 2005, page 25, Figure 2-5. Original sources **A:** From Graff L. A Handbook of Routine Urinalysis. Lippincott Williams & Wilkins, Philadelphia, 1983, page 151, Figure 4-27. **B:** From Graff L. A Handbook of Routine Urinalysis. Lippincott Williams & Wilkins, Philadelphia, 1983, page 173, Figure 4-60. **C:** From Graff L. A Handbook of Routine Urinalysis. Lippincott Williams & Wilkins, Philadelphia, 1983, page 144, Figure 4-16. **D:** From Graff L. A Handbook of Routine Urinalysis. Lippincott Williams & Wilkins, Philadelphia, 1983, page 93, Figure 3-23. **E:** From Wicke L. Atlas of Radiologic Anatomy, 6th ed. Lippincott Williams & Wilkins, Baltimore, 1998, page 133, Figure 88. **F:** From Dunnick NR, et al. Textbook of Uroradiology, 3rd ed. Lippincott Williams & Wilkins, Baltimore, 2001, page 189, Figure 8.17A. **G:** From Eisenberg RL. Clinical Imaging: An Atlas of Differential Diagnosis, 4th ed. Lippincott Williams & Wilkins, Baltimore, 2003, page 651, Figure GU19-1. **H:** From Dunnick NR, et al. Textbook of Uroradiology, 3rd ed. Lippincott Williams & Wilkins, Baltimore, 2001 page 183, Figure 8.8.

Figure 14-5: **A, B, C, D, E, F, and G:** From Dudek RW. High Yield Kidney. Lippincott Williams & Wilkins, Baltimore, 2005, page 31, Figure 2-8.

Figure 14-6: **A:** From Wicke L. Atlas of Radiologic Anatomy, 6th ed. Lippincott Williams & Wilkins, Baltimore, 1998, page 133, Figure 88. **B:** From Wicke L. Atlas of Radiologic Anatomy, 6th ed. Lippincott Williams & Wilkins, Baltimore, 1998, page 135, Figure 89. **C:** From Eisenberg RL. Clinical Imaging: An Atlas of Differential Diagnosis, 4th ed. Lippincott Williams & Wilkins, Baltimore, 2003, page 651, Figure GU 19-3. **D:** From Eisenberg RL. Clinical Imaging: An Atlas of Differential Diagnosis, 4th ed. Lippincott Williams & Wilkins, Baltimore, 2003, page 601, Figure GU 4-4. **E:** From Brandt WE, Helms CA. Fundamentals of Diagnostic Radiology, 2nd ed. Lippincott Williams & Wilkins, Baltimore, 1999, page 778, Figure 33.15.

Figure 14-7: **A:** From Taveras JM. Radiology: Diagnosis, Imaging, Intervention, Vol 4. Lippincott Williams & Wilkins, Baltimore, 1988, page 2, Figure 1. **B:** From Taveras JM. Radiology: Diagnosis, Imaging, Intervention, Vol 4. Lippincott Williams & Wilkins, Baltimore, 1988, page 3, Figure 4. **C:** From Brandt WE, Helms CA. Fundamentals of Diagnostic Radiology, 2nd ed. Lippincott Williams & Wilkins, Baltimore, 1999, page 795, Figure 34.3B. **D:** From Taveras JM. Radiology: Diagnosis, Imaging, Intervention, Vol 4. Lippincott Williams & Wilkins, Baltimore, 1988, page 3, Figure 2.

Figure 14-8: **A:** From Eisenberg RL. Clinical Imaging: An Atlas of Differential Diagnosis, 4th ed. Lippincott Williams & Wilkins, Baltimore, 2003, page 671, Figure GU 22-2. **B:** From Eisenberg RL. Clinical Imaging: An Atlas of Differential Diagnosis, 4th ed. Lippincott Williams & Wilkins, Baltimore, 2003, page 673, Figure GU 23-1.

Figure 14-9: **A:** From Taveras JM. Radiology: Diagnosis, Imaging, Intervention, Vol 4. Lippincott Williams & Wilkins, Baltimore, 1988, page 5, Figure 9. **B:** From Taveras JM. Radiology: Diagnosis, Imaging, Intervention, Vol 4. Lippincott Williams & Wilkins, Baltimore, 1988, page 6, Figure 5. **C:** From Brandt WE, Helms CA. Fundamentals of Diagnostic Radiology, 2nd ed. Lippincott Williams & Wilkins, Baltimore, 1999, page 812, Figure 34.37. **D:** From Brandt WE, Helms CA. Fundamentals of Diagnostic Radiology, 2nd ed. Lippincott Williams & Wilkins, Baltimore, 1999, page 809, Figure 34.31. **E:** From Brandt WE, Helms CA. Fundamentals of Diagnostic Radiology, 2nd ed. Lippincott Williams & Wilkins, Baltimore, 1999, page 811, Figure 34.35.

Figure14-10: **A:** From Daffner RH. Clinical Radiology: The Essentials, 2nd ed. Lippincott Williams & Wilkins, Baltimore, 1999, page 344, Figure 9.2A. **B:** From Daffner RH. Clinical Radiology: The Essentials, 2nd ed. Lippincott Williams & Wilkins, Baltimore, 1999, page 344, Figure 9.2B. **C:** From Laberge JM, Gordon RL, Kerlan RK, Wilson MW. Interventional Radiology Essentials, 1st ed. Lippincott Williams & Wilkins, Baltimore, 2000, page 45, Figure 2. From Laberge JM, Gordon RL, Kerlan RK, Wilson MW. Interventional Radiology Essentials, 1st ed. Lippincott Williams & Wilkins, Baltimore, 2000, page 59, Figure 39.

Figure 14-11: **A:** From Dunnick NR, Sandler CM, Newhouse JH, Amis ES. Textbook of Uroradiology, 3rd ed. Lippincott Williams & Wilkins, Baltimore, 2001, page 63, Figure 3.21. **B:** From Dunnick NR, Sandler CM, Newhouse JH, Amis ES. Textbook of Uroradiology, 3rd ed. Lippincott Williams & Wilkins, Baltimore, 2001, page 63, Figure 3.22. **C:** From Dunnick NR, Sandler CM, Newhouse JH, Amis ES. Textbook of Uroradiology, 3rd ed. Lippincott Williams & Wilkins, Baltimore, 2001, page 64, Figure 3.23.

Figure 14-12: **A:** From Barrett CP, Andersen LD, Holder LE, Poliakoff SJ. Primer of Sectional Anatomy with MRI and CT Correlation, 2nd ed. Lippincott Williams & Wilkins, Baltimore, 1994, page 80, Plate 40. **B:** From Barrett CP, Andersen LD, Holder LE, Poliakoff SJ. Primer of Sectional Anatomy with MRI and CT Correlation, 2nd ed. Lippincott Williams & Wilkins, Baltimore, 1994, page 82, Plate 41. **C:** From Barrett CP, Andersen LD, Holder LE, Poliakoff SJ. Primer of Sectional Anatomy with MRI and CT Correlation, 2nd ed. Lippincott Williams & Wilkins, Baltimore,

1994, page 84, Plate 42. **D:** From Daffner RH. Clinical Radiology: The Essentials, 2nd ed. Lippincott Williams & Wilkins, Baltimore, 1999, page 347, Figure 9.8. **E:** From Daffner RH. Clinical Radiology: The Essentials, 2nd ed. Lippincott Williams & Wilkins, Baltimore, 1999, page 349, Figure 9.11D.

Figure 15-1 A: From Premkumar K. The Massage Connection Anatomy and Physiology. Lippincott Williams & Wilkins, Baltimore, 2004, Figure 6.11.

Figure 15-2: **A:** From Brandt WE, Helms CA. Fundamentals of Diagnostic Radiology, 2nd ed. Lippincott Williams & Wilkins, Baltimore, 1999, page 771, Figure 33.3. **B:** From Rubin E, Farber JL. Pathology, 3rd ed. Lippincott Williams & Wilkins, Baltimore, 1999, page 1193, Figure 21-37. **C:** From Rubin E, Farber JL. Pathology, 3rd ed. Lippincott Williams & Wilkins, Baltimore, 1999, page 1191, Figure 21.34a. **D:** From Weyman PJ, Glazer HS. Adrenals. In: Lee JKT, Sagel SS, Stanley RS, eds. Computed Body Tomography. Raven Press, New York, 1983. 2nd ed., page 111, Figure 13-1A. **E:** From Brandt WE, Helms CA. Fundamentals of Diagnostic Radiology, 2nd ed. Lippincott Williams & Wilkins, Baltimore, 1999, page 770, Figure 33.1. **F:** From Rubin E, Farber JL. Pathology, 3rd ed. Lippincott Williams & Wilkins, Baltimore, 1999, page 1186, Figure 21.31b. **G:** Courtesy of Dr. J. Kitchin, Department of Obstetrics and Gynecology, University of Virginia.

Figure 15-3: **A:** From Sternberg SS. Diagnostic Surgical Pathology, Vol 1, 3rd ed. Lippincott Williams & Wilkins, Baltimore, 1999, page 614, Figure 42. **B:** From Becker KL, Bilezikian JP, Brenner WJ, et al. Principles and Practice of Endocrinology and Metabolism, 3rd ed. Lippincott Williams & Wilkins, Philadelphia, 2001, Figure 7.7A. **C:** From Dudek RW. High Yield Histology, 3rd ed. Lippincott Williams & Wilkins, Baltimore, 2004, page 212, Figure 25-5B. **D:** From Sternberg SS. Diagnostic Surgical Pathology, Vol 1, 3rd ed. Lippincott Williams & Wilkins, Baltimore, 1999, page 609, Figure 33.

Figure 16-1: **A:** From Snell RS. Clinical Anatomy, 7th ed. Lippincott Williams & Wilkins, Baltimore, 2004, page 409, Figure 7-43.

Figure 16-2: **A:** Adapted from Snell RS. Clinical Anatomy for Medical Students, 5th ed. Little Brown, Boston, 1995, page 364, Figure 8-14. **B:** From Moore KL, Dalley AF. Clinically Oriented Anatomy, 5th ed. Lippincott Williams & Wilkins, Baltimore, 2006, page 414, Figure 3.29.

Figure 16-3: **A:** From Rubin E, Farber JL. Pathology, 3rd ed. Lippincott Williams & Wilkins, Baltimore, 1999, page 1009, Figure 18-49A. **B:** From Rubin E, Farber JL. Pathology, 3rd ed. Lippincott Williams & Wilkins, Baltimore, 1999, page 1004, Figure 18-42. **C:** From Sternberg SS. Diagnostic Surgical Pathology, Vol 2, 3rd ed. Lippincott Williams & Wilkins, Philadelphia, 1999, page 2396, Figure 1. **D:** From Sternberg SS. Diagnostic Surgical Pathology, Vol 2, 3rd ed. Lippincott Williams & Wilkins, Philadelphia, 1999, page 2399, Figure 10. **E:** From Rubin E, Farber JL. Pathology, 3rd ed. Lippincott Williams & Wilkins, Baltimore, 1999, page 994, Figure 18-31. **F:** From Rubin E, Farber JL. Pathology, 3rd ed. Lippincott Williams & Wilkins, Baltimore, 1999, page 990, Figure 18-27A. **G:** From Rubin E, Farber JL. Pathology, 3rd ed. Lippincott Williams & Wilkins, Baltimore, 1999, page 999, Figure 18-37A. **H:** From Daffner RH. Clinical Radiology: The Essentials, 2nd ed. Lippincott Williams & Wilkins, Baltimore, 1999, page 401, Figure 10.21A. **I:** From Daffner RH. Clinical Radiology: The Essentials, 2nd ed. Lippincott Williams & Wilkins, Baltimore, 1999, page 402, Figure 10.23B. **J:** From Callahan TL, Caughey AB, Heffner LJ. Blueprints in Obstetrics and Gynecology. Blackwell, Malden, MA, 1998, page 103, Figure 14-5.

Figure 17-1: From Moore KL, Dalley AF. Clinically Oriented Anatomy, 5th ed. Lippincott Williams & Wilkins, Baltimore, 2006, page 407, Figure 3.23.

Figure 17-2: **A:** From Moore KL, Dalley AF. Clinically Oriented Anatomy, 5th ed. Lippincott Williams & Wilkins, Baltimore, 2006, page 223, Figure 2.16. **B:** From Moore KL, Dalley AF. Clinically

Oriented Anatomy, 5th ed. Lippincott Williams & Wilkins, Baltimore, 2006, page 403, Figure 3.20B.

Figure 17-3: **A:** From Moore KL, Dalley AF. Clinically Oriented Anatomy, 5th ed. Lippincott Williams & Wilkins, Baltimore, 2006, page 454, Figure 3.48A. **B:** From Moore KL, Dalley AF. Clinically Oriented Anatomy, 5th ed. Lippincott Williams & Wilkins, Baltimore, 2006, page 455, Figure 3.49B. **C:** From Dudek RW. High Yield Gross Anatomy, 2nd ed. Lippincott Williams & Wilkins, Baltimore, 2002, page 119, Figure 15-1B.

Figure 17-4: **A:** From Fletcher MA. Physical Diagnosis in Neonatology, Lippincott Williams & Wilkins, Baltimore, 1998, Page 378, figure 38C. **B:** From Dudek RW. High Yield Embryology, 3rd ed. Lippincott Williams & Wilkins, Baltimore, 2007, page 75, Figure 10.3E. Courtesy of Dr. T. Ernesto Figueroa. **C:** From Rubin E, Farber JL. Pathology, 3rd ed. Lippincott Williams & Wilkins, 1999, Baltimore, page 950, Figure 17-34, bottom left corner. **D:** From Rubin E, Farber JL. Pathology, 3rd ed. Lippincott Williams & Wilkins, 1999, Baltimore, page 942, Figure 17-24. **E:** From Rubin E, Farber JL. Pathology, 3rd ed. Lippincott Williams & Wilkins, 1999, Baltimore, page 945 Figure 17-27A. **F:** From Sadler TW. Langman's Embryology, 9th ed. Lippincott Williams & Wilkins, Baltimore, 2004, page 352, Figure 14.35B. **G:** From Dudek RW. High Yield Embryology, 3rd ed. Lippincott Williams & Wilkins, Baltimore, 2007, page 75, Figure 10-3B. Courtesy of Dr. T. Ernesto Figueroa. **H:** From Avery GB. Neonatology, Pathophysiology and Management of the Newborn, 5th ed. Lippincott Williams & Wilkins, Baltimore, 1999, page 995, Figure 43-24.

Figure 17-5: **A:** From Dudek RW. High Yield Histology, 3rd ed. Lippincott Williams & Wilkins, Baltimore, 2004, page 240, Figure 27-5A. **B:** From Brandt WE, Helms CA. Fundamentals of Diagnostic Radiology, 2nd ed. Lippincott Williams & Wilkins, Baltimore, 1999, page 825, Figure 35.20. **C:** From Daffner RH. Clinical Radiology: The Essentials, 2nd ed. Lippincott Williams & Wilkins, Baltimore, 1999, page 352, Figure 9.15. **D:** From Brandt WE, Helms CA. Fundamentals of Diagnostic Radiology, 2nd ed. Lippincott Williams & Wilkins, Baltimore, 1999, page 826, Figure 35.21. **E:** From Eisenberg RL. Clinical Imaging, an Atlas of Differential Diagnosis, 4th ed. Lippincott Williams & Wilkins, Baltimore, 2003, page 677, Figure GU 24-4. **F:** From Jarrell BE, Carabasi RA. NMS Surgery, 3rd ed. Lippincott Williams & Wilkins, Baltimore, 1996, page 460, Figure 15-2A, B.

Figure 18-1: **A:** From Rohen JW, Yokochi C, Lutjen-Drecoll E. Color Atlas of Anatomy. 4th ed; Lippincott Williams & Wilkins, Baltimore, 1998, page 409, no figure number. **B:** From Rohen JW, Yokochi C, Lutjen-Drecoll E. Color Atlas of Anatomy, 4th ed. Lippincott Williams & Wilkins, Baltimore, 1998, page 410, no figure number. **C:** From Rohen JW, Yokochi C, Lutjen-Drecoll E. Color Atlas of Anatomy, 4th ed. Lippincott Williams & Wilkins, Baltimore, 1998, page 411, no figure number. **D:** From Rohen JW, Yokochi C, Lutjen-Drecoll E. Color Atlas of Anatomy, 4th ed. Lippincott Williams & Wilkins, Baltimore, 1998, page 412, no figure number.

Figure 18-2 **A:** From Moore KL, Dalley AF. Clinically Oriented Anatomy, 5th ed. Lippincott Williams & Wilkins, Baltimore, 2006, page 368, Figure 3.5.

Figure 18-3: From Moore KL, Dalley AF. Clinically Oriented Anatomy, 5th ed. Lippincott Williams & Wilkins, Baltimore, 2006, page 370, Figure 3.6A.

Figure 18-5: **A:** From Scott DB. Techniques of Regional Anaesthesia. Appleton & Lange, East Norwalk, CT, 1989, page 159. **B:** From Olson TR. ADAM Student Atlas of Anatomy. Lippincott Williams & Wilkins, Baltimore, 1996, page 169, Plate 4.18.

Figure 18-6: **A:** From Snell RS. Clinical Anatomy, 7th ed. Lippincott Williams & Wilkins, Baltimore, 2004, page 407, Figure 7-39. **B:** From Snell RS. Clinical Anatomy, 7th ed. Lippincott Williams & Wilkins, Baltimore, 2004, page 408, Figure 7-40.

Figure 19-1: **A:** From Moore KL, Dalley AF. Clinically Oriented Anatomy, 5th ed. Lippincott Williams & Wilkins, Baltimore, 2006,

page 435, Figure 3.38B. **B:** From Moore KL, Dalley AF. Clinically Oriented Anatomy, 5th ed. Lippincott Williams & Wilkins, Baltimore, 2006, page 435, Figure 3.38A. **C:** From Chung KW. Gross Anatomy, 5th ed. Lippincott Williams & Wilkins, Baltimore, 2005, page 263, Figure 6-3. **D:** From Chung KW. Gross Anatomy, 5th ed. Lippincott Williams & Wilkins, Baltimore, 2005, page 264, Figure 6-4.

Figure 20-1: **C:** Modified from Chung KW. BRS Gross Anatomy, 5th ed. Lippincott Williams & Wilkins, Baltimore, 2005, page 57, Figure 2-21.

Figure 20-2: **A:** From Agur AMR, Dalley AF. Grant's Atlas of Anatomy, 11th ed. Lippincott Williams & Wilkins, Baltimore, 2005, page 485, Figure 6.22A. **B:** From Agur AMR, Dalley AF. Grant's Atlas of Anatomy, 11th ed. Lippincott Williams & Wilkins, Baltimore, 2005, page 531, Figure 6.58A. **C:** From Agur AMR, Dalley AF. Grant's Atlas of Anatomy, 11th ed. Lippincott Williams & Wilkins, Baltimore, 2005, page 552, Figure 6.75A.

Figure 20-3: **A:** Adapted from April EW. NMS Clinical Anatomy, 2nd ed. Lippincott Williams & Wilkins, Baltimore, 1990, page 58, Figure 6-6.

Figure 20-4: **A:** From Moore KL, Dalley AF. Clinically Oriented Anatomy, 5th ed. Lippincott Williams & Wilkins, Baltimore, 2006, page 778, Figure 6.30B. **B:** From Moore KL, Dalley AF. Clinically Oriented Anatomy, 5th ed. Lippincott Williams & Wilkins, Baltimore, 2006, page 779, Figure 6.30C. **C:** From Moore KL, Dalley AF. Clinically Oriented Anatomy, 5th ed. Lippincott Williams & Wilkins, Baltimore, 2006, page 779, Figure 6.30D.

Figure 20-5: **A:** From Agur AMR, Dalley AF. Grant's Atlas of Anatomy, 11th ed. Lippincott Williams & Wilkins, Baltimore, 2005, page 516, Figure 6.47. **B:** From Harris JH, Harris WH. The Radiology of Emergency Medicine, 4th ed. Lippincott Williams & Wilkins, Baltimore, 2000, page 310, Figure 24. **C:** From Chew FS. Musculoskeletal Imaging, The Core Curriculum. Lippincott Williams & Wilkins, Baltimore, 2002, page 63, Figure 2.42A. **D:** From Daffner RH. Clinical Radiology: The Essentials, 2nd ed. Lippincott Williams & Wilkins, Baltimore, 1999, page 417, Figure 11.16. **F:** From Harris JH, Harris WH. The Radiology of Emergency Medicine, 4th ed. Lippincott Williams & Wilkins, Baltimore, 2000, page 304, Figure 10. **G:** From Harris JH, Harris WH. The Radiology of Emergency Medicine, 4th ed. Lippincott Williams & Wilkins, Baltimore, 2000, page 306, Figure 14B. **H:** From Harris JH, Harris WH. The Radiology of Emergency Medicine, 4th ed. Lippincott Williams & Wilkins, Baltimore, 2000, page 327, Figure 60.

Figure 20-6: **A:** From April EW. Anatomy, 2nd ed. Lippincott Williams & Wilkins, 1990, page 62, Figure 7-1. **B and C:** From Slaby F, Jacobs ER. Radiographic Anatomy. Harwal, Media, PA, 1990, page 10, Figure 1-7; page 12, Figure 1-9. **D:** From Harris JH, Harris WH. The Radiology of Emergency Medicine, 4th ed. Lippincott Williams & Wilkins, Baltimore, 2000, page 357, Figure 41. **E:** From Harris JH, Harris WH. The Radiology of Emergency Medicine, 4th ed. Lippincott Williams & Wilkins, Baltimore, 2000, page 352, Figure 28. **F:** From Harris JH, Harris WH. The Radiology of Emergency Medicine, 4th ed. Lippincott Williams & Wilkins, Baltimore, 2000, page 350, Figure 22. **G:** From Harris JH, Harris WH. The Radiology of Emergency Medicine, 4th ed. Lippincott Williams & Wilkins, Baltimore, 2000, page 364, Figure 57.

Figure 20-7: **A:** From Slaby F, Jacobs ER. Radiographic Anatomy. Harwal, Media, PA, 1990, page 22, Figure 1-19. **B:** From Chew FS. Musculoskeletal Imaging, The Core Curriculum, Lippincott Williams & Wilkins, Baltimore, 2002, page 41, Figure 2.9B. **C:** From Harris JH, Harris WH. The Radiology of Emergency Medicine, 4th ed. Lippincott Williams & Wilkins, Baltimore, 2000, page 382, Figure 26A. **D:** From Chew FS. Musculoskeletal Imaging, The Core Curriculum, Lippincott Williams & Wilkins, Baltimore, 2002, page 38, Figure 2.4. **E:** From Harris JH, Harris WH. The Radiology of Emergency Medicine, 4th ed. Lippincott Williams & Wilkins, Baltimore, 2000, page 418, Figure 12. **B:** Modified from Moore KL, Dalley AF. Clinically Oriented Anatomy, 5th ed. Lippincott Williams & Wilkins, Baltimore, 2006, page 670, Figure

5.47A. **C:** Modified from Moore KL, Dalley AF. Clinically Oriented Anatomy, 5th ed. Lippincott Williams & Wilkins, Baltimore, 2006, page 670, Figure 5.47B.

Figure 21-1: A: Modified from Dudek RW. High Yield Gross Anatomy, 2nd ed. Lippincott Williams & Wilkins, Baltimore, 2002, page 149, Figure 19-1. **B:** Modified from Moore KL, Dalley AF. Clinically Oriented Anatomy, 5th ed. Lippincott Williams & Wilkins, Baltimore, 2006, page 670, Figure 5.47A. **C:** Modified from Moore KL, Dalley AF. Clinically Oriented Anatomy, 5th ed. Lippincott Williams & Wilkins, Baltimore, 2006, page 670, Figure 5.47B.

Figure 21-2: From Chung KW. BRS Gross Anatomy, 5th ed. Lippincott Williams & Wilkins, Baltimore, 2005, page 96, Figure 3-11.

Figure 21-3A and B: From Agur AMR, Dalley AF. Grant's Atlas of Anatomy, 11th ed. Lippincott Williams & Wilkins, Baltimore, 2005, page 348.

Figure 21-4: A: From Agur AMR, Dalley AF. Grant's Atlas of Anatomy, 11th ed. Lippincott Williams & Wilkins, Baltimore, 2005, page 380, Figure 5.32. **C:** From Harris JH, Harris WH. The Radiology of Emergency Medicine, 4th ed. Lippincott Williams & Wilkins, Baltimore, 2000, page 780, Figure 112A. **D:** From Chew FS. Musculoskeletal Imaging, 1st ed. Lippincott Williams & Wilkins, Baltimore, 2003, page 107, Figure 4.2A. **E:** From Harris JH, Harris WH. The Radiology of Emergency Medicine, 4th ed. Lippincott Williams & Wilkins, Baltimore, 2000, page 795, Figure 136. **F:** From Chew FS. Musculoskeletal Imaging, 1st ed. Lippincott Williams & Wilkins, Baltimore, 2003, page 109, Figure 4.6. **G:** From Harris JH, Harris WH. The Radiology of Emergency Medicine, 4th ed. Lippincott Williams & Wilkins, Baltimore, 2000, page 801, Figure 146A. **H:** From Eisenberg RL. Clinical Imaging: An Atlas of Differential Diagnosis, 4th ed. Lippincott Williams & Wilkins, Baltimore, 2003, page 889, Figure B24.4.

Figure 21-5: A: From Agur AMR, Dalley AF. Grant's Atlas of Anatomy, 11th ed. Lippincott Williams & Wilkins, Baltimore, 2005, page 400, Figure 5.49. **B:** From Agur AMR, Dalley AF. Grant's Atlas of Anatomy, 11th ed. Lippincott Williams & Wilkins, Baltimore, 2005, page 401, Figure 5.50B. **C:** From Agur AMR, Dalley AF. Grant's Atlas of Anatomy, 11th ed. Lippincott Williams & Wilkins, Baltimore, 2005, page 401, Figure 5.50C. **D:** From Agur AMR, Dalley AF. Grant's Atlas of Anatomy, 11th ed. Lippincott Williams & Wilkins, Baltimore, 2005, page 393, Figure 5.44A.

Figure 21-6: A(2): From Agur AMR, Dalley AF. Grant's Atlas of Anatomy, 11th ed. Lippincott Williams & Wilkins, Baltimore, 2005, page 432, Figure 5.69. **B:** From Agur AMR, Dalley AF. Grant's Atlas of Anatomy, 11th ed. Lippincott Williams & Wilkins, Baltimore, 2005, page 427, Figure 5.68.

Figure 21-7: A(2): From Harris JH, Harris WH. The Radiology of Emergency Medicine, 4th ed. Lippincott Williams & Wilkins, Baltimore, 2000, page 861, Figure 46. **A(3):** From Chew FS. Musculoskeletal Imaging, 1st ed. Lippincott Williams & Wilkins, Baltimore, 2003, page 140, Figure 4.56. **B(2):** From Harris JH, Harris WH. The Radiology of Emergency Medicine, 4th ed. Lippincott Williams & Wilkins, Baltimore, 2000, page 857, Figure 38.

Figure 22-1: Dudek RW. HY Gross Anatomy, 2nd ed. Baltimore, 2002, page 178, Figure 20-6.

Figure 22-2: A. From Sadler TW. Langman's Medical Embryology, 8th ed. Lippincott Williams & Wilkins, Baltimore, 2000, page 169, Figure 8.8C. **B.** From McMillan JA. Oski's Pediatrics, 3rd ed. Lippincott Williams & Wilkins, Baltimore 1999, page 396, Figure 66-8. **C.** From Fletcher MA. Physical Diagnosis in Neonatology. Lippincott Williams & Wilkins, Baltimore, 1997, page 188, Figure 16B. **D.** From McMillan. Oski's Pediatrics, 3rd ed. Lippincott Williams & Wilkins, Baltimore, 1999, page 398, Figure 66-16. **E.** From McMillan. Oski's Pediatrics, 3rd ed. Lippincott Williams &

Wilkins, Baltimore, 1999, page 396, Figure 66-9. **F.** From McMillan. Oski's Pediatrics, 3rd ed. Lippincott Williams & Wilkins, Baltimore, 1999, page 397, Figure 66-10. **G.** From McMillan. Oski's Pediatrics, 3rd ed. Lippincott Williams & Wilkins, Baltimore, 1999, Figure 66-12. **H:** From Swischuk LE. Imaging of the Newborn, Infant and Young Child 5E, Lippincott Williams & Wilkins, Baltimore, 2004, page 1016, Figure 7.52.

Figure 22-3: A: From Dudek RW. HY Gross Anatomy, 2nd ed. Baltimore, 2002, page 178, Figure 20-6. Original source: From Moore KL, Dalley AF. Clinically Oriented Anatomy,. 3rd ed. Lippincott Williams & Wilkins, Baltimore, 1992, page 666. **B:** From Harwood-Nuss A, MD FACEP, Wolfson AB, MD, FACEP, FACP, et al. The Clinical Practice of Emergency Medicine, 3rd ed. Philadelphia: Lippincott Williams & Wilkins, Baltimore, 2001, Figure 47-1. **C:** Dudek RW. HY Gross Anatomy, 2nd ed. Baltimore, 2002, page 165, Figure 20-1E. Original source: Blackbourne LH. Advanced Surgical Recall. Lippincott Williams & Wilkins, Baltimore, 1997, page 787.

Figure 22-4: A: From Fix J. High Yield Neuroanatomy, 3rd ed. Lippincott Williams & Wilkins, Baltimore, 2005, page 37, Figure 3-10. **B:** From Fix J. High Yield Neuroanatomy, 3rd ed. Lippincott Williams & Wilkins, Baltimore, 2005, page 36, Figure 3-9. **C:** From Fix J. High Yield Neuroanatomy, 3rd ed. Lippincott Williams & Wilkins, Baltimore, 2005, page 38, Figure 3-12. **D:** From Fix J. High Yield Neuroanatomy, 3rd ed. Lippincott Williams & Wilkins, Baltimore, 2005, page 37, Figure 3-11. **E:** Jenkins JR, da Costa Lite C. Neurodiagnostic Imaging: Pattern Analysis and Differential Diagnosis. Lippincott-Raven, Baltimore, 1998, page 789, Figure 63-5B.

Figure 22-5: From: Siegel A, Sapru HN. Essential Neuroscience. Lippincott Williams & Wilkins, Baltimore, 2006, page 47, Figure 4-1.

Figure 22-6: A: From: Siegel A, Sapru HN. Essential Neuroscience. Lippincott Williams & Wilkins, Baltimore, 2006, page 53, Figure 4-5A. **B:** From: Siegel A, Sapru HN. Essential Neuroscience. Lippincott Williams & Wilkins, Baltimore, 2006, page 53, Figure 4-5B. **C:** From Moore KL, Dalley AF. Clinically Oriented Anatomy, 5th ed. Lippincott Williams & Wilkins, Baltimore, 2006, page 913, Figure 7.12C.

Figure 22-7: A: From Dudek RW. HY Gross Anatomy, 2nd ed. Baltimore, 2002, page 170, Figure 20-3. **B:** From Haines DE. Neuroanatomy: An Atlas of Structure, Sections, and Systems, 6th ed. Lippincott Williams & Wilkins, Baltimore, 2004, page 48, Figure 2-48B. **C:** From Haines DE; Neuroanatomy An Atlas of Structure, Sections, and Systems. LWW, 6th ed, Baltimore, 2004, page 48, Figure 2-48C. **D:** Daffner RH; Clinical Radiology, 2nd ed, LWW, Baltimore, 1999, page 527, Figure 12.39. **E:** From Haines DE. Neuroanatomy: An Atlas of Structure, Sections, and Systems, 6th ed. Lippincott Williams & Wilkins, Baltimore, 2004, page 51, Figure 2-51A. **F:** From Haines DE. Neuroanatomy: An Atlas of Structure, Sections, and Systems, 6th ed. Lippincott Williams & Wilkins, Baltimore, 2004, page 49, Figure 2-49A.

Figure 22-8 A: From Chung KW. BRS Gross Anatomy, 5th ed. Lippincott Williams & Wilkins, Baltimore, 2005, page 350, Figure 8-3.

Figure 22-9B, C, D: From Scott BD. Techniques of Regional Anaesthesia. Appleton and Lange, Stamford, CT, 1989, pages 77, 93, 209, Figure 77.4, 93.2, 209.4.

Figure 22-10: A, B, D (right): From Rohen JW, Yokochi, Lutjen-Drecoll E. Color Atlas of Anatomy, 4th ed. Lippincott Williams & Wilkins, Baltimore, 1998, page 154, 157. **C (upper):** Redrawn from Moore KL, Dalley AF. Clinically Oriented Anatomy, 5th ed. Lippincott Williams & Wilkins, Baltimore, 2006, page 1090, Figure 8.27A. **C (lower):** From Moore KL, Dalley AF. Clinically Oriented Anatomy, 5th ed. Lippincott Williams & Wilkins, Baltimore, 2006, page 1101, Figure B8.12. **D (left):** Adapted from Moore KL, Dalley AF. Clinically Oriented Anatomy, 5th ed.

Index

Page numbers in italics indicate figures. Page numbers followed by "t" indicate tables.